# Infections in Obstetrics and Gynaecology

# *Infections in Obstetrics and Gynaecology*


***Editors***

**Gauri Gandhi**
MD
Professor
Department of Obstetrics and Gynaecology
MAMC and Lok Nayak Hospital, New Delhi

**Sumita Mehta**
DGO, DNB
Senior Research Associate
Department of Obstetrics and Gynaecology
MAMC and Lok Nayak Hospital, New Delhi

**Swaraj Batra**
MS, FICOG
Director - Professor and Head
Department of Obstetrics and Gynaecology
MAMC and Lok Nayak Hospital, New Delhi



**JAYPEE BROTHERS**
**MEDICAL PUBLISHERS (P) LTD**
New Delhi

*Published by*
Jitendar P Vij
**Jaypee Brothers Medical Publishers (P) Ltd**
EMCA House, 23/23B Ansari Road, Daryaganj
**New Delhi** 110 002, India
Phones: +91-11-23272143, +91-11-23272703, +91-11-23282021, +91-11-23245672
Fax: +91-11-23276490, +91-11-23245683
e-mail: jaypee@jaypeebrothers.com
Visit our website: www.jaypeebrothers.com

*Branches*

- 202 Batavia Chambers, 8 Kumara Krupa Road
  Kumara Park East, **Bangalore** 560 001
  Phones: +91-80-22285971, +91-80-22382956, +91-80-30614073
  Tele Fax : +91-80-22281761 e-mail: jaypeebc@bgl.vsnl.net.in
- 282 IIIrd Floor, Khaleel Shirazi Estate, Fountain Plaza
  Pantheon Road, **Chennai** 600 008
  Phones: +91-44-28262665, +91-44-28269897 Fax: +91-44- 28262331
  e-mail: jpmedpub@md3.vsnl.net.in
- 4-2-1067/1-3, 1st Floor, Balaji Building, Ramkote Cross Road
  **Hyderabad** 500 095, Phones: +91-40-55610020, +91-40-24758498
  Fax: +91-40-24758499 e-mail: jpmedpub@rediffmail.com
- 1A Indian Mirror Street, Wellington Square
  **Kolkata** 700 013, Phones: +91-33-22456075, +91-33-22451926
  Fax: +91-33-22456075 e-mail: jpbcal@cal.vsnl.net.in
- 106 Amit Industrial Estate, 61 Dr SS Rao Road
  Near MGM Hospital, Parel, **Mumbai** 400 012
  Phones: +91-22-24124863, +91-22-24104532, +91-22-30926896
  Fax: +91-22-24160828 e-mail: jpmedpub@bom7.vsnl.net.in

***Infections in Obstetrics and Gynaecology***



*First Edition* : **2006**

ISBN 81-8061-607-X

*Typeset at* JPBMP typesetting unit

Printed and bound in India by Gopsons Papers Ltd., Noida - 201 301

# Contributors

**Raksha Arora**
Professor
Department of Obstetrics and Gynaecology
Maulana Azad Medical College and Lok Nayak Hospital, New Delhi

**Sutopa Banerjee**
Senior Resident
Department of Obstetrics and Gynaecology
Maulana Azad Medical College and Lok Nayak Hospital, New Delhi

**Swaraj Batra**
Director Professor and Head of Department
Department of Obstetrics and Gynaecology
Maulana Azad Medical College and Lok Nayak Hospital, New Delhi

**Chanchal**
Junior Resident
Department of Obstetrics and Gynaecology
Maulana Azad Medical College and Lok Nayak Hospital
New Delhi

**S. Chandra**
Chief Medical Officer
NTPC, New Delhi

**Mona Dahiya**
Senior Resident
Department of Obstetrics and Gynaecology
Maulana Azad Medical College and Lok Nayak Hospital, New Delhi

**Neha Gami**
Senior Resident
Department of Obstetrics and Gynaecology
Maulana Azad Medical College and Lok Nayak Hospital, New Delhi

**Gauri Gandhi**
Professor
Department of Obstetrics and Gynaecology
Maulana Azad Medical College and Lok Nayak Hospital, New Delhi

**Deepti Goswami**
Associate Professor
Department of Obstetrics and Gynaecology
Maulana Azad Medical College and Lok Nayak Hospital
New Delhi

**Sangeeta Gupta**
Assistant Professor
Department of Obstetrics and Gynaecology
Maulana Azad Medical College and Lok Nayak Hospital, New Delhi

**C Jassal**
Senior Resident
Department of Obstetrics and Gynaecology
Maulana Azad Medical College and Lok Nayak Hospital, New Delhi

**Ashok Kumar**
Professor
Department of Obstetrics and Gynaecology
Maulana Azad Medical College and Lok Nayak Hospital, New Delhi

**YM Mala**
Associate Professor
Department of Obstetrics and Gynaecology
Maulana Azad Medical College and
Lok Nayak Hospital, New Delhi

**Usha Manaktala**
Director Professor
Department of Obstetrics and Gynaecology
Maulana Azad Medical College and
Lok Nayak Hospital, New Delhi

**Sumita Mehta**
Senior Research Associate
Department of Obstetrics and Gynaecology
Maulana Azad Medical College and
Lok Nayak Hospital, New Delhi

**Sudha Prasad**
Professor
Department of Obstetrics and Gynaecology
Maulana Azad Medical College and
Lok Nayak Hospital, New Delhi

**Asmita M Rathore**
Professor
Department of Obstetrics and Gynaecology
Maulana Azad Medical College and
Lok Nayak Hospital, New Delhi

**Poonam Sachdeva**
Specialist
Department of Obstetrics and Gynaecology
Maulana Azad Medical College and
Lok Nayak Hospital, New Delhi

**Aparna Sharma**
Junior Resident
Department of Obstetrics and Gynaecology
Maulana Azad Medical College and
Lok Nayak Hospital, New Delhi

**Ruchira Singh**
Junior Resident
Department of Obstetrics and Gynaecology
Maulana Azad Medical College and
Lok Nayak Hospital, New Delhi

**Rimpi Singla**
Junior Resident
Department of Obstetrics and Gynaecology
Maulana Azad Medical College and
Lok Nayak Hospital
New Delhi

**Renu Tanwar**
Senior Resident
Department of Obstetrics and Gynaecology
Maulana Azad Medical College and
Lok Nayak Hospital
New Delhi

**Anjali Tempe**
Professor
Department of Obstetrics and Gynaecology
Maulana Azad Medical College and
Lok Nayak Hospital, New Delhi

**Reva Tripathi**
Professor
Department of Obstetrics and Gynaecology
Maulana Azad Medical College and
Lok Nayak Hospital, New Delhi

**Shakun Tyagi**
Senior Research Associate
Department of Obstetrics and Gynaecology
Maulana Azad Medical College and
Lok Nayak Hospital, New Delhi

**Leena Wadhwa**
Senior Research Associate
Department of Obstetrics and
Gynaecology
Maulana Azad Medical College and
Lok Nayak Hospital, New Delhi

**Vijay Zutshi**
Senior Specialist
Department of Obstetrics and
Gynaecology
Maulana Azad Medical College and
Lok Nayak Hospital, New Delhi

# *Preface*

Infections cause significant morbidity and sometimes mortality in obstetrics and gynaecology as they do in other clinical specialities. Therefore, it is important to have a basic knowledge of the more common causative organisms and their effects on the female genital organs, on the pregnant women and on the foetus and the neonate.

This book describes some of the more important viral, bacterial and parasitic infections relevant to obstetrics and gynaecology.

During pregnancy, some infections have a deleterious effect not only on the pregnant woman but also on the foetus and the newborn. Some viral infections during pregnancy can cause foetal demise and congenital malformations in the foetus. The chapters on viral infections describe these effects on mother and child and also the appropriate counselling and treatment to be given.

The problem of HIV/AIDS has assumed alarming proportions in our country. One chapter has been devoted to HIV in obstetrics and gynaecology and antiretroviral therapy.

Bacterial and parasitic infections need appropriate antimicrobial therapy. This has been described in each chapter. In addition, there is one chapter devoted to antimicrobial therapy in pregnancy, describing the safety profile of these drugs during pregnancy.

Immunisation in pregnancy has been described separately.

The important gynaecological infections like genital tuberculosis, sexually transmitted diseases and pelvic inflammatory disease have been described in different chapters.

Antibiotic prophylaxis is a very important step to prevent infections in elective or emergency surgery. The last chapter describes the evidence based guidelines regarding antibiotic prophylaxis in obstetrics and gynaecology.

We hope this book will help the practising clinicians to treat infections and also judiciously use antibiotics to prevent infections.

**Gauri Gandhi**
**Sumita Mehta**
**Swaraj Batra**

# *Acknowledgements*

The editors would like to express their gratitude to all the contributing authors who have put in a lot of effort to comprehensively present the latest developments in every topic.

We would also like to thank our families who have given us constant support during preparation of this manuscript.

Last, but not the least, we are extremely grateful to Jaypee Brothers Medical Publishers (P) Ltd for their co-operation during the compilation of this book.

# Contents

# Plate 1

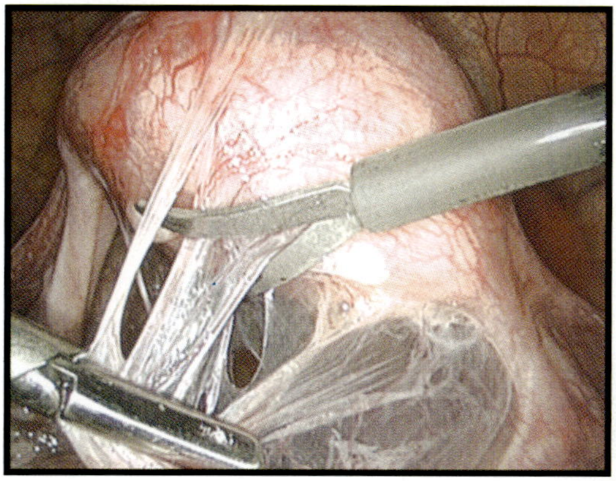

**Fig. 6.1:** Laparoscopy picture showing flimsy adhesions on posterior surface of uterus, involving tubes also

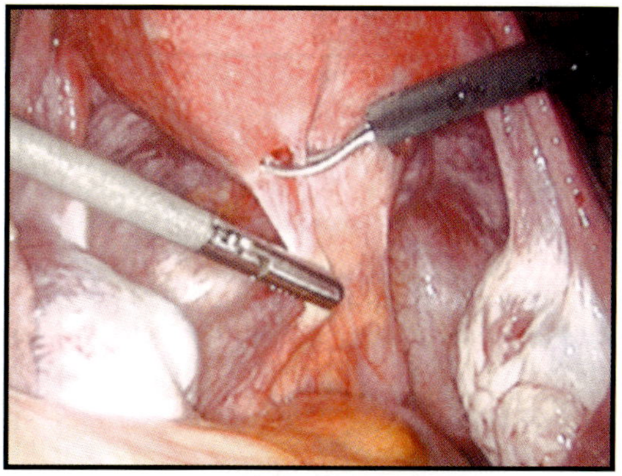

**Fig. 6.2:** Laparoscopy picture showing dense adhesions between uterus and bowel

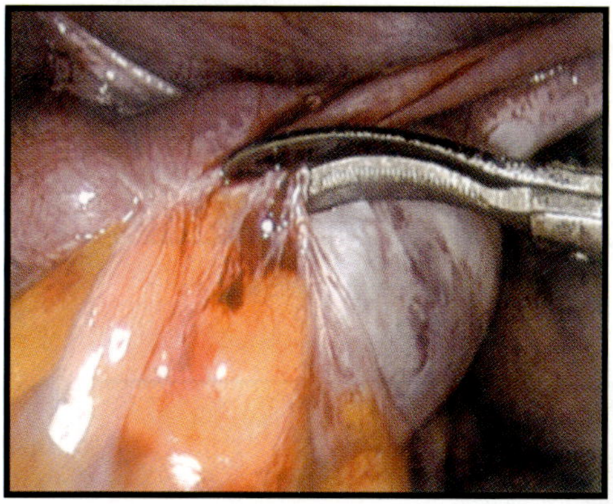

**Fig. 6.3:** Laparoscopy picture showing adhesions leading to distortion of adnexa

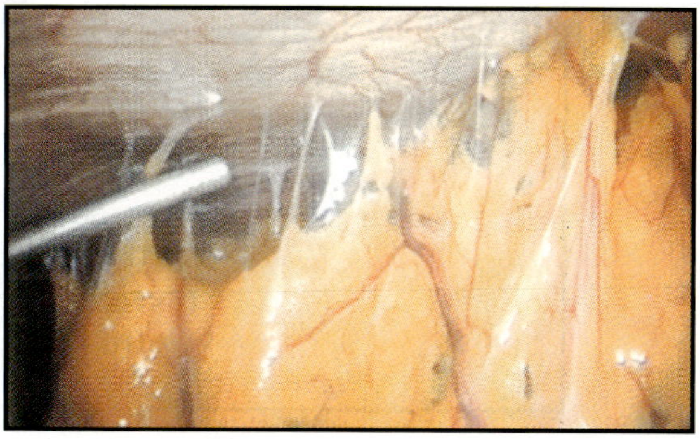

**Fig. 6.4:** Laparoscopy picture showing adhesions between omentum and anterior abdominal wall

# Plate 2

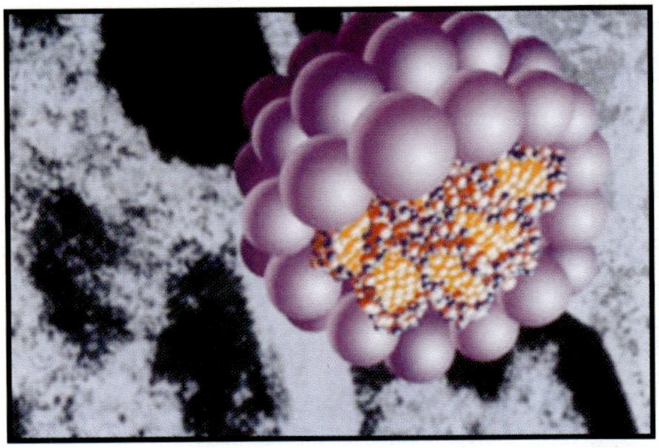

**Fig. 12.1 :** Human papilloma virus

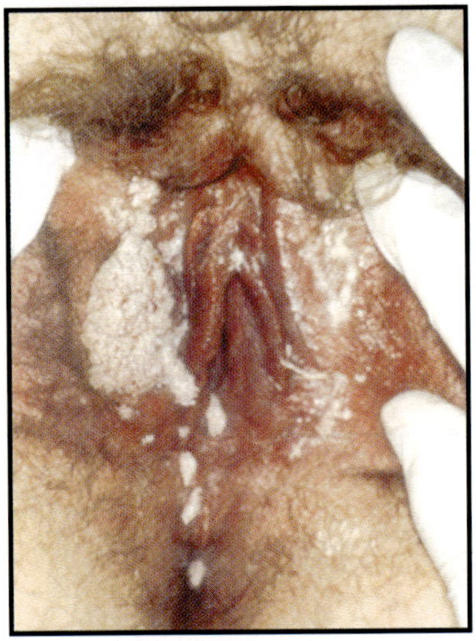

**Fig. 12.2:** Vulval condyloma

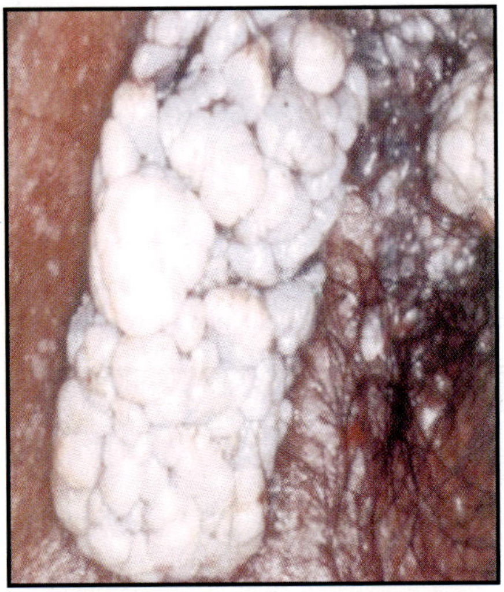

**Fig. 12.3:** Condyloma acuminata of vulva

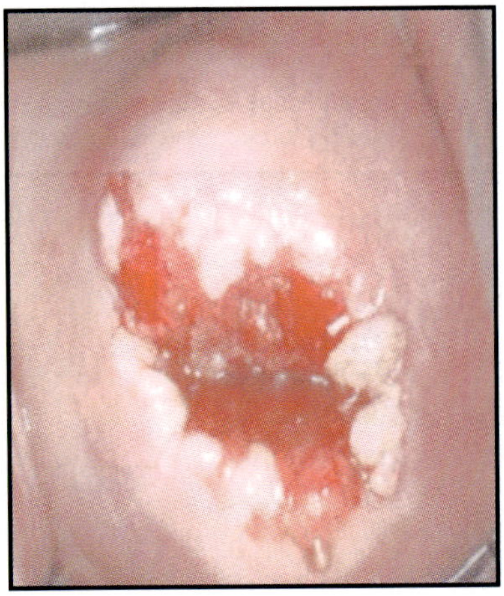

**Fig. 12.4:** Condylomata acuminata of cervix

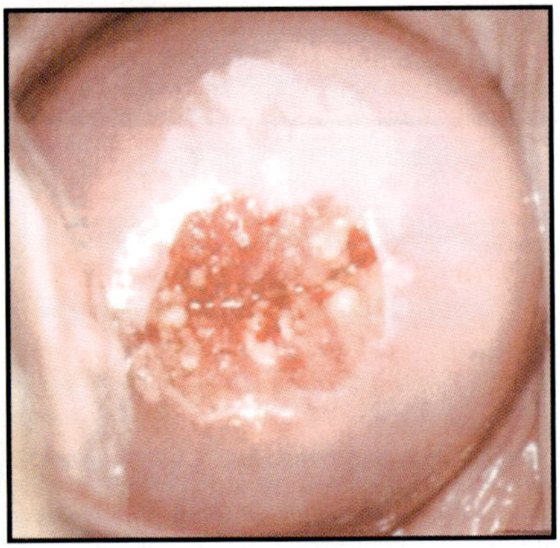

**Fig. 12.5:** Colposcopic view of HPV infection

# Plate 3

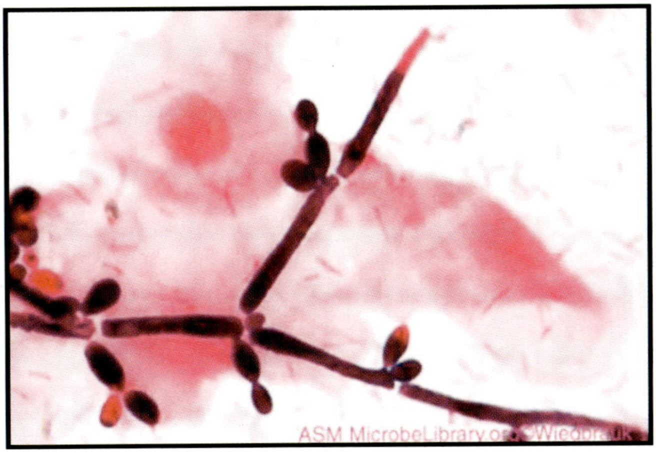

**Fig. 12.6:** Candida mycelia

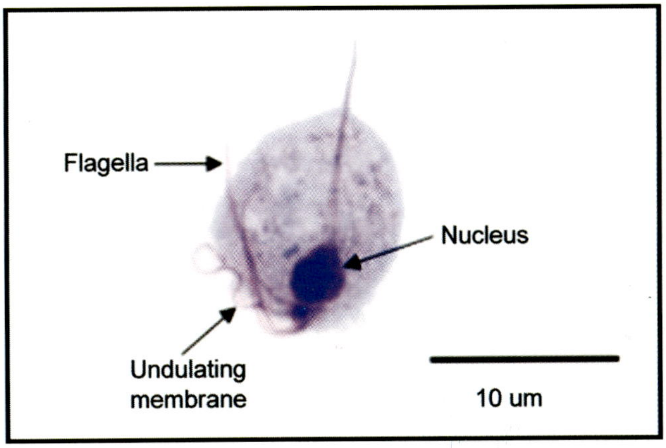


**Fig. 12.7:** *Trichomonas vaginalis* in vaginal discharge

CHAPTER 1

# Viral Infections in Pregnancy

*Sangeeta Gupta, Sutopa Banerjee*

## INTRODUCTION

Viral infections in pregnancy are major causes of morbidity and mortality for both mother and foetus. The viral infections of concern during pregnancy are those caused by cytomegalovirus, rubella virus, herpes simplex virus, varicella-zoster virus, parvovirus, coxsackievirus, measles virus, enterovirus, adenovirus and human immunodeficiency virus.

This chapter will focus on some of these viral infections, except human immunodeficiency virus infection, which is described in another chapter of this book.

## CYTOMEGALOVIRUS (CMV)

## INTRODUCTION

Human cytomegalovirus infection is the most common cause of intrauterine infection resulting in congenital disease and hence, is of particular concern to the obstetrician.

### Causative Agent

CMV infection is caused by a double stranded DNA virus of the herpes family.

### Pathogenesis

CMV has *special affinity for nuclei* of infected cells and multiplies in them to form intranuclear inclusions in the affected tissues and therefore, is also known as cytomegalic inclusion disease. It has the *ability to become latent* following an acute attack and reactivate at a later time.[1] It also exhibits *persistency of viral shedding*; infected children shed the virus in saliva and urine till almost two years of age and adolescents for almost few months after infection. Incubation period is 28 to 60 days.

### Epidemiology

Primary maternal infection occurs in 0.7 to 4 per cent of pregnancies, with 30 to 40 per cent of them resulting in congenital infection.[2] 40-60 per cent women of childbearing age of mid-high socio-economic status and 80 per cent of low socio-economic status are already seropositive.[2,3] But, *preexisting maternal antibodies do not prevent reactivation or recurrent infection in pregnancy* and is essentially not protective against intrauterine CMV infection with around 0.2 to 2 per cent risk of delivering a congenitally infected infant.[2]

**Table 1.1:** Foetal affection in CMV infection

| | *Primary maternal infection* | *Recurrent/Reactivation* |
|---|---|---|
| Incidence | 0.7-4% of pregnancies. (less frequent) | 1-14% (more frequent) |
| Risk to foetus: | | |
| Congenital infection | 30-40% (much more) | Only 0.2-2% (much less) |
| Symptomatic at birth | 10% (much more) | < 1% (much less) |
| Long-term sequel | 10-15% (much more) | 5-10% (much less) |

The above table deduces that in pregnancy, though recurrent/reactivation of CMV infection is more common than primary infection, *risk of foetal transmission, congenital infection and affection are much more and severe with primary maternal infection*. Almost all cases of infants symptomatic at birth are due to primary maternal infection.

CMV infection affects approximately 1 per cent of all births and is the most common infectious cause of childhood deafness.

CMV is not highly contagious. *Horizontal spread* occurs through close contact with saliva, urine, body secretions, contaminated fomites, sexual contact or receipt of infected organs or blood. The most common mode of infection is from a 2 to 3 year-old child attending a day care centre, who usually shed the virus in around 50 per cent cases. *Vertical transmission* occurs by haematogenous spread to the placenta with placental infection and subsequent foetal infection. The virus replicates in the foetal renal tubular epithelium and is excreted into the amniotic fluid. CMV can spread at perinatal period (10-15%) following exposure to infected genital tract secretions during passage through birth canal or from breastfeeding of infected mother's milk. *Recurrent or reactivated infection* transmits by migration of infected leukocytes across the placenta, reactivation of infection locally within the endometrium, ascending infection via the cervical canal due to lower genital tract virus shedding and re-infection with a different strain of CMV.

## Clinical Features

In 90 per cent cases CMV infection in the mother is asymptomatic. Sometimes it may present as a febrile illness mimicking mononucleosis with malaise, fatigue, myalgia, sore throat, lymphadenopathy and hepatosplenomegaly. Rarely, serious complications may occur like interstitial pneumonitis, hepatitis, meningoencephalitis, myocarditis, thrombocytopenia and haemolytic anaemia.[4] Recurrent infection is always asymptomatic.

## Effect of Pregnancy on CMV

Course of disease is not altered or severed due to pregnancy.

## Effect of CMV on Pregnancy

There is no evidence of increase in spontaneous abortions or late pregnancy losses in CMV infection but, it is associated with an increased incidence of premature rupture of membranes and pre-term delivery.

## Foetal Transmission and Prognosis

Transmission of CMV infection to the foetus occurs with equal frequency in all the trimesters (40%), but the infection is more virulent when occurs in early pregnancy (< 20 weeks of gestation) and hence severe sequel occur. Neonates are usually asymptomatic if infection occurred in the third trimester or intrapartum, unless in low birth weight babies. These babies shed the virus for about 2 years in childhood, but, the development is normal with no permanent sequel. Hence, caesarean section in order to avoid intrapartum foetal exposure is not justified.

The mechanisms of development of congenital anomalies due to CMV infection are cell death, resultant ischaemia from vasculitis and immune system mechanisms.

*It is the primary maternal infection in early pregnancy which is of greatest concern* because 10 per cent neonates born to these mothers are symptomatic at birth and have poor prognosis with 25 per cent mortality rate; the survivors develop permanent sequel like mental retardation, neurological symptoms, sensorineural hearing loss and visual impairment. Out of the rest 90 per cent asymptomatic neonates, 10 to 15 per cent develop significant long-term sequel usually within the first 2 years of life; most commonly sensorineural hearing loss[5,6] followed by developmental delay and mental retardation. So, *with primary CMV infection at early gestation, there is 92.7 per cent chance of having a normal infant* while 7.3 per cent chance of neonatal death or sequel. With recurrent/reactivated infection < 1 per cent neonates are symptomatic and only 5 to 10 per cent of the asymptomatic neonates develop long-term sequel: suggesting some but, not all protection by pre-existing maternal antibodies.

The classical tetrad of CMV affection is mental retardation, cerebral calcifications, microcephaly and chorioretinitis. Neonates with severe congenital infections present with thrombocytopenia with petechiae, hepatitis with jaundice, hepatosplenomegaly, microcephaly, pneumonitis, chorioretinitis, optic atrophy, micro-phthalmia, aplasia of various parts of the brain, intrauterine growth retardation and dentine defects. Intracranial calcifications are an indication that the infant will have at least moderate to severe mental retardation.

Structural foetal sequels are common in primary maternal infection in the first trimester (e.g. microcephaly and intracranial calcifications), whereas functional abnormalities are more common in primary maternal infections closer to delivery (e.g. hepatitis, thrombocytopenia and pneumonia).[3]

## Diagnosis

Diagnosis of CMV infection in *antenatal women* clinically is difficult because mostly it is asymptomatic or has non-specific symptoms. *Routine antenatal screening of CMV infection is not recommen-ded* because neither it influences the management nor it is cost effective. In primary infection IgM antibodies become positive but, may persist for 6 to 9 months and even upto 18 months. Therefore it is difficult to say if the infection has been acquired during the pregnancy or before. *A four-fold rise in IgG antibody titres at 4 to 6 weeks interval is suggestive of a recent or recurrent infection.* CMV IgG antibody avidity test is useful in diagnosing primary infection when the IgG antibodies produced have low affinity for the CMV antigens whereas on reactivation or re-infection the antibodies have high avidity. Viral culture or PCR (polymerase chain reaction) will diagnose CMV infection but, they do not differentiate between primary and recurrent/reactivated infection.

*Prenatal diagnosis* of CMV infection of foetus is best done by analysis of amniotic fluid by PCR after 21 weeks of gestation when it is 100 per cent sensitive. Hence, *amniocentesis* should be done after 21 weeks of gestation and atleast 4 weeks after maternal serological diagnosis. A positive amniotic fluid test suggests foetal infection (excreting virus into urine) but, not the degree of fetal affection or its prognosis. A single negative amniotic fluid test does not exclude intrauterine infection and a repeat test should be done 4 to 8 weeks later. Viral culture of amniotic fluid can also be used. *Ultrasound* is also useful in prenatal diagnosis but positive findings like microcephaly, ventriculomegaly, intracerebral calcifications, hydrops, IUGR and oligohydramnios are limited to those foetuses with severe symptoms.

Foetal blood culture has low sensitivity and hence, is not recommended. IgM antibodies in foetal blood are not present until after 20 weeks of gestation and may not appear even in later gestation despite long infection. Therefore, cordocentesis is not justified.

Diagnosis of congenital CMV infection *in neonates* is best done by PCR or viral culture from urine, saliva or cord blood in first 2 weeks of life. A positive test on cerebrospinal fluid suggests high risk for abnormal neurological development.

## Management

*Preconceptional counselling* is required in women with unknown serostatus who come in contact with CMV infected individuals more often like health care personnel or day care workers. They should be advised to prevent infection by maintaining proper hygiene, frequent hand washing and taking universal precautions or change occupation. Counselling may also be sought by a lady who has delivered a CMV affected infant previously. She should be told that there is no increased risk of vertical transmission. Chances of delivering an infected infant is small (about 2%) and the neonate is usually asymptomatic with very low risk of developing long term sequel. Usually the risk of clinically symptomatic neonate is 0.2 per cent. No prophylactic measures to prevent transmission are required and prenatal diagnosis is impractical. There is no data to indicate how long conception should be delayed after a primary infection.

*Routine maternal screening* of primary CMV infection is not recommended because in seronegative women, serial samples have to be taken to exclude seroconversion and is not cost effective; hygiene and sanitation instructions can be given to all women irrespective of knowledge of her serostatus; no vaccine is available; less than 25 per cent of infected foetus will be affected and hence it is difficult to advice how to proceed in the pregnancy, above all there is no therapy available to prevent the fetal damage and pregnancy termination is the only alternative to expectant management.

*The management options* for women with presumed primary CMV infection are as follows:

Treatment of an affected neonate with ganciclovir or forscarnet has considerable haematotoxicity and is recommended only in CMV retinitis in immunocompromised host. Acyclovir is not useful in CMV infection because the virus does not induce its own thymidine kinase enzyme. There is no data to indicate how congenital compilations can be delayed.

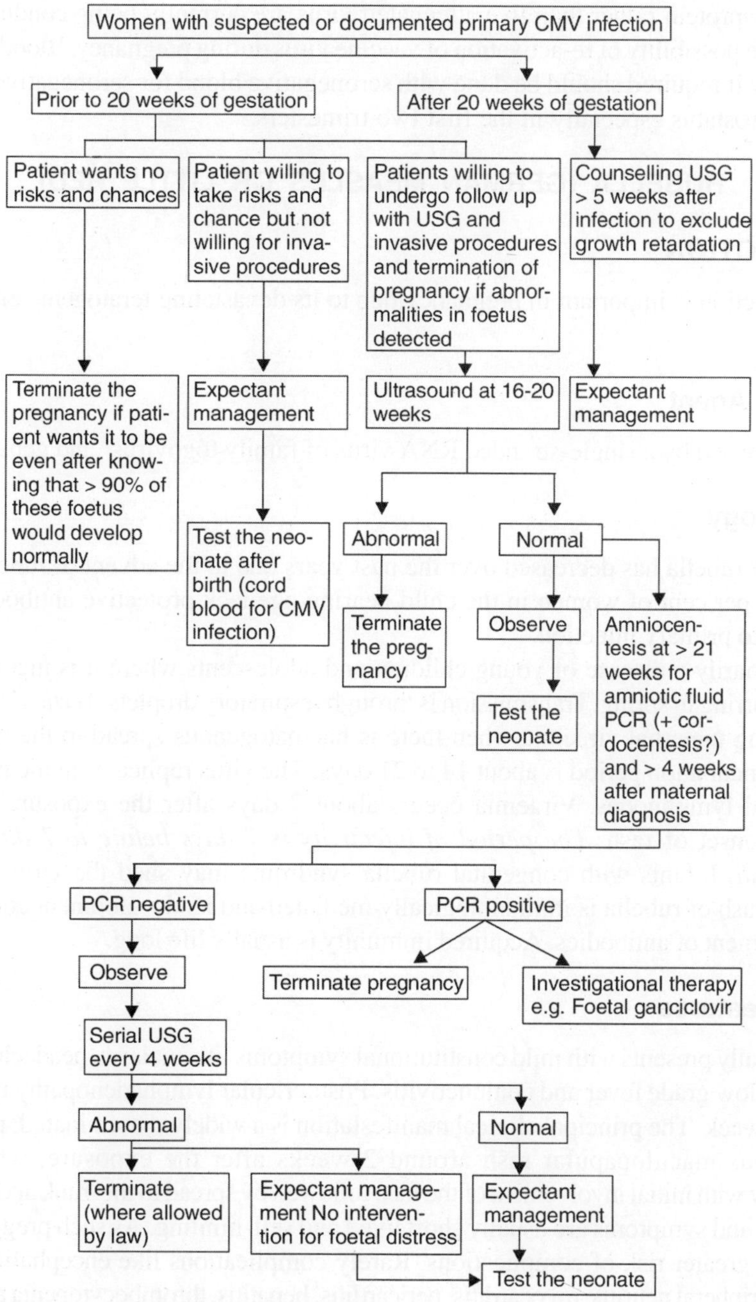


## Prevention

Prevention of CMV infection in pregnancy is through *health education* regarding maintaining hygiene. There are no controlled trials till date to support the use of passive immunization with hyperimmune plasma or globulin after a primary infection. Vaccination trials using CMV surface glycoprotein rather than live attenuated virus are currently being conducted. These will avoid the possibility of re-activation of vaccine virus during pregnancy. Blood transfusion in pregnancy if required should be done with seronegative blood for seronegative lady or for unknown serostatus especially in the first two trimesters.

## RUBELLA (GERMAN MEASLES OR LITTLE RED)

## INTRODUCTION

Rubella infection is important in pregnancy due to its devastating teratogenic effects on the foetus.

### Causative Agent

Rubella is caused by a single-stranded RNA virus of family togovirus[7] and genus rubivirus.

### Epidemiology

Incidence of rubella has decreased over the past years due to the advent of rubella vaccine; still 5 to 25 per cent of women in the child bearing age lack protective antibodies and are susceptible to primary infection.

It is primarily a disease of young children and adolescents where it is inconsequential; usually occurring in spring. Transmission is through respiratory droplets. *Vertical transmission* occurs during maternal viraemia when there is haematogenous spread to the placenta and the foetus. Incubation period is about 14 to 21 days. The virus replicates in the nasopharynx and regional lymphnodes. Viraemia occurs about 7 days after the exposure and 7 days before the onset of rash. *The period of infectivity is 7 days before to 7 days after the onset of rash*. Infants with congenital rubella syndrome may shed the virus for about 2 years. The rash of rubella is immunologically mediated and its development coincides with the development of antibodies. Acquired immunity is usually life long.

### Clinical Features

Rubella usually presents with mild constitutional symptoms like malaise, headache, myalgias, arthralgias, low grade fever and conjunctivitis. Postauricular lymphadenopathy may occur in the second week. The principal clinical manifestation is a widely disseminated, non-pruritic, erythematous maculopapular rash around 2 weeks after the exposure, which affects centrifugally with initial involvement of the face followed by spread to the trunk and extremities. These signs and symptoms are usually short lived and self-limiting. As such pregnant women are not at a greater risk of complications. Rarely complications like encephalitis, myelitis, optic and peripheral neuritis, myocarditis, pericarditis, hepatitis, thrombocytopenia and Guillain-Barré syndrome may occur.

### Effect of Pregnancy on Rubella

Disease course is not altered or severed. As such pregnant women are not at a greater risk of complications.

## Effect of Rubella on Pregnancy

Rubella may lead to spontaneous abortions and congenital rubella syndrome (CRS) in early pregnancy and stillbirths in late pregnancy.

## Foetal Transmission and Prognosis

Many a times the foetus may escape the infection with or without placental infection and may show no clinically detectable lesion.

The various *mechanisms of teratogenecity* of rubella are direct cellular destruction causing altered formation or function of developing tissues, blood vessel obliteration with hypoxic damage, chromosomal injury, immunopathologic damage to tissues, formation of antigen-antibody complexes with deposition into certain tissues and interference with cell mitosis. Rubella virtually affects every organ.[8] The foetal consequences relate directly to the gestational age at the time of maternal infection:

**Table 1.2:** Foetal consequences in Rubella

| *Period of gestation* | *Risk of infection* | *Consequence* |
|---|---|---|
| 0-12 weeks | 40-50% | 100% risk of major congenital abnormalities |
| 13-16 weeks | 30-35% | Deafness and retinopathy in 15%. Spontaneous abortion in 20%. |
| After 16 weeks | 10% | Usually normal development with slight risk of deafness and retinopathy. |

*The clinical manifestations of CRS are:*

**Table 1.3:** Clinical manifestations of CRS

| *Classical triad* | *Cataract, heart defects, sensorineural deafness.* |
|---|---|
| Others | |
| a. Transient (Present at birth but resolve spontaneously) | Low birth weight, hepatosplenomegaly, thrombocytopenic purpura, meningo-encephalitis, hepatitis, haemolytic anaemia, pneumonitis, myocarditis lymphadenopathy, blue berry muffin spots. |
| b. Permanent | • Sensorineural deafness (most common manifestation; 80% CRS children are affected).<br>• Eye defects like salt and pepper retinopathy, cataract, microphthalmia, glaucoma and severe myopia-(10-30%).<br>• CNS anomalies like microcephaly and mental retardation -(10-25%).<br>• CVS defects like patent ductus arteriosus (most common cardiac defect), pulmonary artery and valve stenosis (most pathognomonic of rubella) and VSD- (10-20%). |
| c. Developmental (appear and progress with age) | Sensorineural deafness, mental retardation, IDDM (autoimmune mechanism), thyroid disorders and hypertension. |

## Diagnosis

Diagnosis of rubella *in mother* is done by *serology*; ELISA for IgG and IgM antibodies. *Demonstration of serocoversion is suggestive of recent infection*, i.e. a four-fold or greater rise in IgG titres in paired acute and convalescent sera samples taken at 3 to 4 weeks interval. IgG antibody appears within 7 to 10 days of exposure and persists for life. IgM antibody usually peaks within 7 to 10 days after the onset of illness and then declines over a period of 4 weeks. Presence of rubella specific IgM also suggests recent infection. But, false positive and false negative results may occur. Moreover it may persist for many months and may not suggest a recent infection. It may also be present with re-infection. IgG avidity testing may help to differentiate recent from long ago infection. Viral culture is time consuming, costly and difficult.

*Prenatal diagnosis* of congenital rubella is investigational. Foetal infection can be diagnosed by PCR of amniotic fluid for rubella antigen or culture for rubella virus. Cordocentesis for PCR and to detect rubella specific IgM is not useful since before 22 weeks the foetus is not immunocompetent and even after that appropriate immune response may not occur. Prenatal diagnosis on USG is not reported but, cerebral ventriculomegaly, intracranial calcifications, cardiac malformations, and foetal growth retardation can be looked for in suspected first trimester exposure.

*Diagnosis of CRS* is by PCR in nasal secretions, urine or CSF. IgM in serum and postnatal persistence of IgG supports the diagnosis of CRS. Imaging studies for periventricular calcifications, leukomalacia or subependymal cystic lesions can be done.

## Management Options of Rubella in Pregnancy

a. *Women coming for preconceptional counselling* should be tested for susceptibility to rubella by IgG testing:

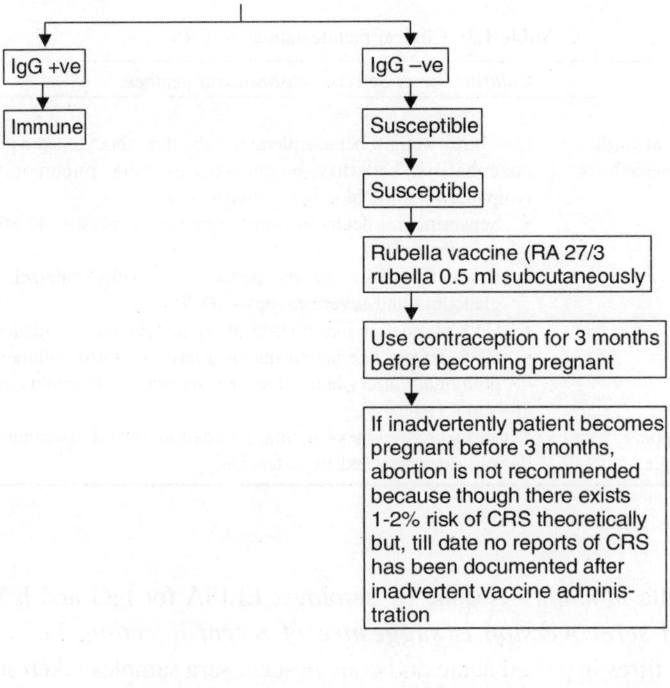

b. *All women in their first antenatal visit* should undergo rubella testing

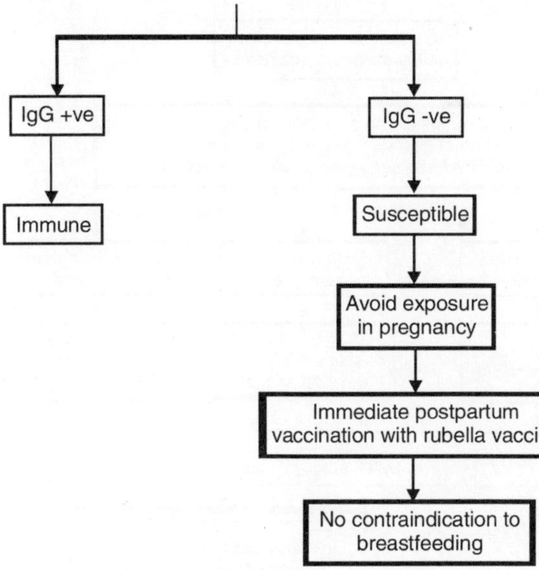


C. Test for primary infection in pregnant women exposed to rubella with demonstration of seroconversion or presence of IgM antibody (see Flow chart on next page).

*Postexposure prophylaxis* with immunoglobulins does not prevent infection or viremia; therefore, not routinely recommended. But, it may be considered for women exposed to rubella in the first 16 weeks of gestation who, under no circumstances would terminate their pregnancy. Suggested dose is 20 ml.

Protection for fetal infection is also not guaranteed.

*Women with known immunity when exposed to natural rubella or vaccination may develop asymptomatic re-infection with viremia.*

They generally do not have congenital infection in their foetus and risk of CRS is too low to justify pregnancy termination. For the same reason, serological testing for all women exposed to rubella to exclude re-infection is not recommended.

### *Prevention*

Prevention is the key to rubella management in pregnancy. It can be done by universal MMR (mumps-measles-rubella) vaccination of children and selective vaccination of women in childbearing age.

## HERPES GENITALIS

## INTRODUCTION

Herpes simplex virus (HSV) is important to the obstetrician because it causes neonatal herpes which is a severe viral infection with significant morbidity and mortality.

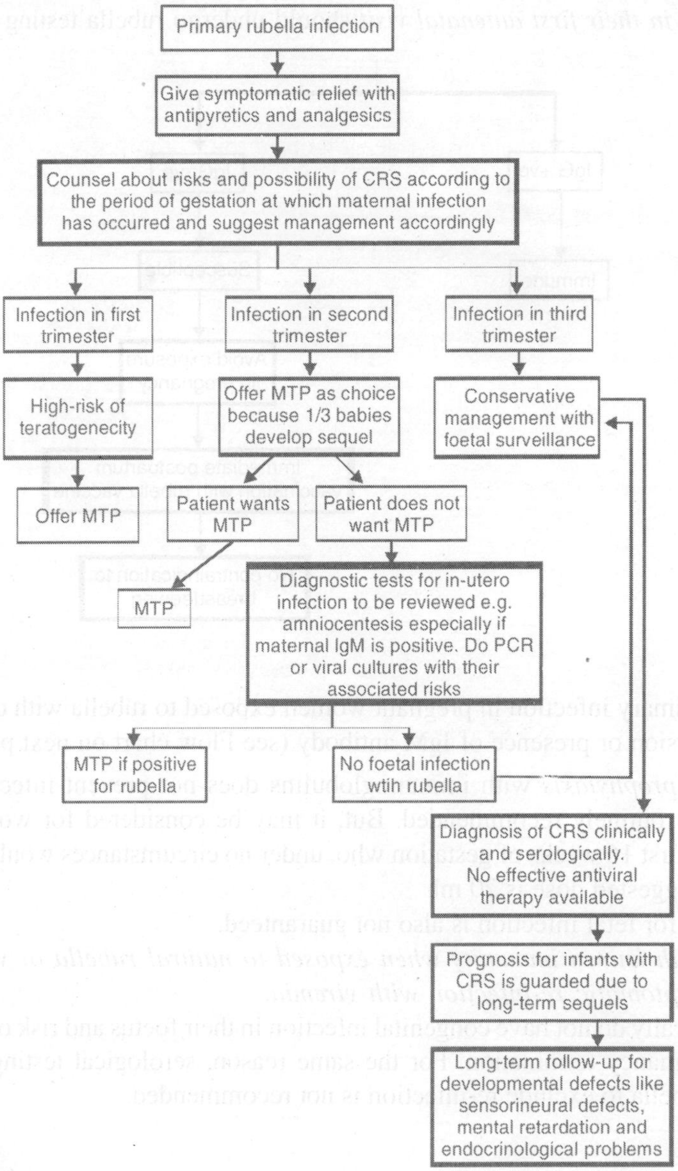


## Causative Agent

HSV is a double stranded DNA virus of the herpes family. In humans there are two serotypes: HSV-1 and HSV-2. HSV-1 primarily causes oropharyngeal infection whereas HSV-2 primarily causes genital herpes; but, both can cause genital herpes with equal severity. 3/4 cases of neonatal herpes infection is caused by HSV-2 while ¼ cases by HSV-1.

## Epidemiology

0.5 to 1 per cent of reproductive age group women have clinically evident disease and 25 to 30 per cent have sub-clinical disease with the rate of asymptomatic shedding during pregnancy between 0.2 to 7.4 per cent and at the time of delivery 0.1 to 4 per cent. Asymptomatic shedding is episodic and lasts for approximately 1.5 days with less viral load.

Transmission of herpes genitalis virus is via sexual contact or through fomites. *Vertical transmission* is maximum during intrapartum period via direct contact of the infant with virus infected maternal secretions while passing through the birth canal. The virus gains entry into the foetus through the eyes, upper respiratory tract, scalp and cord. Vertical transmission can also occur rarely by haematogenous dissemination or ascending infection from the cervix. Infection may be transmitted post delivery from contact with infected caregivers.

## Clinical Features

Pregnant women may present with any of the three types of presentations as given in the table.

**Table 1.4:** Clinical presentations of genital herpes

| *Classification* | *Criteria* |
|---|---|
| Primary genital herpes | First clinical infection. No pre-existing antibody. |
| Non-primary first episode | No history of genital tract infection.Positive antibody for the other strain of the virus (HSV-1 or HSV-2) |
| Recurrent | Prior history of clinical infection. Positive antibody for the same strain of virus causing the present infection. |

*Primary genital herpes* presents with multiple painful vesicles on the vulva, vagina, cervix and urethra between 2 to 14 days of exposure which rupture to form shallow eroded ulcers with erythematous bases resolving in 4 to 6 weeks without scarring. It is accompanied by constitutional symptoms, regional lymphadeno-pathy, dysuria, haematuria, and vaginal discharge; very rarely viral meningitis, encephalitis and hepatitis may occur.

*First episode of non-primary infection* is characterized by fewer systemic manifestations, lesser pain, briefer duration of viral shedding and more rapid resolution of clinical lesion.

*Recurrent genital herpes* occurs due to reactivation of the virus lying dormant in the neuronal ganglia. The infection is much milder and shorter with viral shedding lasting an average of only 3 to 5 days.

Many of the times, the maternal infection is asymptomatic or unrecognised, and it may be difficult to distinguish clinically between recurrent and primary genital HSV infections.

## Effect of Pregnancy on HSV

Disease course is not altered or severed. As such pregnant women are not at a greater risk of complications.

## Effect of HSV on Pregnancy

Primary herpes simplex infection but, not recurrent genital herpes in early pregnancy is associated with an increased rate of spontaneous abortions (50%)[9], whereas in later pregnancy it manifests as stillbirth, pre-maturity and IUGR.

### Foetal Transmission and Prognosis

The transmission rates, and incidence of neonatal herpes depend on the type of infection, e.g. with primary genital herpes it is greatest upto 50 per cent, with non-primary first episode infection it is 33 per cent, with recurrent HSV infection it is 0 to 3 per cent due to pre-existing protective antibodies and with asymptomatic shedding it is only 0.94 per cent. Risk factors for increased intrapartum transmission of HSV are maternal first episode infection with HSV, multiple genital lesions, maternal infection acquired at or just before onset of labour, pre-term delivery, premature rupture of membranes, rupture of membranes for more than 4 hours,[9] placement of foetal scalp electrodes, prolonged second stage of labour and instrumental vaginal delivery. Infection in utero by haematogenous transmission is rare and may cause skin vesicles or scarring, retinitis or keratoconjunctivitis, microcephaly or hydranencephaly.[10] Routine termination of pregnancy is not recommended if genital herpes occurs during first or second trimester of pregnancy.

Neonatal herpes is a severe viral infection with significant morbidity and mortality especially without antiviral treatment. It is most commonly acquired during intrapartum period with active genital lesions in the mother. It presents within the first 1-2 weeks of life with three distinct syndromes.

i. Involving mainly the skin, eyes and mouth (45% cases)
ii. CNS symptoms with or without mucocutaneous involvement (35% cases)
iii. Disseminated infections where multiple organs are involved like visceral infection, meningitis, encephalitis with high mortality rates (20% cases).

Infants with topical disease show 100 per cent survival with antiviral treatment; 5 per cent survivors have long-term complications. 85 per cent infants with CNS disease survive; but, 85 per cent of these survivors suffer serious sequel like mental retardation, chorioretinitis and seizures. The risk of serious sequel is more if treatment is delayed, severely affected CNS or multiple recurrences in first six months of life. Disseminated disease results in 20 per cent survival rates; 40 per cent out of them have serious morbidity.

Five per cent of neonatal herpes is acquired in utero by haematogenous transmission which presents at birth or within 24 to 48 hours of life.

### Diagnosis

Diagnosis is *clinical* and confirmed best by *PCR* of HSV DNA or viral culture from vulva, cervix and anal canal.

Serology is of limited value because of often poor and slow antibody response, pre-existing antibodies and cross-reacting antibodies to both HSV-1 and HSV-2. In primary infection, seroconversion from negative to positive serology in noted in 2 to 3 weeks. Presence of antibody titre in the initial specimen is suggestive of non-primary first episode infection or recurrent infection.

*Cytology* for demonstration of intranuclear inclusion bodies and multinucleated giant cells in scrapings from base of lesions in Tzanck smear, Wright's staining or Papanicolaou's staining can be done with 20 to 25 per cent false positive rates.

*Electron microscopy* can demonstrate herpes virus in vesicular fluid and scrapings from the base of an active lesion by negative contrast.

## Management

The management options for herpes genitalis mainly aim at prevention of neonatal herpes which is a serious infection with great morbidity and mortality and is as follows:

a. Management of *women presenting with first episode of genital herpes in pregnancy*:
   - The woman should be managed in association with a genitourinary physician. Screen for other sexually trans-mitted diseases. Treatment with acyclovir is recommended for all women who develop a first episode of genital herpes in pregnancy in doses of 400 mg TDS or 200 mg five times a day for five days. In cases of severe infection the duration of treatment is 7 to 14 days. Life threatening herpes genitalis or herpes encephalitis require intravenous acyclovir 10 mg/kg over 1 hour every 8 hourly for 14-21 days. Acyclovir reduces the duration and severity of symptoms and decreases the duration of viral shedding. Acyclovir is well tolerated in late pregnancy and there are no clinical or laboratory evidence of maternal or foetal toxicity.[11,12]
   - Consider daily suppressive therapy with oral acyclovir 200 mg QID in the last four weeks of pregnancy (36 weeks of gestation to term) which may prevent genital herpes recurrences at term and the potential of continuous viral shedding to prevent neonatal herpes and reduce the need for caesarean sections. However, there is insufficient evidence to recommend this practice routinely. Moreover, in recurrent genital herpes, transmission to foetus is very low and women may be delivered vaginally.
   - *Caesarean section* is recommended for all women presenting with first episode genital herpes lesions at the time of delivery to reduce intrapartum transmission of infection to the foetus but, is not indicated for women who develop first episode genital herpes lesions during the first or second trimester. Even in the presence of rupture of membranes for more than 4 hours, caesarean section should be done because it significantly decreases the size of viral inoculation to the foetus. For women who present with first episode genital herpes lesions within 6 weeks of the expected date of delivery or onset of pre-term labour, elective caesarean section may be considered at term, or as indicated, and the paediatricians should be informed. For women like this, who opt for a vaginal delivery, invasive procedures like fetal scalp electrode monitoring , foetal blood sampling and instrumental deliveries should be avoided. In these women, intravenous acyclovir given intrapartum to the mother and subsequently to the neonate may reduce the risk of neonatal herpes by minimising maternal viraemia and reducing exposure of the foetus to HSV.
   - Earlier it was said that weekly viral cultures should be taken in the last six weeks of pregnancy in women with a history of genital herpes to detect recurrent herpes episodes, both symptomatic and asymptomatic and positive cultures near term were an indication for caesarean section. However, this practice is no longer recommended because antenatal swabbing did not predict the shedding of virus at the onset of labour.[13]

b. Management of *women presenting with a recurrent episode of genital herpes during pregnancy*.

   For women presenting with recurrent genital herpes lesions at the onset of labour, the risk to the baby of neonatal herpes during vaginal delivery is small (only 0-3%),[14,15] and should be set against the risks to the mother of caesarean section. Caesarean section to prevent this small per centage of neonatal transmission is not cost effective.[16] A recurrent episode of genital herpes occurring at any other time during pregnancy is not an indication for delivery by caesarean section.

*Neonates* born to mothers with herpes genitalis infection should be observed for the development of neonatal herpes. Cultures should be obtained from the conjunctiva, skin and pharynx at birth and repeated after 24 hours.

Women with prior history of genital herpes can be reassured that in the event of HSV recurrence during pregnancy, the risk of transmission to the neonate is very small, even if genital lesions are present at delivery.[9,11,14,15]

Type specific antibody testing to identify women susceptible to acquiring genital herpes in pregnancy as a routine screening has not been found to be cost effective.

### Prevention

All women should be asked in their first antenatal visit if they or their male partners have ever had genital herpes. Prevention of herpes genitals in pregnancy in women with no prior history of genital herpes can be attempted by avoiding sexual intercourse at times when their partner with previous history of genital herpes has an HSV recurrence. However, the impact of this intervention is limited because sexual transmission of HSV commonly results from sexual contact during periods of asymptomatic viral shedding.[17] Use of condoms throughout pregnancy has also been proposed.

For prevention of postnatal HSV transmission to the neonate, mothers with symptomatic infection do not need to be isolated from their babies. She should wash her hands carefully before handling the infant and shield the baby from any contact with the vesicular lesions. Breastfeeding is permissible as long as no skin lesions are present on the breasts. Health care workers and family members with active HSV infection, such as orolabial herpes or herpetic whitlow should avoid direct contact between lesions and the neonate.

## VARICELLA-ZOSTER VIRUS

### INTRODUCTION

Primary infection with Varicella zoster virus (VZV) causes chickenpox and reactivation of latent virus causes shingles (Zoster).

### Causative Agent

VZV is a double stranded DNA virus of herpes family.

### Epidemiology

Primary VZV infection in pregnancy is uncommon (3/10,000 pregnancies)[18] because 90 per cent of antenatal population is seropositive for VZV IgG antibodies due to infection acquired in childhood.[19]

It is a highly contagious infection transmitted by respiratory droplets, direct personal contact with vesicle fluid, fomites and *vertical transmission* by haematogenous dissemination of virus across the placenta. Incubation period is 10 to 21 days. *The disease is infectious 48 hours before the rash appears and continues until the vesicles crust over 6 to 10 days later*. Once infection is acquired, antibodies to VZV develops within 2 weeks and persist for life offering lifelong immunity. Presence of IgG antibody within a week of exposure reflects prior immunity.

## Clinical Features

Primary infection of a pregnant women is characterised by fever, malaise and pruritic rash that develops into crops of maculopapules which become vesicular and crust over before healing; first on the trunk and then centripetally to the extremities.

Reactivation of latent virus in the sensory nerve root ganglia after a primary infection causes a vesicular erythematous skin rash in a dermatomal distribution known as herpes zoster or shingles. Shingles in pregnancy does not pose major risk either to the mother or to the baby. It is usually mild and viraemia is uncommon unless immunocompromised. There are no foetal or neonatal risks due to transplacentally acquired maternal antibodies.

## Effect of Pregnancy on Chickenpox

In pregnancy chickenpox is associated with greater maternal morbidity and mortality due to varicella pneumonia (10% incidence) whose severity increase in later gestation,[20] hepatitis and encephalitis (< 1%). Delivery during the viraemic period is extremely hazardous and maternal risks are bleeding, thrombocytopenia, DIC and hepatitis.

## Effect of Chickenpox on Pregnancy

There are no increased risks of spontaneous miscarriages if infection occurs in the first trimester. It is the primary infection which poses risk to the foetus and the newborn.

## Foetal Transmission and Prognosis

Presentations in the foetus and newborn vary according to the time when maternal primary infection occurred, and is as follows:

a. *Before 20 weeks of gestation*:

Only 1 to 2 per cent of primary maternal VZV infection occurring before 20 weeks of gestation present with foetal varicella syndrome (FVS)[21,22] (previously called congenital varicella syndrome) characterised by one or more of the following: skin scarring in dermatomal distribution; eye defects like microphthalmia chorioretinitis, cataracts; hypoplasia of the limbs distal to the skin involvement; neurological abnormalities like microcephaly, cortical atrophy, mental retardation and dysfunction of bowel and bladder sphincter. FVS doesn't occur at the time of initial foetal infection but results from a subsequent herpes zoster reactivation *in utero*. It also does not occur if infection occurs after 20 weeks of gestation. FVS can be diagnosed prenatally by detailed ultrasound revealing limb deformity, microcephaly or hydrocephalus, soft tissue calcifications and IUGR. VZV DNA can be detected by PCR in amniotic fluid but, only 3.7 per cent of those having VZV infection develop FVS.

b. *After 20 weeks of gestation and before 36 weeks*:
   1. Primary infection during this period is not associated with adverse foetal effect but, may present as shingles in the first few years of infant life due to reactivation of primary infection *in utero*.
   2. There may be an increased incidence of pre-term labour and delivery due to production of inflammatory mediators.

c. *After 36 week of gestation and immediate postpartum*:
   Primary maternal infection during this period leads to varicella infection of the newborn which occurs within 10 days of birth. Upto 50 per cent babies are infected and approximately 23 per cent of these develop clinical varicella despite high titres of passively acquired maternal antibodies. Most severe neonatal infection occurs when onset of maternal rash happens 5 days before and 2 days after delivery, resulting in significant morbidity and mortality (30%) of neonates.[23,24] This is because it takes atleast 5 days after the onset of maternal disease for the antibodies to be transferred to the foetus and the disease is infectious from 2 days prior to the onset of rashes.

## Prevention

Prevention of primary infection of mother is done as follows:

a. In a non-immune lady who plans to become pregnant, e.g. a seronegative lady undergoing infertility treatment or coming for preconceptional counselling may be offered vaccination (two doses) with live attenuated varicella vaccine at 4 to 8 weeks interval followed by avoidance of pregnancy for one month after receiving each vaccine with appropriate contraceptive method. Otherwise, they may be advised to avoid contact with chickenpox.
b. In a pregnant lady who has come for her *first antenatal visit*, inquire about previous history of chickenpox. If no such history is present, advise to avoid contact and report immediately if exposure occurs.
c. In a pregnant lady with a *history of contact with chickenpox*, a careful history should be taken to confirm (i) the certainty of infection and infectiousness, e.g. a vesicular rash or rash within 48 hours of contact. (ii) the significance of contact or the degree of exposure, e.g. household or face to face contact for atleast five minutes or indoor contact for more than fifteen minutes or for that matter, any close contact during the period of infectiousness. (iii) the susceptibility of the patient e.g. she is immune if past history of chickenpox is present or if no such definite history is present but, her serum is positive for VZV IgG antibodies.

Prevention of chickenpox in a pregnant lady with history of contact with chickenpox is as follows:

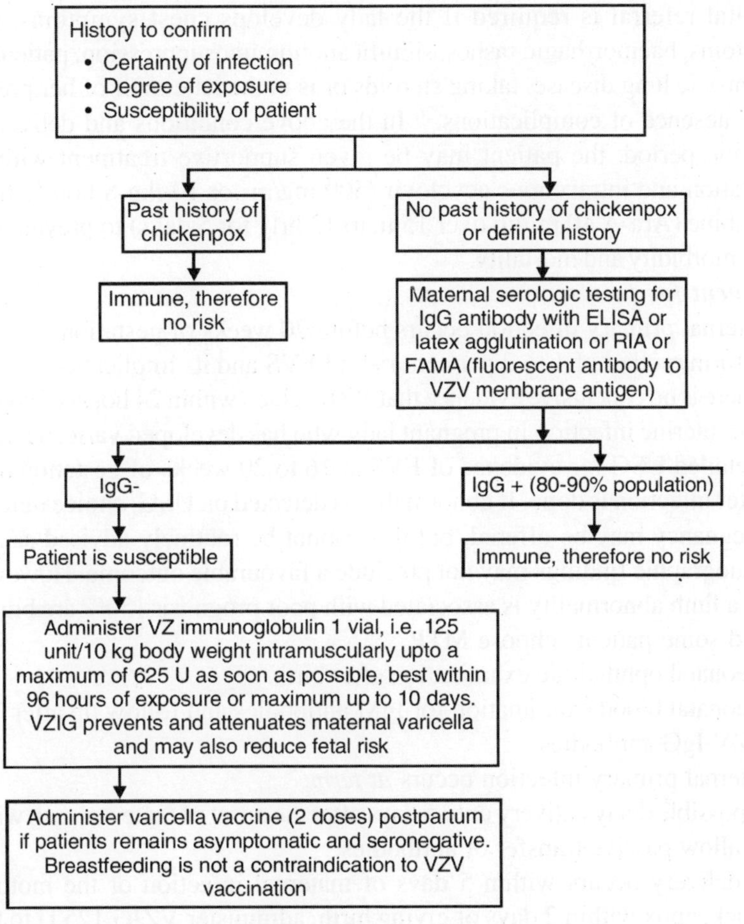


## Management Options for Chickenpox in Pregnancy

a. *Management for mother*:

- Initial management on OPD basis.
  - *Report* to the doctor immediately because varicella in pregnancy is associated with serious complications like pneumonia, hepatitis and encephalitis.
  - Avoid contact with other pregnant ladies and neonates until 5 days of onset of rash or until the lesions have encrusted.
  - Symptomatic treatment with antipruritic, analgesics and hygiene to prevent secondary bacterial infection of the lesions.
  - Oral acyclovir, (800 mg orally five times a day for 5 to 7 days) after an informed consent is started within 24 hours of onset rash if pregnancy is of > 20 weeks of gestation. It reduces the duration of fever and symptoms of VZV infection.[25] Data to support its role on serious complications like pneumonia is insufficient. No adverse foetal or neonatal effect of oral acyclovir in pregnancy has been reported.
  - VZIG has no therapeutic benefit once chickenpox has developed.[26]

- Hospital referral is required if the lady develops chest symptoms, neurological symptoms, haemorrhagic rashes, significant immunosuppression, patient is a smoker, has chronic lung disease, taking steroids or is in the latter half of her pregnancy even in the absence of complications.[26] In the above conditions and delivery during the viraemic period, the patient may be given supportive treatment with mechanical ventilation and intravenous acyclovir (500 mg/m$^2$ or 10-/kg 8 hourly for 7 days) or vidarabine (Ara-A 10 ml/kg over 15 m to 12 hrly for 5 days) to prevent maternal and foetal morbidity and mortality.

b. *Management for foetus or neonate*:
- If maternal primary infection occurs before 20 weeks of gestation:
  - Inform mother of 1 to 2 per cent risk of FVS and its implications.
  - There is no conclusive evidence that VZIG given within 24 hours of contact prevents intrauterine infection in pregnant lady who has developed varicella despite VZIG.
  - Detailed USG for evidence of FVS at 16 to 20 weeks of gestation or at 5 weeks after infection is done. If abnormality is detected on USG, choice of termination of pregnancy may be offered, but this cannot be routinely advised as all abnormal sonographic findings may not preclude a favourable outcome. However, presence of a limb abnormality is associated with poor prognosis (50% are brain damaged) and some patients choose MTP.
  - Neonatal ophthalmic examination after birth.
  - Neonatal blood examination for IgM antibodies and follow up after 7 months for VZV IgG antibodies.
- If maternal primary infection occurs *at term*:
  - If possible delay delivery until 5 days after the onset of maternal rash with tocolytics to allow passive transfer of antibodies.
  - If delivery occurs within 5 days of maternal infection or the mother develops chickenpox within 2 days of giving birth, administer VZIG 125 U to the newborn and observe for the signs of infection for 14 to 16 days. VZIG does not prevent neonatal infection but decreases its severity.
  - Isolate the infant from the mother until all vesicles are encrusted.
  - Breastfeeding is permissible in the absence of vesicles on the nipples.
  - If neonatal infection occurs, treat with acyclovir. VZIG is of no benefit once neonatal chickenpox has developed.[26]

Herpes zoster requires no specific treatment in pregnancy. It is not associated with adverse foetal or maternal outcomes, which would justify the routine use of acyclovir except, for patients with zoster involving the ophthalmic branch of the trigeminal nerve to reduce the risks of serious ocular and central nervous system complications.

## Prevention of Spread of Infection

a. If a neonate is exposed within the first 7 days of life; no due to passively acquired maternal antibodies; administer VZIG to the neonate if the mother is non-immune or if the baby is premature or very low-birth weight. The mother does not require VZIG because she is no longer a high-risk for complications of chickenpox once she has delivered; acyclovir prophylaxis may be considered for her as it provides some protection from the infection with an associated reduction in the chance of transmission to the newborn.

B. Non-immune health workers who are exposed to the infection should be warned that they may develop chickenpox and therefore minimise patient contact from day 8 to 21 post contact. VZIG is not recommended for exposed non-immune health workers.

## HUMAN PARVOVIRUS B19 INFECTION

## CAUSATIVE AGENT

Human parvovirus B19 is a small (20-25 nm diameter with 5.5 kilo base genome) single stranded DNA virus of genus parvoviridae.

### Epidemiology

Parvovirus infection is usually a disease of children of elementary school age. Outbreaks are usually in spring. Fifty per cent of women by the childbearing age are already seropositive and therefore immune to the infection.[27] Rest 50 per cent are susceptible, especially those who work at day care centres or primary schools.

Parvovirus infection is transmitted through respiratory droplets and infected blood components and fomites. Incubation period is 4 to 20 days. Serum and respiratory secretions are infective several days prior to onset of clinical symptoms. Once symptoms appear, respiratory secretions and serum are free of virus, as antibodies have already formed. Symptoms occur due to immune complex formation.

### Clinical Features

Parvovirus infection in 25 per cent pregnant women is asymptomatic. Others may present with erythema infectiosum or fifth disease; most commonly low grade fever, malaise, adenopathy, polyarthritis and arthralgia of hands, wrists and knees[28] and occasionally characteristic pruritic erythematous "slapped cheek" rash on the face and finely reticulated erythematous rash on the trunk and extremities. It is usually self limiting with no serious long-term sequel. Patients with chronic haemolytic anaemias such as thalassaemia or sickle cell disease may present with a transient aplastic crisis due to destruction of the red cell precursors. Overall risk of parvovirus infection in pregnancy is 1 to 5 in 1000 pregnancies. The probability of infection is based on the prevalence of seronegativity in reproductive age population (50%), occupational risk of infection (20% for teachers, 30% for day care personnel), and the risk of foetal infection if the mother develops the disease (10%).

### Pathogenesis

Parvovirus B19 has a predilection for the haematopoietic system by binding to a specific cellular receptor, erythrocyte P antigen, thus destroying the erythroid progenitor cells. It also infects the endothelial cells and the myocardium.

## Foetal Transmission and Prognosis

Parvovirus B19 infection in foetus present as non-immune hydrops with ascites, pleural and pericardial effusions and subcutaneous oedema due to destruction of the foetal erythroid stem cells, resulting in aplastic anaemia and high output congestive heart failure. Also infection of myocardium results in myocarditis and congestive heart failure.[29] Non-immune hydrops may lead to intrauterine death especially when the foetal affection is severe and in early gestation; before 20 weeks.

Risk of foetal infection is greatest if the maternal illness occurs in the first trimester (19%). Between 13 to 20 weeks gestation 15 per cent foetus are infected and in more than 20 weeks gestation around 6 per cent. Affection of foetus is most common between 16 to 28 weeks gestation because this is a period of very active erythropoiesis causing red cell aplasia; foetal immune system is relatively immature before 22 weeks of gestation with inability to produce significant foetal IgM response; maternal IgG antibodies cross the placenta most readily in the third trimester; during the third trimester red cells begin to contain more adult type haemoglobin and less of foetal haemoglobin thus, red cell life span is longer. Teratogenecity of parvovirus infection has not been clearly established but, has rarely caused ocular abnormalities detected in abortus. The risk of foetal growth restriction may be slightly increased.

Neonates born to parvovirus B19 infected mothers rarely present with hepatic disease, transfusion dependent anaemia, myocarditis, CNS abnormalities like arthrogryposis, ventriculomegaly, periventricular calcifications and cerebral atrophy. Long-term prognosis of neonate is usually excellent.

## Diagnosis

Serological testing is recommended in pregnant women with nonspecific flue like syndrome with rashes or joint pains, those with foetal hydrops with no other obvious cause, who had contact with children with erythema infectiosum or have abnormally raised maternal serum alpha-fetoprotein in absence of other causes (marker of hydrops foetalis associated with parvovirus infection). Maternal serum IgG and IgM should be done. IgM appears by the third day of symptoms and typically disappears by 30 to 60 days, but, may persist upto 120 days. IgG antibodies appear by day seven of illness and persist for life, offering life long immunity. Immuno-compromised women may not mount an antibody response to the virus and PCR testing may be necessary to determine infection.

Diagnosis of foetal affection is by ultrasound examination for the development of hydrops. Since the incubation period may be longer in the foetus and most IUDs occur within 6 to 8 weeks of infection, serial weekly ultrasounds for 8 to 10 weeks after acute illness in mother should be done to see the development of hydrops. On development of hydrops, cordocentesis is to be done to detect foetal anaemia. PCR on foetal blood can be done to detect parvovirus antigens or characteristic nuclear clearing and inclusions in nucleated RBCs can be seen. Cordocentesis to detect IgM antibodies is not useful because it may not be positive before 22 weeks of pregnancy after which, foetus becomes immunocompetent or even after that immune response may not be mounted.

It is routinely not required to determine foetal infection with invasive testing like cordocentesis or amniocentesis for PCR testing of parvovirus DNA because, only infection without hydrops has no adverse sequel on the foetus.

## Management Options for Parvovirus B19 Infection in Pregnancy

Intrauterine blood transfusion with packed red blood cells in hydrops foetus with anaemia and low reticulocyte count prevents intrauterine death and mostly causes resolution of foetal

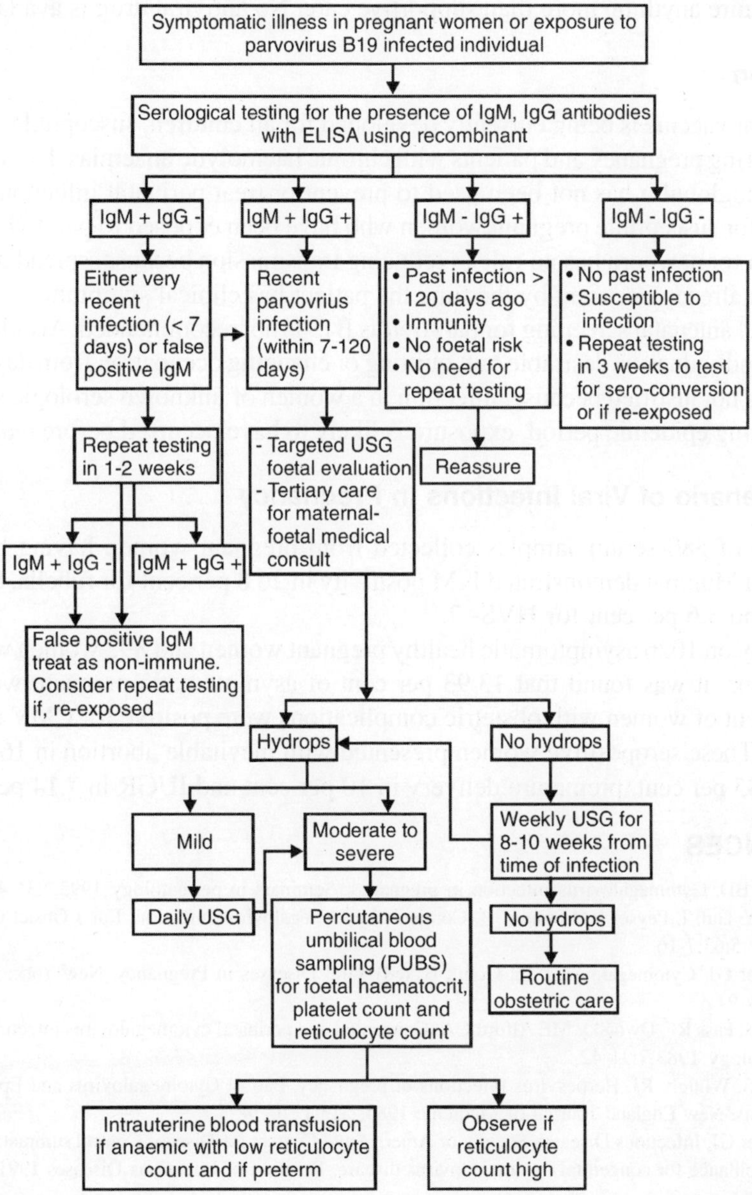

hydrops.[30] A single transfusion to raise the foetal haematocrit to 45 per cent may suffice because foetal red blood cell aplasia is transient and related to the period of viraemia. The foetus should further be followed up with biophysical profile. Hydrops with anaemia and high reticulocyte count suggests resolution stage of transient marrow aplasia and hydrops may resolve without transfusion. Current status of digitalisation to counteract myocarditis induced hydrops is unknown. Maternal administration of intravenous immunoglobulin has been proposed as an alternative to foetal transfusion but no guidelines have been set yet.

Parvovirus infection in the mother is usually self limiting without serious sequel. They may not require anything more than supportive care. No antiviral drug is available till date.

## Prevention

Recombinant vaccine is being currently developed for all children, susceptible adult women before or during pregnancy and patients with chronic haemolytic anaemias. Passive immunity with immunoglobulin has not been used to prevent or treat perinatal infection. It could be considered for susceptible pregnant women who have been exposed to parvovirus infection.

Isolation for newborn has no role in reducing transmission because, spread of respiratory droplets has already occurred by the time the patient has clinical symptoms.

Universal antenatal screening for parvovirus B19 is not recommended. Avoiding exposure to infected individuals is desirable but, quitting or changing occupation from daycare centres or schools is not justified because, infection in a women of unknown serologic status is very low and during epidemic period, exposure is likely to have occurred before realisation.

## Indian Scenario of Viral Infections in Pregnancy

In a survey of 380 serum samples collected from pregnant women having bad obstetric history from Mumbai demonstrated IgM positivity in 26.8 per cent for rubella, 8.42 per cent for CMV and 3.6 per cent for HVS- 2.[31]

In a study on 1026 asymptomatic healthy pregnant women and 892 women with obstetric complications, it was found that 13.93 per cent of asymptomatic pregnant women, while 18.27 per cent of women with obstetric complications were positive for CMV specific IgM antibodies. These seropositive women presented with inevitable abortion in 16.83 per cent, IUD in 28.85 per cent, premature delivery in 10 per cent and IUGR in 7.14 per cent.[32]

## REFERENCES

1. Raynor BD. Cytomegalovirus infection in pregnancy. Seminars in perinatology 1993;7:31-42.
2. Daniel Y, Gull I, Peyser R, Lessing JB. Congenital cytomegalovirus infection. Eur J Obstet Gynecol Reprod Biol 1995;63:7-16.
3. Demmler GJ. Cytomegalovirus. In: Gonik B, (ed) Viral Diseases in Pregnancy. New York: Springer Verlag 1994;69-91.
4. Stagno S, Pass RF, Dworsky ME Alford CA. Congenital and perinatal cytomegalovirus infections. Seminars in perinatology 1983;7:31-42.
5. Stagno S, Whitely RJ. Herpesvirus infections of pregnancy. Part 1: Cytomegalovirus and Epstein-Barr virus infections. New England Journal of Medicine 1985; 313:1270-74.
6. Demmler GJ. Infectious Diseases Society of America and Centers for Disease Control summary of a workshop on surveillance for congenital cytomegalovirus disease. Reviews of Infectious Diseases 1991;13:315-29.

7. Gershon AA. Rubella virus (german measles). In Mandell GL, Douglas RG Bennett JE (eds). Principles and Practice of Infectious Diseases, New York: Churchill Livingstone 1990;3:1242-47.
8. Freij BJ, South MA, Sever JL. Maternal rubella and the congenital rubella syndrome. Clinics of perinatology 1988;15:247-57.
9. Nahmias AJ, Josey WE, Naib ZM, Freeman MG, Fernanderz RJ,Wheeler JH. Perinatal risk associated with maternal genital herpes simplex virus infection. Am J Obstet Gynecol 1971;110:825-37.
10. Hutto C, Arvin A, Jacobs R, et al. Intrauterine herpes simplex virus infections. J Pediatr 1987;110:97-101.
11. Brocklehurst P, Kinghorn G, Carney O, Helsenky, Ross E, Ellis, et al. A randomised placebo controlled trial of suppressive acyclovir in late pregnancy in women with recurrent genital herpes infection. Br J Obstet Gynecol 1998; 105:275-80.
12. Reiff-Eldrige R, Heffener CR, Ephross SA, Tennis PS, White AD, Andrews EB. Monitoring pregnancy outcomes after prenatal drug exposure through prospective pregnancy registries: a pharmaceutical company commitment. Am J Obstet Gynecol 2000;182:159-63.
13. Arvin AM, Hensleigh PA, Prober CG, Au DS, Yasukawa LL, Wittek AE, et al. Failure of antepartum maternal cultures to predict the infants risk of exposure to HSV at delivery. New England Journal of Medicine 1986;315:796-800.
14. Prober CG, Sullender WM, Yasukawa LL, Au DS, Yeager AS, Arvin AM. Low- risk of HSV infections in neonates exposed to the virus at the time of vaginal delivery to mothers with recurrent genital herpes infections. New England Journal of Medicine 1987; 316:240-44.
15. Brown ZA, Benedetti J, Ashley R, Burchetts, Selkes, Berry S, et al. Neonatal HSV infection in relation to asymptomatic maternal infection at the time of labor [see comments]. New England Journal of Medicine 1991;324:1247-52.
16. Randolph AG, Washington AE, Prober CG. Caesarean delivery for women presenting with genital herpes lesions. Efficacy, risks and cost. [see comments]. JAMA 1993;270:77-82.
17. Mertz GJ, Benedetti J, Ashley R, Selke SA, Coreyl. Risk factors for the sexual transmission of genital herpes. Ann Intern Med 1992;116:197-202.
18. Miller E, Marshall R, Vurdien JE. Epidemiology, outcome and control of varicella zoster infection. Rev Med Microbiol 1993;4:222-30.
19. O' Riordan M, O' Gorman C, Morgan C, et al. Sera prevalence of varicella zoster virus in pregnant women in Dublin. Ir J Med Sci 2000;169:288.
20. Smego RA, Asperilla MO. Use of acyclovir for varicella pneumonia during pregnancy. Obstet Gynecol 1991;78:1112-6.
21. Enders G, Miller E, Cradock-Watson JE, Bolley I, Ridehalgh. Consequences of varicella and herpes zoster in pregnancy: Prospective study of 1739 cases. Lancet 1994;343:1548-51.
22. Pastuszak AL, Levy M, Sehick RN, Zuber C, Feld Kamp M, Gladstone J, et al. Outcome after maternal varicella infection in the first 20 weeks of pregnancy. New England Journal of Medicine 1994;330:901-05.
23. Miller E, Cradock-Watson JE, Ridehalgh MK. Outcome in newborn babies given anti-varicella zoster immunoglobulin after perinatal maternal infection with varicella zoster virus. Lancet 1989;2:371-73.
24. Meyers JD. Congenital varicella in term infants: risks reconsidered. J Infect Dis 1974;129:215-17.
25. Wallace MR, Bowler WA, Murray NB, Brodine SK, Oldfield EC III. Treatment of adult varicella with oral acyclovir. A randomised placebo controlled trial. Ann Intern Med 1992;117:358-63.
26. Nathwani D, Maclean A, Conway S, Carrington D. Varicella infections in pregnancy and the newborn. J Infect 1998;361:59-71.
27. Cohen BJ, Buckley MM. The prevalence of antibody to human parvovirus B19 in England and Wales. Med Microbiol 1988;25:151-53.
28. Woolf AD. Human parvovirus B19 and arthritis. Behring Inst Mitt 1990;85: 64-68.
29. Chao WT. Human parvovirus B19: infection in pregnancy and fetal manifestations. Res Med 1990;5:28-32.
30. John F, Rodis. Parvovirus infection. Clinical Obst and Gynae 1999;42(1):107-20.
31. Subhaskar D, Mathur M, Rele M. Seroprevalence of TORCH infection in BOH. Ind J of Med Microbiol 2003;21(2):108-10.
32. Lone R, Bashin A, Phokar M, Vani P, Kakru D, Shahin R, Nazir A. Seroprevalence for CMV in Kashmir valley: a preliminary study. JK Practitioner 2004;11(4):261-62.

CHAPTER 2

# Viral Hepatitis in Pregnancy

Ashok Kumar, Mona Dahiya

Viral hepatitis is a diffuse necro-inflammatory disease of the liver, which develops as a result of infection by primary hepatotropic viruses namely hepatitis A, B, C, D, E, and G viruses, cyto-megalovirus, Epstein-Barr virus and herpes simplex virus. Although taxonomically, it should encompass infection caused by exotic viruses such as yellow fever, Ebola Marburg and Lassa fever, the term viral hepatitis is conventionally used only for few diseases caused by the above mentioned primary hepatotropic viruses.

Viral hepatitis during pregnancy may present itself in two different clinical forms either as Acute Viral Hepatitis (AVH) or Fulminant Hepatic Failure (FHF).

## ACUTE VIRAL HEPATITIS (AVH)

It is defined as those cases, which have acute self-limited disease and a serum aspartate aminotransferase elevation of atleast five fold or clinical jaundice or both.[1] The differentiation of acute viral hepatitis from chronic viral hepatitis is based on the duration of the disease using 6 months for distinction. The natural course of the disease may be divided into three phases:

### Prodromal Phase

The mildest attack is without any symptoms and is marked only by a rise in serum transaminase levels. Alternatively the patient may be an icteric but suffer from gastrointestinal and influenza likes symptoms.

The usual icteric attack in adults is marked by a prodromal period, usually of about 3-4 days, even up to 2-3 weeks, during which the patient feels generally unwell, suffers from digestive symptoms, particularly anorexia and nausea and may in later stages have a mild pyrexia.

### Icteric Phase

The prodromal period is followed by darkening of the urine and lightening of the faeces. This heralds the development of jaundice and symptoms decrease in severity. The temperature returns to normal. Pruritis may appear transiently for a few days. The liver is palpable with a smooth, tender edge in 70 per cent of patients.

### Recovery Phase

After an icteric period of about 1-4 weeks, the adult patient usually makes an uneventful recovery. The stools regain their colour. After apparent recovery, lassitude and fatigue persist for some weeks. Clinical and biochemical recovery is usual within six weeks of onset.

The signs and symptoms of acute viral hepatitis are the same in pregnant and in non-pregnant patients. Fewer subclinical cases without jaundice are detected during gestation since nausea, vomiting, anorexia and malaise are common complaints among pregnant women.

## FULMINANT HEPATIC FAILURE (FHF)

Fulminant hepatic failure is considered when the patient after having a typical acute hepatitis develops hepatic encephalopathy within four weeks after the onset which is characterised by mental changes progressing from confusion, to stupor and coma as a result of severe impairment of hepatic function, without any history of pre-existing liver disease.[2]

### Clinical Features of FHF

Altered mental status in a jaundiced patient is the hallmark of FHF. Deep jaundice, violent behaviour, 'flapping tremors' with fetor hepaticus are the other features.

Cerebral oedema is seen in advanced stages and associated with deep coma. This is the commonest cause of death in FHF, being found in 81 per cent of the fatal cases.[3] Infections are the second most common cause of death. Hypolglycaemia is found in upto 40 per cent of patients with FHF. Functional renal failure (Hepatorenal syndrome) develops in about 55 per cent with or without acute tubular necrosis.[4] At least 80 per cent of the patients have platelet counts of less than 1 lakh per cu mm. The total leukocyte count is high. The prothrombin time is the best indicator of prognosis. Serum bilirubin level and serum aminotransferase are markedly elevated.

The viral hepatitis in pregnancy may be caused by viruses A, B, C, D, E, and G. With regard to the aetiological agent, the spectrum of viral hepatitis, as was evident from our study in Lok Nayak Hospital,[5] is as follows:

| | *A* | *B* | *C* | *E* | *A+B* | *B+E* | *A+E* | *A–E* | *Total number* |
|---|---|---|---|---|---|---|---|---|---|
| AVH | 14% | 7.2% | 0% | 36.2% | 1.4% | 2.8% | 0% | 57.9% | 69 |
| FHF | 14.3% | 7.1% | 0% | 75% | 0% | 7.1% | 10.7% | 21.4% | 28 |

## HEPATITIS A VIRUS (HAV)

It is a non-enveloped RNA virus belonging to the PICORNAVIRI-DAE family. Transmission occurs by the faeco-oral route and person-to-person spread is common. In developing countries, the infection usually occurs is childhood. The incubation period is 15 to 45 days.

The infection is usually self-limiting and chronicity or carrier state is not seen. Pregnant women with hepatitis A infection may have higher incidence of pre-term births. Vertical transmission of the virus is negligible, although, isolated instances have been reported. However, no teratogenic effects have been reported. Pregnant females, who have come in contact with infected patients, may be given 1 ml of immunoglobulin. Management of hepatitis A infection in pregnant women is usually conservative by rest and balanced diet.

## HEPATITIS B VIRUS (HBV)

It is DNA virus belonging to HEPADNAVIRIDAE family. It is 42 nm spherical double-layered DNA particle. It has three antigens namely HBsAg, HBcAg and HBeAg, all three of which are capable of stimulating antibody production.

### Mode of Infection

Hepatitis B virus is present in the blood in last stages of incubation period (30-180 days) and during active episodes of acute and chronic hepatitis. It is also detected in all physiological and pathological body fluids: whole blood, semen, saliva, breast milk, amniotic fluid, cord blood, sweat and tears.

### Mode of Transmission

It is mainly via:

1. Blood and blood products
2. Sexual contact
3. Vertical transmission.

### Epidemiology

The estimated prevalence of hepatitis B virus infection in India is 3 to 7 per cent. In pregnant women, it ranges from 2.26 to 5 per cent, average being 2.8 per cent. HBV is responsible for nearly 30 per cent of acute sporadic hepatitis cases, however, it is seen is <5 per cent of endemic viral hepatitis.

### Pregnant Women at High Risk for HBsAg Positivity are:

1. Acute/chronic liver disease
2. With homosexual partners
3. Drug abusers
4. Spouses of patient with chronic/ acute hepatitis B
5. Repeated blood transfusions
6. Health care workers (1) medical (2) dental (3) laboratory technicians (4) dialysis unit
7. Endemic areas.

Hepatitis B virus infection can result in acute hepatitis, chronic non-progressive hepatitis, chronic disease ending in cirrhosis, fulminant hepatitis, asymptomatic carrier state or hepato-cellular carcinoma (Fig. 2.1).

### Clinical Presentation

There is no difference in clinical presentation in the pregnant state. Acute infection results in the flu-like symptoms in 25 per cent cases and is asymptomatic in the rest. Other symptoms

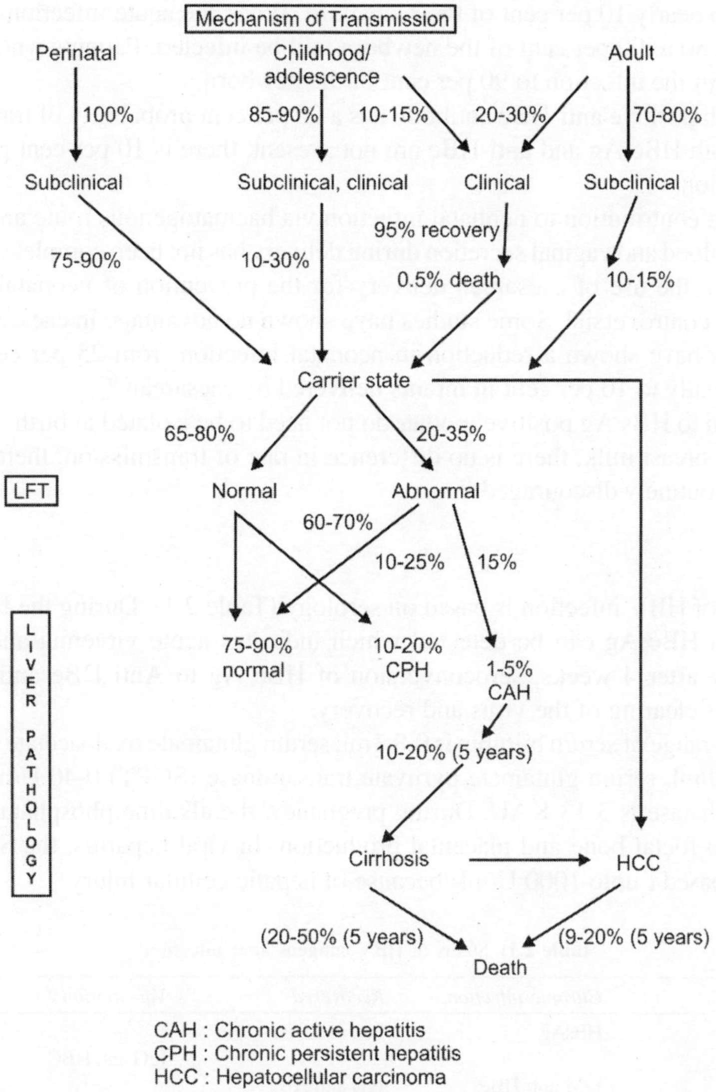


**Fig. 2.1:** Acute hepatitis B infection

include malaise, anorexia, nausea and few develops arthralgia and rashes. There is marked rise in the level of serum transminases (300-800 U/L) Approximately 50 per cent of patients develop jaundice. Persistent HBV infection occurs with varying frequency depending on time of exposure.

## Perinatal Transmission

Most of the infection occurs at the time of delivery due to contact with the maternal blood/ lochia. Incidence of transmission depends on acute/chronic state, period of gestation and HBe Ag status. Mother with acute infection during the first and second trimester transmits the infection to nearly 10 per cent of their newborn. When the acute infection occurs in the third trimester, 80 to 90 per cent of the newborn will be infected. Patients who are HBe Ag positive transmit the infection to 90 per cent of the newborn.

Mother with positive anti-HBe antibody has a 25 per cent probability of transmitting the infection. If both HBe Ag and anti-HBe are not present, there is 10 per cent probability of neonatal infection.

The relative contribution to neonatal infection via haematogenous route and the contact with maternal blood and vaginal secretion during delivery has not been completely elucidated. For that reason, the use of caesarean delivery for the prevention of neonatal infection in HBV carrier is controversial. Some studies have shown no advantage in caesarean delivery, whereas others have shown a reduction in neonatal infection from 25 per cent in infants delivered vaginally to 10 per cent in infants delivered by caesarean.[6]

Infants born to HBs Ag positive mother do not need to be isolated at birth. Though HBs Ag is found in breast milk, there is no difference in rate of transmission; therefore, breast-feeding is not routinely discouraged.

## Diagnosis

The diagnosis of HBV infection is based on serology (Table 2.1). During the first month of acute infection HBe Ag can be detected which indicates acute viraemia and infectivity. Approximately after 4 weeks, seroconversion of HBe Ag to Anti HBe antibody occurs which indicates clearing of the virus and recovery.

The normal range of serum bilrubin is 0.8-1ml; serum glutamate oxaloacetate transaminase (SGOT) 0-40U/ml, serum glutamate pyruvate transaminase (SGPT) 0-40 U/ml and serum alkaline phosphatase is 3-13 KAU. During pregnancy, the alkaline phosphatase is slightly elevated due to foetal bone and placental production. In viral hepatitis, the SGOT/PT are markedly increased ( upto 1000 U/ml) because of hepatic cellular injury.

**Table 2.1:** Status of HBV antigens after infection

| *Acute infection* | *Chronic infection* | *Recovered* | *Vaccination* |
|---|---|---|---|
| HBsAg | HBsAg | IgG anti HBs | IgG anti HBC |
| IgG anti HBs | IgM anti HBe | IgG anti HBe | |

## MANAGEMENT

The following investigations are needed:

| *To confirm liver involvement* | *For diagnosing pathology* | *For identifying complication* |
|---|---|---|
| 1. LFT | Viral markers | KFT |
| 2. Prothrombin time(PT) | Liver biopsy | Coagulation profile |
| 3. USG abdomen | — | Upper GI endoscopy |

The management of acute hepatitis is usually conservative. The patients are followed monthly till HBs Ag is cleared and they have developed anti HBs antibodies.

### Care of HBs Ag Positive Mother and Newborn During Delivery

- Universal precautions to be followed
- I.V. line to be maintained, arrange blood and FFP
- BT, CT, CRT and PT
- Active management of 3rd stage to minimise the risk of PPH
- Vit. K injection to mother (10-20 mg intramuscularly) and baby
- Avoid morphine/pethidine/hepatotoxic drugs
- Caesarean not indicated to prevent transmission
- Handle blood/lochia with gloved hands
- Dispose placenta with incineration
- Separation of mother and newborn not indicated.
- Infants of Hbs Ag positive mothers should receive both active and passive immunisation at birth in the form of recombinant vaccine and hepatitis B immunoglobulin (0.5 ml) within 12 hours after birth.

### Hepatitis B Vaccine

It is a genetically engineered recombinant vaccine. It is a recombinant DNA vaccine obtained from culture of yeast cloned with HBs Ag. It is safe, effective, immunogenic and cost effective. The protective efficacy is 95 per cent after 3 doses. The goal of administering the vaccine is to reduce the incidence of and possibly eliminate hepatocellular carcinoma and chronic liver disease by reducing the number of carriers in the population. Since the administration of hepatitis B vaccine is safe during any stage of pregnancy, nonimmune, uninfected pregnant women with risk factors should be immunised.

The dosage of vaccine is:

| | |
|---|---|
| Age > 10 years: | 1 ml (20 μg) at 0,1,6 months |
| Age < 10 years: | 0.5 ml (10 μg) at 0,1,6 months |

### Hepatitis B Immunoglobulin (HBIG)

It is given for immediate post exposure prophylaxis as in:

- Needle stick injuries
- Newborns born to carrier mothers
- Sexual contacts of hepatitis B patient

HBIG should be given as soon as possible after accidental inoculation.

(Ideally within 6 hours, preferably 48 hours)
0.005-0.007 ml/kg

↓

Simultaneously victims blood drawn to test for viral markers

| HBs Ag +ve | HBs Ag –ve |
|---|---|
| ↓ | ↓ |
| No further intervention | Active immunisation |

## HEPATITS C VIRUS (HCV)

It was discovered in 1989. It is an RNA virus belonging to the group FLAVIVIRIDAE. It has two structural proteins $E_1$ and $E_2$.

### Transmission

1. Blood borne
2. Sexual transmission
3. Vertical transmission

### Risk Factors Associated with Hepatitis C Infection

- Injecting drug abuse
- Transfusion of blood products
- Tattooing and body piercing

### Diagnosis

1. Detection of antibody against $E_2$ protein by ELISA
2. Detection of RNA

### Prevalence

The prevalence of HCV infection in the general population is 1.5 per cent. In one of our studies, the prevalence of HCV infection among pregnant women was estimated to be 0.73 per cent.[7]

### Long-term Complications

HCV infection is associated with the development of cirrhosis (20% cases over 1-2 decades), hepatocellular carcinoma (1-4%) and liver failure.

## HEPATITIS C IN PREGNANCY

Majority of the cases are asymptomatic. Elevated liver enzymes are seen in 10 per cent of the cases. Vertical transmission of HCV from mother to child is seen in 5.2 per cent of the cases. When HCV infection is associated with HIV infection, the vertical transmission ranges from 8.9 to 70.4 per cent (average 23.4%).

To date, the clinical course of pregnancy and the mode of delivery have not been changed by HCV infection. A screening for HCV markers is required 18 months after delivery for infants born to HCV positive mothers. Because of the relatively low rate of HCV vertical transmission, pregnancy can be allowed in infected women. The definitive management of HCV with interferon and ribavarin is withheld during pregnancy due to the teratogenicity and side-effects of these drugs. It is therefore, carried out after delivery.

## HEPATITS E VIRUS (HEV)

Hepatitis E virus is an RNA virus. The earliest recorded epidemic was in Delhi in 1955 in which 29,000 people were affected. It was recognised as a distinct clinical entity in 1980.

## Clinical Features

Hepatitis E produces acute icteric self-limited disease, which may occur in epidemic outbreaks or in sporadic forms. It is faeco-orally transmitted, therefore, epidemics usually occur in the monsoon especially in areas with inadequate sanitation.
*Incubation period*: Varies from 2 to 9 days (average 40 days).

## Diagnosis

1. Ig M antibodies
   - Detected by ELISA
   - Early phase
   - Appears at 1 week to 2 months of infection
   - Disappears by 4 to 5 months.
2. Ig G antibodies:
   Appears shortly after IgM.
3. HEV RNA-detected by reverse transcriptase PCR.

## Incidence

In a prospective Indian study on 97 consecutive pregnant females in 3rd trimester with jaundice, the incidence of HEV infection was 47.7 per cent.[5] It was the aetiological agent in 36.2 per cent cases of AVH and 75 per cent cases of FHF.

## HEPATITIS E IN PREGNANCY

Reports from Europe and United States have shown the course of viral hepatitis during pregnancy to be in no way different from that in non-pregnant women. However, studies carried out in India, Iran, Africa and Middle East[8-10] have found the incidence of fulminant hepatitis to be higher during pregnancy. Alteration in the hormonal status and of T and B cells ratios during pregnancy are postulated to be contributing factors.[11] Fatality rates among pregnant women, especially those infected in third trimesters range between 15 to 25 per cent.[12-14] Poor antenatal care services and poor maternal nutrition are some of the factors responsible for high maternal and foetal mortality in developing countries. Malnutrition has been postulated to explain the increased severity of viral hepatitis in pregnant women. In our study from Lok Nayak Hospital on 21 pregnant females with acute viral hepatitis fulminant hepatic failure, there was no definite correlation between malnutrition (nutrition status assessed by body mass index and haemoglobin) and increased severity of viral hepatitis (under publication).

## Vertical Transmission of HEV

Little is known about vertical transmission of HEV. Ten consecutive women infected with HEV in the third trimester were studied by Khuroo, et al.[15] HEV RNA was detected in cord blood samples of five infants. In another study from UAE,[16] 26 infants born to the 26 HEV RNA positive mothers developed acute/ongoing clinical infection and were HEV RNA positive. Six of the 18 cord blood samples collected in our study were HEV positive therefore, accounting for a vertical transmission rate of 33 per cent.[14] Vertical transmission of HEV is associated with complication like an icteric hepatitis, hypothermia, hypoglycaemia in the newborn and neonatal death.

Thus, HEV is one of the most common identifiable hepatropic viruses causing hepatitis in pregnant women. In the fulminant form in pregnancy, it is associated with high mortality.

## MANAGEMENT OF PREGNANT PATIENT WITH HEPATITIS

### Acute Viral Hepatitis

1. The management of these patients is usually conservative
2. Most of the patients do not need admission
3. Hospitalise patient with severe symptoms like anorexia, vomiting or raised PT
4. Rest: usually not needed, allow activity as per tolerance
5. Nutrition: high calories 3000 K cal/day, avoid fatty foods
6. Drugs: No specific drugs.

### Fulminant Hepatic Failure

1. ICU setting is required
   - Avoid precipitating factors
   - Correct hypokalaemia
   - Avoid morphine, pethidine and diuretics.
2. Discontinue oral proteins
3. Administration of fluid, electrolytes, calories
   - 3000 K cal/day in form of 20-25 percent dextrose and hypo-kalaemia to be corrected (60 mg/day KCL).
   - Correct acidosis with sodium bicarbonate.
4. Measures that affect intestinal bacteria
   - Ampicillin 2-4 g/day to sterilise bowel and to decrease endogeneous ammonia production.
   - Lactulose 30-45 ml 6 hourly
   - High bowel wash
5. Control infections with antibiotics
6. Mannitol if intracranial tension is raised
7. Steroids have no role.

Usually the pregnant patients go into spontaneous labour if they develop fulminant hepatic failure. It is believed that labour may further aggravate the hepatic dysfunction. There is also a risk of coagulopathy. Therefore, obstetricians usually do not interfere in cases of AVH/FHF and prefer to manage them conservatively.

### Key Points

- Viral hepatitis in pregnancy may present itself either in acute or fulminant form.
- HEV is one of the commonest identifiable viruses causing viral hepatitis in pregnancy.

- Fulminant hepatic failure associated with HEV infection has high mortality (15-20 %).
- Management of the patient is usually on conservative lines.
- Induction of labour is usually avoided.

## REFERENCES


1. Smedile A, Carcil, Verma G, et al. Influence of delta infection on severity of hepatitis B. Lancet 1982;2:945-47.
2. Trey C, Davidson LS. The management of fulminant hepatic failure. In : Popper H. Schaffner eds. Progress in liver disease NY Greene and Stration 1970;282-98.
3. Sallie R , Tibcs, Salva AE, Sheron N, Eddelstron A , Willians R. Detection of hepatitis E but not C in sera of patient with fulminant NANB hepatitis. Hepatology 1991;14:68 A.
4. Ring Larson H, Palazzo V. Renal failure in fulminant hepatic failure and terminal cirrhosis : A comparison between incidence, type and prognosis. NEJM 1981; 22:585.
5. Beniwal M, Kumar A, Kar P, Jilani N, Sharma JB. Prevalence and severity of acute viral hepatitis and fulminant hepatitis during pregnancy. A prospective study from North India. Indian J of Medical Microbiology 2003;21(3):184-85.
6. Lees SD, Lo KJ, Tsai yT, et al. Role of cesarean section in prevention of mother -infant transmission of hepatitis B virus. Lancet 1988;1:833-34.
7. Kumar A, Sharma KA, Gupta RK, Kar P, Murthi NS. Hepatitis C virus infection during pregnancy in North India, Intl J Gynaecol Obstet 2005;88(1):55-56.
8. Vishwanathan R. Infectious hepatitis in Delhi (1955-56). A critical study and epidemiology. Ind J Med Res 1957;45 (Supl):1-30.
9. Tandon BM, Joshi YK, Jain SK, Gandhi BM, Mathisen LR, Tandon HD. An epidemic of NANB Hepatitis in North India. Ind J Med Res 1982;75:739-44.
10. Borhan Manish F, Heaghigli P, Hkmat K, Rezaizadeh K, Ghavani AJ. Viral hepatitis during pregnancy-severity and effect on gestation. Gastroenterology 1973;64:304-12.
11. Sterl Haus Kas AJ, Dartes IJ, Dray S. Longitudinal studies showing alteration in levels and functional response of T and B lymphocytes in human pregnancy. Clin Exp Journal 1978;32:531-39.
12. Tsega E, Hanson BG, Krawezynski K, Nordenfelt E. Acute sporadic viral hepatitis in Ethiopia : Causes, risk factors and effects on pregnancy. Clinical Infect Dis 1992;14:961-65.
13. Sreenivasan MA, Banerjee K, Panday PG, Kotak PR, Pandaya FM, Desai NS. Epidemiological investigations of an outbreak of infectious hepatitis in Ahemdabad city during 1975-76. Ind J Med Res 1978;67:197-206.
14. Kumar A, Beniwal M, Kar P, Sharma JB, Murthi NS. Hepatitis E in pregnancy. Int J Gynaecol Obstet 2004;85 (3):240-44.
15. Khuroo MS, Kamilis, Jameel S. Vertical transmission of hepatitis E virus. Lancet 1995;315:1025-26.
16. Kumar RM, Uduman S, Rama S, Kochiyil YK, Umani A, Thomas L. Seroprevalence and mother to infant transmission of E virus among pregnant women in United Arab Emirates. Eur J of Obstet Gynaecol Reprod Biol 2001; 100(1):9-15.

# CHAPTER 3

# HIV in Obstetrics and Gynaecology

*Reva Tripathi, Shakun Tyagi, Chanchal*

## INTRODUCTION

The Human Immunodeficiency Virus (HIV) pandemic continues to spread and steady increases are reported in number of infected women and children. AIDS has killed more than 20 million people till date. Worldwide about 40 million adults aged between 15 to 45 years are currently living with HIV. Although the situation is steadily improving in developed world, reverse is true regarding India and most of the developing world. Same situation prevails regarding incidence of vertical transmission. In 2003 an estimated 7,00,000 children were newly infected with HIV worldwide; about 90 per cent of these infections occurred in sub-Saharan Africa.[1] New HIV cases in children are becoming increasingly rare in many parts of the world with the advent of Highly Active Antiretroviral Therapy (HAART). In 2003, less than 1000 children were estimated to have become infected with HIV in North America and Western Europe and less than 100 in Australia and New Zealand.[1]

Officially, 5.1 million people are infected with HIV in India, although the unofficial figures are estimated to be much higher. In six high prevalence states of Maharashtra, Tamil Nadu, Andhra Pradesh, Karnataka, Manipur and Nagaland the HIV prevalence rates exceed 5 per cent among high-risk groups and exceed 1 per cent among antenatal women. According to HIV surveillance report 2003 prepared by NACO, males account for 73.5 per cent of AIDS cases and females 26.5 per cent.[2] In India with 27 million pregnancies a year and an overall estimated 0.3 per cent prevalence rate of HIV infection among pregnant women, it is estimated that about 100,000 HIV infected women deliver every year. Using a conservative vertical transmission rate of 30 per cent, about 30,000 infants acquire HIV infection each year.

Although currently, India has an overall low prevalence of HIV among pregnant women, with further progression of the epidemic in general population it is bound to rise in women in reproductive age group and thereby increasing chances of mother-to-child transmission (MTCT) of HIV infection. Therefore, the challenge for future is to keep the prevalence of HIV infection among women low and reduce mother to child transmission.

## VIROLOGY

The Human Immunodeficiency Virus (HIV) is an RNA virus characterised by the enzyme reverse transcriptase. It exists in two structurally similar forms HIV-1 and HIV-2, sharing approximately 50 per cent of their nucleotide sequence. HIV-1 is found mostly in North, Central and South America, Europe and Asia. HIV-2 is closely related to simian immunodeficiency virus and is concentrated primarily in West Africa although occasional cases have also been reported from other parts of the world. In man, the target host cells are CD4 antigen bearing T helper lymphocytes. The virus infects these key immune cells by attaching to the CD4 receptors and other cell membrane molecules and introduces its RNA into the cell. The viral enzyme reverse transcriptase uses this RNA as a template to effect a backward transcription of viral genome from RNA into DNA, which is then incorporated into the host's genome and subsequently transcribed to produce viral RNA. The genetic material of next generation of viral particles and the blueprint required for their proteins is contained within this RNA. As the new viral particles mature, the enzyme viral protease cleaves the precursor proteins to generate viral enzymes and structural proteins. The mature viral particles bud from the host cell and can infect other cells. The rapid and continuous replication of HIV impairs and eventually depletes the patient's CD4 and T cell population. This progressive debilitation of the immune system and its network renders the patient susceptible to opportunistic infections and neoplasia that characterise AIDS. During replication mutations may occur in the DNA copies incorporated into the host's DNA because reverse transcriptase is inherently inaccurate. With each cycle of viral replication, which takes 48 hours, single point mutations arise, which may confer resistance to drugs.

## EFFECT OF PREGNANCY ON DISEASE

Plasma HIV viral load and CD4 cell count are the laboratory markers for severity of HIV infection. Its range in healthy adult is 500-1,500 cells/cum. In all women, the absolute CD4 count decreases to 543±169 cells/cum during pregnancy irrespective of whether they are HIV-positive or negative. Pregnancy is not associated with worsening of the disease.

## EFFECT OF DISEASE ON PREGNANCY

Increased incidence of IUGR and preterm delivery has been observed in HIV positive women with low CD4 count and advanced disease. No increased risk of congenital malformations has been observed.

## ANTENATAL CARE IN WOMEN WITH HIV

- All pregnant women who are HIV positive should be screened and treated for genital infections during pregnancy. This should be done as early as possible in pregnancy and repeated at around 28 weeks.
- Plasma viral load and CD4 T-lymphocyte measurements should be reviewed by the HIV physicians at four to six monthly interval during pregnancy in order to advise regarding choice and timing of anti-retroviral therapy and the need for prophylaxis of *Pneumocystis carinii* pneumonia (PCP). PCP prophylaxis is usually administered when the CD4 T-lymphocyte count is below $200 \times 10^6$/l in the form of Tab Cotrimoxazole (Sulfamethoxazole 800 mg and Trimethoprim 160 mg) once daily.
- Women taking anti-retroviral drugs should be monitored for drug toxicity (full blood count, urea and electrolytes, liver function tests, lactate and blood glucose). Presentation with symptoms or signs of pre-eclampsia, cholestasis or other signs of liver dysfunction

during pregnancy may indicate drug toxicity and early liaison with HIV physician should be sought.

- A detailed ultrasound scan for foetal anomalies is important especially after first-trimester exposure to HAART and folate antagonists used for prophylaxis against PCP.
- Intensive foetal monitoring, including assessment of foetal anatomy with a level II ultrasound and continued assessment of foetal growth and well-being during the third trimester should be considered for mothers receiving combination antiretroviral therapy as scant literature is available regarding the effect of such therapy on the foetus.

## VERTICAL TRANSMISSION

Mother-to-child transmission (MTCT) of HIV can occur during pregnancy, parturition, or during breastfeeding. In women who do not breastfeed, it is estimated that, in the absence of intervention, over 80 per cent of HIV transmissions from mother to child occur late in the third trimester (from 36 weeks), during labour and at delivery, with fewer than 2 per cent of transmissions occurring during the first and second trimesters.[5]

### Rate

In the absence of any intervention the risk of MTCT of HIV varies between 15 and 20 per cent in non-breastfeeding women and between 25 and 40 per cent in breastfeeding populations.[3] Interventions such as antiretroviral therapy, caesarean section and avoidance of breastfeeding can reduce the risk of mother-to-child HIV transmission from 25 to 30 per cent to less than 2 per cent.[17-19]

### Risk Factors for Vertical Transmission

Factors Increasing the Risk of Vertical Transmission of HIV

| *Maternal factors* | *Intrapartum events* |
|---|---|
| Low CD4+ lymphocyte count | Artificial rupture of membranes |
| High viral load | Rupture of membranes for longer than 4 hours |
| Preterm delivery | Use of foetal scalp monitor |
| Chorioamnionitis | Foetal scalp pH measurement |
| Advanced AIDS | Instrumental delivery |
| Presence of p24 core antigen in maternal serum | Use of DeLee suctioning |
| | Other events increasing foetal exposure to maternal blood |

It is well established that advanced maternal HIV disease, low antenatal CD4 T lymphocyte counts and high maternal plasma viral loads are associated with an increased risk of mother-to-child transmission.[4]

The principal obstetric risk factors for mother-to-child HIV transmission are vaginal delivery, duration of membrane rupture, chorioamnionitis and preterm delivery.[6]

- Viral load in cervicovaginal secretions has been shown to correlate with mother-to-child HIV transmission. Usually, the genital tract viral load will mirror the plasma viral load,[7,8] but discordance may occur, notably in the presence of inflammatory genital infections (*Chlamydia trachomatis* and *Neisseria gonorrhoeae*)[9] or ulceration.[10]

- Organisms associated with bacterial vaginosis have been shown to stimulate HIV-1 *in vitro*.[11,12] There is a strong association between bacterial vaginosis and preterm birth,[13,14] and preliminary data suggest that bacterial vaginosis may be associated with an increased risk of MTCT.[15]
- Chorioamnionitis, prolonged rupture of membranes and preterm birth have been independently associated with mother-to-child HIV transmission and may be interlinked.[13-16] If there is preterm rupture of membranes, with or without labour, the risk of HIV transmission should be set against the risk of preterm delivery. Preterm infants are more likely to be infected with HIV. This may be attributable to underlying chorioamnionitis[16] or to increased susceptibility of preterm infants to HIV transmission because of immature immune function, incompe-tent mucosal barriers or reduced levels of acquired maternal antibody. Studies conducted before the advent of HAART found that ruptured membranes for more than four hours were associated with double the risk of HIV transmission. These studies also demonstrated a 2 per cent incremental increase in transmission risk for every hour of ruptured membranes up to 24 hours.[16] The relevance of these studies for women taking HAART who have undetectable viral loads is uncertain.
- There is no known contraindication to the use of short-term steroids to promote foetal lung maturation.

## Screening for HIV Infection in Pregnant Women

All pregnant women should be offered screening for HIV early in pregnancy because appropriate antenatal interventions can reduce maternal-to-child transmission of HIV infection.

Detection of anti-HIV antibodies is the mainstay of screening and diagnosis of HIV. Tests to detect specific HIV antibodies can be classified into:

## Screening Tests

- ELISA (2-3 hours)
- Rapid/Simple tests (<30 Minutes) based on principle of agglutination and ELISA
- Dot-blot assays
- Particle agglutination
- HIV Spot and Comb tests
- Fluorimetric microparticle techniques

When a serum specimen is reactive by any one of the screening tests it has to be tested again by a different system using different HIV antigens or different principle of test to confirm the diagnosis. If a specimen is reactive in 2 different systems it has to be tested again using one of the supplemental tests.

### *Supplemental (Confirmatory) Assays*

A supplemental test may be

- ELISA with different antigen system (recombinant or synthetic peptides) or with different principle of test which makes the test more specific;
- Rapid(R)/Simple(S) test
- Western Blot test(WB)

- Immunoblot (IB);
- Line immunoassay;
- Indirect fluorescent antibody test (IFA);
- Radioimmunoprecipitation test (RIPA).

A healthy individual reactive in three different systems of testing, usually (ELISA/S/R) is confirmed to be having HIV infection. The supplemental tests like WB/IF are used to resolve discordant results of ELISA and for research and are expensive, time-consuming and need expertise.

## PRESCRIBING ANTI-RETROVIRAL THERAPY IN PREGNANCY

Women may receive ARV drugs during pregnancy as part of combination regimens used to treat their HIV infection or as prophylaxis to prevent HIV infection in infants.

Initially Zidovudine was the only drug being used for MTCT prevention. Although it still remains the mainstay, various combination regimens mentioned below have been studied and are being used to further reduce the risk of MTCT.[1,20,21] The details of various studies are provided in Table 3.6.

Observational studies in industrialised countries, where MTCT rates are now below 2 per cent, have shown that triple-ARV combinations given to HIV-infected women during pregnancy and labour are highly effective in reducing MTCT.[17-19]

However, the increased complexity of these triple-combination regimens (especially Protease Inhibitor-based regimens), increased exposure to potential drug toxicity and lack of evidence on the efficacy and safety of these regimens for preventing MTCT in resource-constrained settings need to be considered.

Therefore in resource-constrained settings, efforts to prevent MTCT have mostly focused on reducing MTCT around the time of labour and delivery, which accounts for one to two-thirds of overall transmission, depending on whether or not breastfeeding occurs.

ARV prophylaxis around the time of delivery alone can reduce the risk of MTCT in a breastfeeding population almost two-fold following vaginal delivery (41-47% reduction in risk).[22,23] If ARV prophylaxis is extended to include the last month of pregnancy, efficacy at six weeks postpartum can be as high as 63 per cent.[24]

WHO convened a Technical Consultation on Antiretroviral Drugs and the Prevention of Mother-to-child Transmission of HIV Infection in Resource-limited Settings in Geneva, Switzerland on 5-6 February 2004. Key recommendations in the guidelines are as follows:

1. Women who need ARV treatment for their own health should receive it in accordance with the WHO guidelines on ARV treatment. (Criteria for starting ARV treatment of HIV positive adults are listed in Table 3.2). The use of ARV treatment, when indicated, during pregnancy substantially benefits the health of the woman and decreases the risk of HIV transmission to the infant.
2. HIV-infected pregnant women who do not have indications for ARV treatment, or do not have access to treatment should be offered ARV prophylaxis to prevent MTCT using one of following ARV regimens:
   - ZDV from 28 weeks of pregnancy plus single-dose NVP during labour to the mother and single-dose NVP and one-week ZDV for the infant.

- Alternative regimens based on ZDV alone, short-course ZDV + 3TC or single-dose NVP alone are also recommended.

3. Although expanding access to programmes to prevent MTCT presents many challenges and single-dose maternal and infant NVP is the simplest regimen to deliver, programmes should consider introducing more complex ARV regimens where possible.[25]

In India NACO has recommended following strategies as components of its Prevention of Mother to Child Transmission (PMTCT) Program.

1. Provision of quality antenatal services
2. Strategies to enhance acceptance of antenatal services and make the clinics husband-friendly.
3. Offering comprehensive health education including nutrition, exclusive breastfeeding, RTIs/STIs, HIV/AIDS.
4. Implementing peer-based strategies (community participation) for promoting exclusive breastfeeding with mothers informed about risk of transmission of HIV through breast milk and its consequences and be helped for making informed choice regarding infant feeding. Reduction of stigma and preventive measures for STIs, HIV/AIDS.
5. Promotion of rational use of blood and blood products.
6. Provision of services to counsel for birth-spacing methods.
7. Voluntary counselling and testing (VCT) for HIV infection.
8. Interventions to reduce MTCT including antiretroviral drug chemoprophylaxis and drugs for prompt and effective treatment of opportunistic infections are the mainstay of the package, Training of physicians, obstetricians and pedi-atricians in management of HIV disease using antiretroviral drugs; to institute a regimen and monitor patient, if they can afford these drugs themselves.
9. Care and support for HIV infected persons especially women and children.
10. Strengthening of well baby clinics.

    Additionally, establishment of support groups will be critical in maintaining infant feeding practices through training and reducing psychosocial impact.[2]

The main classes of antiretroviral drugs are:

- Nucleoside Reverse Transcriptase Inhibitors (NRTIs).
- Non-nucleoside Reverse Transcriptase Inhibitors (NNRTIs).
- Protease Inhibitors (PIs).

The details of the drugs in these groups are given in Tables 3.6 to 3.8.

## Side Effects/Toxicity of Antiretroviral Drugs

Research is still ongoing regarding the safety of various antiretroviral drugs and it will take time before the long-term effects become known. The major short-term toxicity among infants exposed to prophylactic ZDV to reduce MTCT is anaemia, which is greater for longer exposures. However the effect is usually mild and reversible after treatment is interrupted.[21, 26-29] Whenever possible, the didanosine (ddI) + stavudine(d4T) combination is to be avoided in ARV treatment regimens as several case reports of lactic acidosis among pregnant women receiving ARV combinations including ddI + d4T, some resulting in maternal and in some cases, also foetal, death. Efavirenz has been classified as Class D (positive evidence of human foetal risk) and hence contraindicated. Women, particularly those with CD4+ counts > 250 cells/mm$^3$, have an increased risk of developing symptomatic, often rash associated, nevirapine-related hepatotoxicity, which can be severe, life threatening, and in some cases fatal and therefore requires careful monitoring of transaminase levels. Single dose regimen is not associated with any such side effect but may result in development of resistant strains. Viral resistance was detected among 33-53 per cent of HIV-infected infants who were exposed to single-dose maternal and infant NVP.[30,31]

## MODE OF DELIVERY

- The risk of MTCT can be reduced to below 2 per cent by interventions that include antiretroviral (ARV) prophylaxis given to women during pregnancy and labour and to the infant in the first weeks of life, obstetrical interventions including elective caesarean delivery (prior to the onset of labour and membrane rupture) and completely avoiding breastfeeding.
- Women with, or who are expected to have, a viral load of <50 copies/ml on HAART at 36 weeks, may be offered the option of a vaginal delivery. This is provided there are no complications such as previous uterine surgery or caesarean section, concurrent genital infection or indication of a difficult or prolonged labour as no transmissions with planned vaginal delivery births have been observed for women with undetectable viral load.[35]
- For women who are HIV positive, but not taking HAART during pregnancy and for women with a detectable plasma viral load, delivery by elective caesarean section is of clear benefit in reducing the risk of mother to child HIV transmission[34] and they may be offered this option. However, an increased risk of postoperative complications following caesarean section have been observed among HIV-infected women with more advanced disease as measured by CD4+ lymphocyte count.[32,33] Moreover, in resource-constrained settings, elective caesarean delivery is seldom available and/or safe, and refraining from breastfeeding is often neither acceptable, feasible or safe.
- Therefore, HIV-1 infected women should be counseled regarding the increased risks and potential benefits associated with caesarean delivery based on their HIV-1 RNA levels/ CD4 count, current antiretroviral therapy and any obstetric indication for caesarean section and decision regarding mode of delivery should be taken accordingly.
- Caesarean section is indicated if there is any obstetric indication.

## INTRAPARTUM MANAGEMENT

### In Case of a Vaginal Delivery

Women who opt for a planned vaginal delivery should have their membranes left intact for as long as possible. Use of foetal scalp electrodes and foetal blood sampling should be avoided.

1. If already on HAART women should continue their regimen throughout labour.
2. If an intravenous infusion of zidovudine is planned it should be commenced at the onset of labour and continued until the umbilical cord has been clamped. Dose is one-hour

initial dose of 2 mg/kg body weight, followed by a continuous infusion of 1 mg/kg body weight/hour until delivery.

3. Tablet nevirapine 200 mg single dose orally should be administered in early labour. Repeating nevirapine in case delivery does not take place within 48 hours of drug intake is controversial as repeated dosages increase the chances of emergence of drug resistance.

The cord should be clamped as early as possible after delivery and the baby should be bathed immediately after the birth.

An emergency caesarian section should be performed for the usual obstetric reasons and to avoid a prolonged labour and prolonged rupture of membranes.

### In Case of Elective Caesarean Section

Prophylactic antibiotics should be administered. A zidovudine infusion should be started four hours before beginning the caesarean section and should continue until the umbilical cord has been clamped. A maternal sample for plasma viral load may be taken at delivery. The cord should be clamped as early as possible after delivery and the baby should be bathed immediately after the birth.

## POSTPARTUM MANAGEMENT

Where safe infant feeding alternatives are available, women who are HIV positive are advised not to breastfeed. If the woman is HIV-positive and chooses to breastfeed, exclusive breastfeeding for 6 months should be promoted. She should be advised regarding contraception.

## MANAGEMENT OF THE NEONATE

All infants born to women who are HIV positive should be treated with anti-retroviral therapy from birth. Unless the mother started anti-retroviral therapy late in pregnancy (within four weeks of delivery) treatment of the infant may be discontinued after four to six weeks. Infants of mothers who received zidovudine antenatally and intrapartum, either as single-agent therapy or as part of a HAART regimen, should be given single-agent oral zidovudine till six weeks.

Syrup Nevirapine should be administered to the neonate if the mother received it during intrapartum period.

- If infant weighs 2000 grams or more, give nevirapine solution 0.6 mL (6 mg) by mouth.
- If infant weighs less than 2000 grams, give nevirapine solution 0.2 mL/kg (2 mg/kg) by mouth.

The concentration of nevirapine syrup is 50 mg/5 mL (10 mg/mL).

HAART for neonates may be considered in the case of mothers who started anti-retroviral therapy late in pregnancy. Maternal antibodies crossing the placenta are detectable in most neonates of mother who are HIV-positive. For this reason, direct viral amplification by polymerase chain reaction (PCR) is used for the diagnosis of infant infections. Tests may be carried out at birth, then at three weeks, six weeks and six months. For non-breastfed babies, over 99 per cent of those testing HIV negative by PCR at six months will be uninfected. The definitive test is the HIV antibody test: a negative result at 18 months of age confirms that the child is uninfected.

## PREPREGNANCY COUNSELLING

For couples wishing to conceive where one or both partners is HIV positive, prepregnancy counselling should be undertaken by an appropriately trained health professional. For couples discordant for HIV infection who wish to conceive, appropriate advice should be given to optimise the chance of conception while minimising the risk of sexual transmission. For HIV discordant couples where the woman is HIV positive, the couple should be advised on how to perform artificial insemination at the time of ovulation.[36] Where a woman who is HIV negative has an HIV-positive partner, the risk of transmission to the woman, estimated as approximately 1:500 per sexual act, can be reduced by limiting sexual intercourse to around the time of ovulation. 'Sperm washing,' whereby spermatozoa are separated from surrounding HIV-infected seminal plasma by a sperm swim-up technique can also be tried.[37] To date, there have been no seroconversions in women inseminated with washed sperm.[38] HIV positive men with low sperm counts may be offered intracytoplasmic sperm injection following sperm washing. IVF is now considered ethically acceptable in view of vertical transmission rates of less than 2 percent and increased life expectancy for parents taking HAART.[39]

## GYNAECOLOGICAL PROBLEMS IN HIV POSITIVE WOMEN

- Sexually transmitted infections: Syphilis, gonorrhoea, chlamydia infection, herpetic genital ulcers and trichomoniasis may be coexistent and the frequency of these increases in HIV infected individuals. All HIV infected patients should be screened for these infections and appropriately treated.
- Recurrent vulvovaginal candidiasis defined as at least four discrete episodes in one year: Frequency of vulvovaginal candidiasis increases when CD4+ cell count decreases to less than 100/mm$^3$. Fluconazole at the dose of 200 mg weekly for prevention of mucosal candidiasis in women infected with HIV is safe, efficacious and does not precipitate clinical resistance.
- A rare manifestation described in women with advanced HIV disease is the presence of idiopathic vulvar or vaginal ulcers defined by either negative herpes simplex virus and syphilis testing or non-diagnostic ulcer biopsy, that can be intractable, progress to fistula formation, and cause severe bleeding. This condition has been found to be associated with low CD4 count. It may respond to corticosteroid treatment or initiation of antiretroviral treatment.
- Hormonal changes: Variable effect of HIV infection on menstrual cycle has been reported. Few studies found no effect, while others have reported three-fold increase in risk of amenorrhoea and rise in frequency of hormonal dysfunction with fall in CD4+ cell count.[40]
- Women infected with HIV are two to three times more likely than non-infected women to have HPV DNA detected in cervico-vaginal specimens and five times as likely to

have squamous intraepithelial lesions, vulvovaginal condyloma acuminata or anal intraepithelial neoplasia. Prevalence of cervical Squamous Intraepithelial Lesion(SIL) among women infected with HIV has been reported to range between 12 and 40 per cent.[41] Multifocal extensive cervical and lower genital tract lesions may be present. Cervical and associated lower genital tract neoplasia tend to appear at a younger age and have a higher grade of malignant potential and take a more aggressive course in HIV infected patient. Pap smear should be performed when a woman is found to be infected with HIV. It should be repeated after six months. HIV positive women who have never had an abnormal pap and have had at least two normal pap smears can undergo pap screening every 12 months. If inflammation/ atypia is present, the pap smear should be repeated in 3 months. Colposcopy should be performed in women with SIL, HPV findings, and persistent atypia.

- The natural course of other neoplasia such as ovarian carcinoma and choriocarcinoma may be altered with resistance to conventional therapy, rapid deterioration and poor prognosis.
- Some other neoplasia such as Non-Hodgkin's Lymphoma and Kaposi's sarcoma, which are "AIDS- defining neoplasia", may rarely present as a primary gynaecological malignancy.

## CONTRACEPTION

Contraception in HIV positive patients poses a challenge as the method most effective in preventing further spread is the least efficient one as contraceptive. The use of intra-uterine contraceptive is debatable as it increases the incidence of PID. Moreover, IUD causes cervicitis in HIV-infected women and causes increased viral load in vaginal secretions.

The World Health Organization's *Medical Eligibility Criteria for Contraceptive Use* states that women at risk of HIV infection or those whom are HIV-infected may use hormonal contraception with no restrictions.[42] However, the use of DMPA at the time of infection has been reported to hasten HIV-related deterioration of the immune system and the natural course of HIV infection.[43]

Therefore, it is recommended that while continuing to promote hormonal contraception for family planning when appropriate, providers should counsel hormonal contraceptive users who are HIV positive or at risk of HIV to restrict to a single sexual partner and to use a condom correctly and consistently during each act of sexual intercourse.

## PREVENTION OF OCCUPATIONAL EXPOSURE AND UNIVERSAL PRECAUTIONS

An occupational exposure may place a worker at risk of HIV infection. This can be a percutaneous injury, contact of mucous membrane or contact of skin with blood, tissue or other body fluids from an HIV infected individual. Risk is increased when the skin is chapped, abraded or afflicted with dermatitis or the contact is prolonged or involving an extensive area. In most of the cases the HIV status of the patient is not known. Therefore, following universal precautions should be applied in order to prevent exposure.

- Wash hands after patient contact and after removing gloves.
- Wash hands immediately if hands contaminated with body fluids. Wear gloves when contamination of hands with body substances anticipated
- Protective eyewear and masks should be worn when splashing with body fluids is a possibility, e.g. During vaginal delivery/caesarean section.
- All health care workers should take precautions to prevent injuries during procedures, when cleaning or during disposal of needles and other sharp instruments.
- Needle should **NOT** be-
  - Recapped
  - Purposely bent or broken by hand
  - Removed from disposable syringe nor manipulated by hand
- After use, disposable syringes and needles, scalpel blades and other sharp items should be placed in a puncture resistant container
- Health care workers who have exudative lesions or dermatitis should refrain from direct patient care and from handling equipment
- All needle stick injuries should be reported to infection control officer
- Handling and disposal of sharps safely is essential
- Cleaning and disinfection of blood / body substance spills should be performed with appropriate agents
- Adhere to disinfection and sterilisation standards
- Regard all waste material soiled with blood/body substance as contaminated and dispose of according to relevant standards
- Vaccinate all clinical and laboratory workers against hepatitis B
- Other measures include double gloving, changing surgical techniques to avoid " exposure prone" procedures, use of needle-less systems and other safe devices.

## Body Fluids to which Universal Precautions Apply

- Blood and-or its components
- All body fluids containing visible blood
- Semen
- Vaginal secretions
- Cerebrospinal fluid (CSF)
- Synovial fluid
- Pleural fluid
- Peritoneal fluid
- Pericardial fluid
- Amniotic fluid

Body fluids to which Universal Precautions do not apply. The risk of HIV transmission is extremely low or negligible unless these contain visible blood. These include:

- Nasal secretions
- Sputum
- Sweat
- Tears
- Urine
- Vomitus
- Saliva

*Use of Protective Barriers*: Protective barriers reduce the risk of exposure of the health care worker's skin or mucus membrane to potentially infective materials. Protective barriers include gloves gowns, masks, protective eye wears. Selection of protective barriers depends on the type of exposure

**Type of exposure**: **Low Risk** (contact with skin but with no visible blood)

*Examples*: Administering injections

- Dressing of minor wound

*Protective barriers*: Gloves helpful but not essential.

**Type of exposure: Medium Risk** (probable contact with blood)

*Examples*:

- Vaginal examination
- Insertion or removal of intravenous canulae
- Handling of laboratory specimens
- Dressing of large open wounds
- Venipuncture, spills of blood

*Protective barriers*: Gloves ,Gowns and Aprons may be necessary;

**Type of exposure: High Risk** (probable contact with blood, splashing, uncontrolled bleeding)

*Examples*: Major surgical procedures, particularly in orthopaedic surgery and oral surgery;

- Vaginal delivery

Protective barriers Gloves, Water proof Gown or Apron, Eye wear, Mask Heavy duty rubber gloves should be worn for cleanings instruments, handling soiled linen or when dealing with spills.

## POST EXPOSURE PROPHYLAXIS (PEP) GUIDELINES FOR OCCUPATIONAL EXPOSURE

### Factors Affecting Transmission from HIV Positive Patient

- Amount of blood in the exposure
- Amount of virus in patient's blood
- Whether PEP taken or not

## What to Do on Exposure to HIV Infected Blood?

*Prompt measures*

- Do not panic
- Do not put cut/pricked finger into your mouth
- Wash with soap and water
- No added advantage with antiseptic/bleach

Next step should be prompt reporting.

Post-exposure treatment should begin as soon as possible and preferably within two hours. Late PEP may be initiated in certain situations, which should be individualised. PEP is not needed for all types of exposures.

1. *Post Exposure Prophylaxis*:
   The decision to start PEP is made on the basis of degree of exposure to HIV (Exposure code-EC) and the HIV status of the source (Source code-SC) from whom the exposure/infection has occurred.
2. *Determination of the Exposure Code (EC)*
   Exposure code can be defined as per the flow chart given below. It may be classified into three categories, EC1, EC2 and EC3, depending upon the nature of exposure.

## Exposure Code

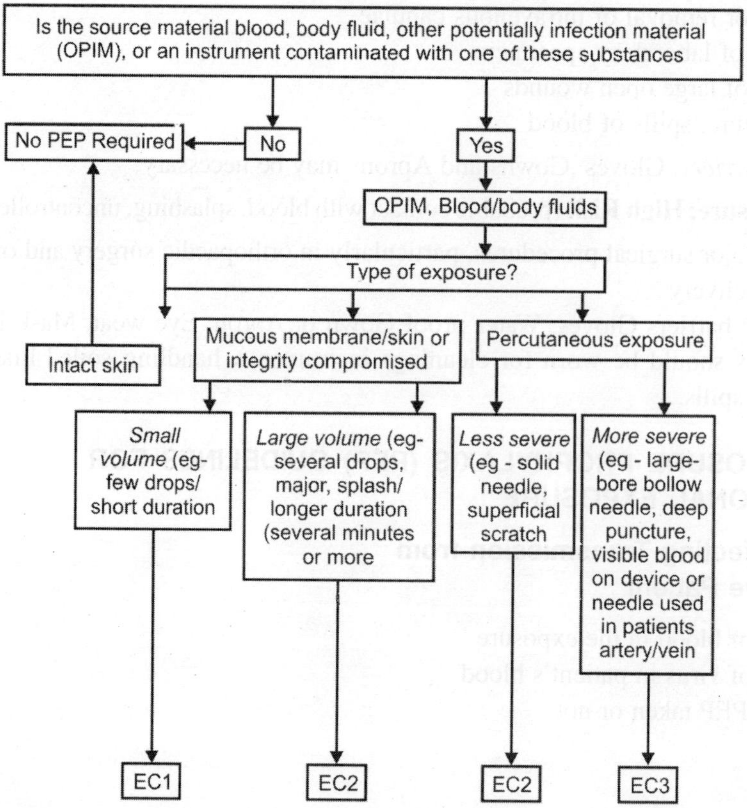

**Source Code**

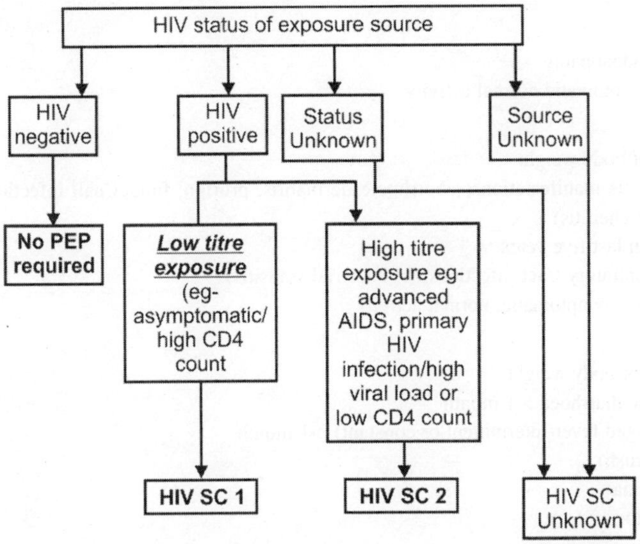


3. Determination of the source code (SC): It can be classified as SC1, SC2 or SC unknown according to HIV status of the exposure source.
4. Determination of PEP Recommendation :This is done using a combination of exposure code(EC) and HIV status code(SC) and recommendations are enumerated below:

| EC | HIV SC | PEP Recommendation |
|---|---|---|
| 1 | 1 | PEP may not be warranted |
| 1 | 2 | Consider Basic Regimen |
| 2 | 1 | Recommend Basic Regimen (most exposures are in this category) |
| 2 | 2 | Recommend Expanded Regimen |
| 3 | 1 or 2 | Recommend Expanded Regimen |

2/3 unknown If setting suggests a possible risk (epidemiological risk factors) and EC is 2 or 3, consider basic regimen

*Basic regimen*: Zidovudine (AZT) –600 mg in divided doses (300 mg/twice a day or 200 mg/thrice a day for 4 weeks + Lamivudine (3TC) – 150 mg twice a day for 4 weeks.

*Expanded regimen (4 weeks therapy)*: Basic regimen + Indinavir – 800 mg/thrice a day. Any other protease inhibitor can be used if Indinavir is not available.

5. *Testing and Counselling*: The health care provider should be tested for HIV as per the following schedule-
   i. Base-line HIV test - at time of exposure
   ii. Repeat HIV test - at six weeks following exposure
   iii. 2nd repeat HIV test - at twelve weeks following exposure. On all three occasions, HCW must be provided with a pre-test and post-test counselling. HIV testing should be carried out on three ERS (ELISA/Rapid/Simple) test kits or antigen preparations. The HCW should be advised to refrain from donating blood, semen or organs/tissues

**Table 3.1:** WHO staging system for HIV infection and disease in adults and adolescents

**Clinical Stage I**

1. Asymptomatic
2. Generalised lymphadenopathy

Performance scale: 1: asymptomatic normal activity

**Clinical Stage II**

3. Weight loss<10% of body weight
4. Minor mucocutaneous manifestations(seborrhoeic dermatitis, prurigo, fungal nail infections, recurrent oral ulcerations, angular cheilitis)
5. Herpes zoster within last five years
6. Recurrent upper respiratory tract infections(i.e. bacterial sinusitis)

And/or performance scale 2:symptomatic, normal activity

**Clinical stage III**

7. Weight loss, >10% of body weight
8. Unexplained chronic diarrhoea > 1 month
9. Unexplained prolonged fever(intermittent or constant) ,>1 month
10. Oral candidiasis(thrush)
11. Oral hairy leukoplakia
12. Pulmonary tuberculosis
13. Severe bacterial infections(i.e.pneumonia, pyomyositis)

And/or performance scale 3: bedridden < 50% of the days during last month

**Clinical stage IV**

14. HIV wasting syndrome(1)
15. Pnemocystis carinii pneumonia
16. Toxoplasmosis of the brain
17. Cryptosporidiosis with diarrhoea >1month
18. Cryptococcosis, extrapulmonary
19. Cytomegalovirus disease of an organ other than liver spleen or lymph node(eg. Retinitis)
20. Herpes simplex virus infection, mucocutaneous(>1 month) or visceral
21. Progressive multifocal leukoencephalopathy
22. Disseminated endemic mycosis
23. Candidiasis of oesophagus, trachea, bronchi
24. Atypical mycobacteriosis, disseminated or lungs
25. Non-typhoid salmonella septicemia
26. Extrapulmonary tuberculosis
27. Lymphoma
28. Kaposi's sarcoma
29. HIV encephalopathy

And/or performance scale 4: bedridden more than 50% of the day during last month

**Table 3.2:** WHO criteria for starting ARV

After confirmation of HIV infection one of the following conditions should be present:

- WHO clinical stage IV: HIV disease irrespective of CD4 count
- WHO clinical stage III: HIV disease with consideration of using CD4 cell counts < 350/mm$^3$
- WHO stage I, II or III disease with CD4 cell count < 200/mm$^3$

**Table 3.3:** Characteristics of nucleoside reverse transcriptase inhibitors (NRTIs)

| *Generic name trade name* | *Zidovudine (AZT, ZDV) retrovir* | *Didanosine (ddI) videx* | *Zalcitabine (ddC) HIVID* | *Stavudine (d4T) zerit* | *Lamivudine (3TC) epivir* |
|---|---|---|---|---|---|
| Dosing Recommendations | 200 mg tid or 300 mg bid or with 3TC as combivir, 1 bid | Tablets >60kg: 200 mg bid < 60 kg: 125 mg bid | 0.75 mg tid | >60 kg: 40 mg bid < 60 kg: 30 mg bid | 150 mg bid <50 kg: 2 mg/ kg bid or with ZDV as combivir 1 bid |
| Oral bioavailability | 60% | Tablet: 40% Powder: 30% | 85% | 86% | 86% |
| Serum half-life | 1.1 hour | 1.6 hour | 1.2 hour | 1.0 hour | 3-6 hours |
| Adverse events | Bone marrow suppression: Anaemia and/ or neutropenia Subjective complaints: GI intolerance, headache, insomnia, asthenia lactic acidosis with hepatic steatosis is a rare but potentially life-threatening toxicity with the use of all NRTIs | Pancreatitis Peripheral neuropathy nausea diarrhoea Lactic acidosis with hepatic steatosis is a rare but potentially life-threatening toxicity with the use of all NRTIs. | Peripheral neuropathy Stomatitis Lactic acidosis with hepatic steatosis is a rare but potentially life-threatening toxicity with the use of all NRTIs. | Peripheral neuropathy Lactic acidosis steatosis is a rare but potentially life-threatening toxicity with the use of all NRTIs. | (Minimal toxicity) Lactic acidosis with hepatic steatosis is a rare but potentially life-threatening toxicity with the use all NRTIs. |

**Table 3.4:** Non-nucleoside reverse transcriptase inhibitors (NNRTIs)

| *Generic name* | *Nevirapine* | *Delavirdine* | *Efavirenz* |
|---|---|---|---|
| Form | 200 mg tabs | 100 mg tabs | 50, 100, 200 mg capsules |
| Dosing Recommendations | 200 mg po qd × 14 days, then 200 mg po bid | 400 mg po tid (Four 100 mg tabs in > = 3 oz water to produce slurry) | 600 mg po qHS |
| Oral bioavailability | > 90% | 85% | 42% (increased with high fat content |
| Serum half-life | 25-30 hrs | 5.8 hrs | 40-55 hours |
| Adverse events | Rash[1] Increased transaminase levels Hepatitis | Rash[1] Headaches | Rash[1] Central nervous systems symptoms[2] Increase transaminase levels False positive cannabinoid test Teratogenic in monkeys[3] |

1. Severe rash may occur in up to 5% of patients; cases of Stevens-Johnson Syndrome have been reported.
2. May include dizziness, somnolence, insomnia, abnormal dreams, confusion, abnormal thinking, impaired concentration, amnesia, agitation, depersonalisation, hallucinations, and euphoria. The overall frequency of any of these symptoms associated with use of efavirenz was 52% compared with 26% in controls; 2.6% of those on efavirenz discontinued the drug due to these symptoms.
3. No data are available regarding teratogenicity of other NNRTIs in non-human primates.

**Table 3.5:** Characteristics of protease inhibitors

| *Generic name* | *Indinavir* | *Ritonavir* | *Saquinavir* | *Nelfinavir* | |
|---|---|---|---|---|---|
| Form | 200, 400 mg caps | 100 mg caps 600 mg/7.5 ml po solution | 200 mg caps | 200 mg caps | 250 mg 50 mg/g oral powder |
| Dosing recommendations | 800 mg q8h Take 1 hr before or 2 hrs after meals; may take with skim milk or low fat meal | 600 mg q 12h Take with food | 600 mg TID* Take with high fat meal | 1200 mg TID Take with large meal | 750 mg TID Take with food (meal light snack) |
| Oral bioavailability | 30% | (not determined) | Hard gel capsule: 4%, erratic | Soft-gel capsule (not determined) | 20-80% |
| Serum half-life | 1.5-2 hrs | 3-5 hours | 1-2 hours | 1-2 hours | 3.5-5 hours |
| Adverse effects | Nephrolithiasis, GI intolerance, nausea Lab: increased indirect bili-rubinaemia (in-consequential) Misc: headache, asthenia, blurred vision, dizziness, rash, metallic taste, thrombocytopenia hyperglycaemia* fat redistribution and lipid abnor-malities** Possible increased bleeding episodes in patients with haemophilia | GI intolerance, nausea, vomiting, diarrhoea Paresthesias - circumoral and extremities Hepatitis asthe-nia taste per-version Lab: Triglycerides increase > 200%, transaminase elevation, elevated CPK and uric acid hypergly-caemia* fat redistribution and lipid abnor-malities** Possible increased bleeding episodes in patients with haemophilia | GI intolerance, nausea and diarrhoea head-ache elevated transaminase enzymes hyper-glycaemia* fat redistribu-tion and lipid abnormalities** possible incre-ased bleeding episodes in patients with haemophilia | GI intolerance, nausea diarrhoea, abdominal pain and dyspepsia headache elevated elevated transaminase enzymes hypergly-mia* Fat redistribution and lipid abnormalities** possible increased bleeding episodes in patients with haemophilia | Diarrhoea Hyperglycaemia* Fat redistribution and lipid abnor-malities** Possible increased bleeding episodes in patients with haemophilia |

* Cases of worsening glycaemia control in patients with pre-existing diabetes, and cases of new-onset diabetes including diabetic ketoacidosis have been reported with the use of all protease inhibitors (50-52).

** Fat redistribution and lipid abnormalities have become increasingly recognised with the use of protease inhibitors. Discontinuation of PIs may be required to reverse fat redistribution. Patients with hypertriglyceridemia or hypercholesterolemia should be evaluated for risks for cardiovascular events and pancreatitis. Possible interventions include dietary modification, lipid lowering agents, or discontinuation of PIs.

and abstain from sexual intercourse. In case sexual intercourse is undertaken a latex condom be used consistently. In addition, women HCW should not breast-feed their infants till the situation is clarified. If HIV status of the patient from whom exposure occurred is unknown it may be worthwhile to get HIV test done of that patient immediately after pre- and post- test counselling. This will help to allay fears in the

**Table 3.6:** Characteristics of protease inhibitors

| *Study* | *Drugs* | *Antenatal and intrapartum* | *Postpartum* | *Maternal CD4+ count at enrolment $10^6$ cells/L* | *Mode of infant feeding* | *Vertical transmission rate and efficacy* |
|---|---|---|---|---|---|---|
| PACIG 075/ANRS 024 trial, USA, France 1994 | ZDV versus placebo | Long (from 14 weeks), intravenous intraparutm | Long (six weeks), infant only | 550 | Replacement feeding | 8.3% in intervention arm versus 29.5% In placebo arm at 18 months (68% efficacy) |
| Bangkok CDC short course ZDV trial, Thailand 1999 | ZDV versus placebo | Short (from 26 weeks intrapartum) | None | 419 | Replacement feeding | 9.4% in intervention arm versus 18.9% in placebo arm at 6 months (50% efficacy) |
| Ditrame (ANRS 049a) Trial, Cole D'Ivoire, Burkina Faso 1999, 2002 | ZDV versus placebo | Short (from 26 weeks intrapartum) | Short (one week), mother only | 551 | Breastfeeding | 18.0% in ZDV arm, 27.5% in placebo arm at 6 months (38% efficacy); 21.4% versus 30.6% (30% efficacy) at 15 months 22.5% versus 30.2% (26% efficacy) at pooled analysis at 24 months |
| Petratrial, South Africa, Tanzania and Uganda 2002 | Antenatal, intrapartum and postpartum ZVD+3TC versus placebo | Short (from 26 weeks intrapartum) | Short (one week), mother and infant | 448 | Breastfeeding | 5.7% at six weeks for antenatal, intrapartum and postpartum ZDV + 3TC, only and 15.3% for placebo efficacy compared with placebo; 63%, 42% and 0% respectively) 14.9% at 18 months for antenatal, intrapartum and postpartum ZDV + 2TC, 18.1% for intrapartum and postpartum ZDV + 3TC, 20.0% for intrapartum ZDV + 3TC only and 22.2% for placebo (efficacy |
| compared | | | | | | with placebo: 34%, 18% and 0% respectively) |
| Hivnet 012 trial, Uganda 1999, 2003 | NVP versus ZDV | No antenatal ARV, intrapartum: single-dose NVP 200 mg versus oral ZDV | Single-dose NVP 2 mg/kg within 72 hours of birth (infant only) versus ZDV (one week), infant only | 443 | Breastfeeding | The placebo arm was stopped vertical transmission rate 13.1% in NVP arm versus 25.1% in ZDV arm (47% efficacy) at 14-16 weeks; 15.7% in NVP arm versus 25.8% in ZDV arm (41% efficacy) at months |

Contd...

*Contd...*

| *Study* | *Drugs* | *Antenatal and intrapartum* | *Postpartum* | *Maternal CD4+ count at enrolment $10^6$ cells/L* | *Mode of infant feeding* | *Vertical transmission rate and efficacy* |
|---|---|---|---|---|---|---|
| SAINT, South 2003 | NVP versus + 3TC | No antenatal ARV: Intrapartum: single dose NVP 200 mg versus ADV+3TC | Single NVP dose within 48 hour of birth (mother and infant) versus ZDV + 3TC (one week), mother and infant | 394 | Breastfeeding (42% and replacement feeding | 12.3% in NVP arm versus 9.3% in ADV + 3TC arm at eight weeks (difference not statistically significant) |
| PAGTG 316 trial, Bahainas, Belgium, Brazil, France, Germany, Italy, Spain, Sweden, Switzerland, United Kingdom, United States 2002 | NVP versus placebo among women already reveiving ZDV or ZDV plus other ARV drugs | Antenatal non-study ARV regimen; intrapartum: placebo versus single NVP dose 200 mg, plus intravenous ZDV | Placebo versus single NVP dose 2 mg/kg within 72 hours of birth plus non-study ARV drugs including ZDV (infant only) | 432 | Replacement feeding | S77% of women received dual or triple combination ARV regimens during pregnancy Trial stopped early due to very low vertical transmission rate in both arm (53% of the vertical transmission rate in utero)<br><br>Vertical transmission rate 1.4% in intervention arm versus 1.6% in placebo arm. |
| Thai Perinatal HIV presentation Trial (PHPT-2) Thailand 2004 | ZDV alone versus ZDV plus maternal and infant NVP versus ZDV plus maternal NVP | Antenatal ZDV from 28 weeks. Intrapartum: ZDV alone o ZDV plus single dose NVP at onset of labour | ZDV for one week with or without single dose NVP (infant only) | Not reported | Replacement feeding | ZDV-alone arm was stopped due to a to a higher transmission rate than the NVP-NVP arm (6.3% versus 1.1%); in arms in which the mother received single dose NVP, the vertical transmission rate did nto differ significantly between the infant receiving or not receiving single dose NOVP (2.0% versus 2.8%) |
| Ditrative plus (ANRS 1201.01) trial, abidjan, cote d'ivoire 2003 | Open lable, ADV plus single-dose NVP | ZDV from 36 weeks plus single-dose NVP at onset of labour | Single-dose NVP, plus ZDV fro one week (infant only) | 370 | Breastfeeding and replacement feeding | 4.7% at six weeks |

mind of exposed HCW. It could also be repeated after six weeks if initial test is negative but risk is presumed to be high in order to cover window period.

6. *Duration of PEP*: PEP should be started, as early as possible, after an exposure. The optimal course of PEP is not unknown, but 4 weeks of drug therapy appears to provide protection against HIV. If the HIV test is found to be positive at anytime within 12 weeks, the HCW should be referred to a physician for treatment.
7. *Pregnancy and PEP*: Based on limited information, anti-retroviral therapy taken during 2nd and 3rd trimester of pregnancy has not caused serious side effects in mothers or infants. There is very little information on the safety in the 1st trimester. If the HCW is pregnant at the time of exposure to HIV, the designated authority/physician must be consulted about the use of the drugs for PEP. Usually decision to provide PEP has to be individualised in these situations. Termination of pregnancy is not mandatory unless seroconversion is documented.
8. *Monitoring during PEP*: Most of the drugs used for PEP have usually been tolerated well except for nausea, vomiting, tiredness, or headache. Haemogram and Liver Function Test may be monitored during PEP.

## REFERENCES


1. UNAIDS and World Health Organization. AIDS epidemic update: 2003. Geneva, UNAIDS, 2003.
2. Current NACO Guidelines for the Prevention of Mother to Child Transmission of HIV.
3. Working Group on Mother-To-Child Transmission of HIV. Rates of mother-to-child transmission of HIV-1 in Africa,America, and Europe: results from 13 perinatal studies. J Acquir Immune Defic Syndr Hum Retrovirol 1995;8;506-10.
4. Maternal viral load and vertical transmission of HIV-1: an important factor but not the only one.The European Collaborative Study. AIDS 1999;13:1377-85.
5. Garcia PM, Kalish LA, Pitt J, Minkoff H, Quinn TC, Burchett SK, et al. Maternal levels of plasma human immunodeficiency virus type 1 RNA and the risk of perinatal transmission.Women and Infants Transmission Study Group. N Engl J Med 1999;341: 394-402.
6. Mofenson LM, Lambert JS, Stiehm ER, Bethel J, Meyer WA,Whitehouse J, et al. Risk factors for perinatal transmission of human immunodeficiency virus type 1 in women treated with zidovudine. Pediatric AIDS Clinical Trials Group Study 185 Team. N Engl J Med 1999;341:385-93.
7. Ioannidis JP,Abrams EJ,Ammann A, Bulterys M, Goedert JJ,Gray L, et al. Perinatal transmission of human immunodeficiency virus type 1 by pregnant women with RNA virus loads <1000 copies/ml. J Infect Dis 2001;183:539-45.
8. Kourtis AP, Bulterys M, Nesheim SR, Lee FK. Understanding the timing of HIV transmission from mother to infant. JAMA 2001;285:709-12.
9. Risk factors for mother-to-child transmission of HIV-1. European Collaborative Study. Lancet 1992;339:1007-12.
10. Dunn DT, Newell ML, Ades AE, Peckham CS. Risk of human immunodeficiency virus type 1 transmission through breastfeeding. Lancet 1992;340:585-88.
11. NHS Executive. Reducing mother to baby transmission of HIV. Health Service Circular. HSC1999/183.2002. London: Department of Health; 1999.
12. Cliffe S, Tookey PA, Nicoll A. Antenatal detection of HIV: national surveillance and unlinked anonymous survey. BMJ 2001;323:376-7.
13. Brocklehurst P. Interventions for reducing the risk of mother-to-child transmission of HIV infection. Cochrane Database Syst Rev 2002;CD000102.
14. National Institute for Clinical Excellence. Antenatal Care: Routine Care for the Healthy Pregnant Woman. London: RCOG Press; 2003.

15. Lyall EG, Blott M, de Ruiter A, Hawkins D, Mercy D, Mitchla Z, et al. Guidelines for the management of HIV infection in pregnant women and the prevention of mother-to-child transmission. HIV Med 2001;2:314-34.
16. General Medical Council. Serious Communicable Diseases. London: GMC; 1997.
17. Cooper ER, Charurat M, Mofenson L, Hanson IC, Pitt J, Diaz C, et al. Combination antiretroviral strategies for the treatment of pregnant HIV-1-infected women and prevention of perinatal HIV-1 transmission. J Acquir Immune Defic Syndr 2002;29:484-94.
18. Elective caesarean-section versus vaginal delivery in prevention of vertical HIV-1 transmission: a randomised clinical trial.The European Mode of Delivery Collaboration. Lancet 1999;353:1035-9. AIDS Clinical Trials Group Protocol 076 Study Group. N Engl J Med 1994;331:1173-80.
19. Thorne C, Newell ML. Are girls more at risk of intrauterine-acquired HIV infection than boys? AIDS, 2004;18(2):344-47.
20. Mofenson LM, Lambert JS, Stiehm ER, et al. Risk factors for perinatal transmission of human immunodeficiency virus type 1 in women treated with zidovudine. Pediatric AIDS Clinical Trials Group Study 185 Team. N Engl J Med, 1999;341(6):385-93.
21. United States Public Health Service Task Force. Recommendations for use of antiretroviral drugs in pregnant HIV-1-infected women for maternal health and interventions to reduce perinatal HIV-1 transmission in the United States. Washington, DC, United States Department of Health and Human Services, 2003.
22. Jackson JB, et al. Intrapartum and neonatal single-dose nevirapine compared with zidovudine for prevention of mother-tochild transmission of HIV-1 in Kampala, Uganda: 18-month follow-up of the HIVNET 012 randomised trial. Lancet 2003;362(9387):859-68.
23. Guay LA, et al. Intrapartum and neonatal single-dose nevirapine compared with zidovudine for prevention of mother-tochild transmission of HIV-1 in Kampala, Uganda: HIVNET 012 randomised trial. Lancet 1999;354 (9181):795-802.
24. The Petra study team. Efficacy of three short-course regimens of zidovudine and lamivudine in preventing early and late transmission of HIV-1 from mother to child in Tanzania, South Africa, and Uganda (Petra study): a randomised, double-blind, placebo-controlled trial. Lancet 2002;359(9313):1178-86.
25. Antiretroviral drugs for treating pregnant women and prevention HIV infection in infants : guidelines on care, treatment and support for women living with HIV/AIDS and their children in resource-constrained settings. WHO, Geneva, 2004.
26. Shaffer N, et al. Short-course zidovudine for perinatal HIV-1 transmission in Bangkok, Thailand: a randomised controlled trial. Bangkok Collaborative Perinatal HIV Transmission Study Group. Lancet 1999;353(9155):773-80.
27. Dabis F, et al. Six-month efficacy, tolerance, and acceptability of a short regimen of oral zidovudine to reduce vertical transmission of HIV in breastfed children in Côte d'Ivoire and Burkina Faso: a double-blind placebocontrolled multicentre trial. DITRAME Study Group. DIminution de la Transmission Mere-Enfant. Lancet 1999;353(9155):786-92.
28. European Collaborative Study. Exposure to antiretroviral therapy in utero or early life: the health of uninfected children born to HIV-infected women. Journal of Acquired Immune Deficiency Syndromes and Human Retrovirology, 2003;32(4):380-87.
29. Taha TE, et al. Effect of HIV-1 antiretroviral prophylaxis on hepatic and hematological parameters of African infants. AIDS 2002;16(6):851-58.
30. Sullivan J. South African Intrapartum Nevirapine Trial: selection of resistance mutations. 14th International Conference on AIDS, Barcelona, Spain, 7-12 July 2002 (Abstract LbPeB9024).
31. Jourdain G, et al. Exposure to intrapartum single-dose nevirapine and subsequent maternal 6-month response to NNRTI based regimens. 11th Conference on Retroviruses and Opportunistic Infections, San Francisco, California, USA, 8-11 February 2004 (Abstract 41LB).
32. Read JS, Tuomala R, Kpamegan E, et al. Mode of delivery and postpartum morbidity among HIVinfected women: the Women and InfantsTransmission Study. J Acquir Immune Defic Syndr 2001;26(3):236-45.
33. Marcollet A, Goffinet F, Firtion G, et al. Differences in postpartum morbidity in women who are infected with the human immunodeficiency virus after elective cesarean delivery, emergency cesarean delivery, or vaginal delivery. Am J Obstet Gynecol, 2002;186(4):784-89.

34. Brocklehurst P. Interventions for reducing the risk of mother-to-child transmission of HIV infection. Cochrane Database Syst Rev 2002;CD000102.
35. Browne R, Lyall EG, Penn Z, et al. Outcomes of planned vaginal delivery of HIV-positive women managed in a multi-disciplinary setting. 11th BHIVA Conference, Dublin 2005. Abstract P45.
36. Smith JR, Forster GE, Kitchen VS, Hooi YS, Munday PE, Paintin DB. Infertility management in HIV positive couples: a dilemma. BMJ 1991;302:1447-50.
37. Mandelbrot L,Heard I,Henrion-Geant E,Henrion R.Natural conception in HIV-negative women with HIV-infected partners. Lancet 1997;349:850-51.
38. Gilling-Smith C. HIV prevention. Assisted reproduction in HIVdiscordant couples. AIDS Read 2000;10:581-87.
39. Gilling-Smith C, Smith JR, Semprini AE. HIV and infertility: time to treat. There's no justification for denying treatment to parents who are HIV positive. BMJ 2001;322:566-67.
40. Cohen M,Greenblatt R, Minkokoff H, et al. Menstrual abnormalities in women with HIV infection. Proceedings XI International conference on AIDS, Vancouver, Canada, 1996 (absrtract no. Mo.B.540).
41. Del Mistro A, Cheico Bianchi L. HPV-related neoplasia in HIV-infected individuals. Europian Journal of Cancer 2001;37:1227-35.
42. World Health Organization (WHO). Improving Access to Quality Care in Family Planning: Medical Eligibility Criteria for Contraceptive Use. Second Edition. Geneva, Switzerland: WHO, 2000; WHO.
43. Lavreys L, Baeten JM, Kreiss JK, et al. Injectable contraceptive use and genital ulcer disease during the early phase of HIV-1 infection increase plasma virus load in women. J Infect Dis 2004;189:303-11.

# CHAPTER 4

# Protozoal Infections in Pregnancy

YM Mala

Protozoal infections which are commonly encountered during pregnancy and can have deleterious effects on the foetus are toxoplasmosis and malaria.

## TOXOPLASMOSIS

Toxoplasmosis is caused by *Toxoplasma gondii*, an obligate intracellular protozoan that infects one-third of the world population. It has a predilection for central nervous system and can infect all mammals, who serve as intermediate hosts. Although adult acquired toxoplasmosis is usually mild to asymptomatic, the disease can be severe in the immunocompromised, leading to encephalitis.

Congenital toxoplasmosis is caused by transplacental transmission of the parasite in women who acquire the infection during pregnancy. In Western countries approximately 1 to 10,000 children are born with congenital toxoplasmosis.[1] The incidence in the United States is about 400 to 4000 cases per year. In a study from Northern India by Saxena et al, it was observed that 27 per cent of women with bad obstetric history was positive.[2] However, the incidence of seropositivity in general population in India is reported to be much lower. Most infected infants have no apparent physical abnormalities at birth, but, without treatment, most of the infected infants will have significant morbidity that is related to chorioretinitis, hydrocephalus, or neurologic damage by the end of adolescence.[3] Therefore, strategies for prevention and early recognition of maternal or infant infection and the institution of effective treatment could have a substantial impact on the incidence and morbidity that are associated with this congenital infection.

### Pathophysiology

Toxoplasma can exist in three forms in its life cycle: the oocyst, the tachyzoite and the cyst. Members of the cat family are the definite hosts where sexual division of the parasite occurs following ingestion of tissue cysts by the cat, usually in uncooked meat. Replication of the parasite occurs in the intestine of the cat, resulting in the production of oocysts. During acute infection, several million oocysts are shed in the faeces of the cat for 7 to 21 days. After sporulation takes place, which occurs between 1 and 21 days, oocysts containing sporozoites are infective which, when ingested by mammals (including man) give rise to tachyzoite stage.

Tachyzoites are the rapidly dividing products of asexual reproduction, which occurs in macrophages following invasion of the host intestinal wall by either sporozoites (from oocysts) or bradyzoites (from tissue cysts). Once within the host cell, they multiply and develop a protective vacuole. In an active infection, replication continues, the cell ruptures and the tachyzoites invade adjacent cells including CNS, eye, skeletal and heart muscle and placenta. Replication leads to cell death and rapid invasion of neighbouring cells. The tachyzoites are responsible for the strong inflammatory response and tissue destruction and therefore, causes clinical manifestations of disease. Due to immune response tachyzoites are transformed into bradyzoites and form cysts.

The tissue cysts contain hundreds and thousands of bradyzoites and form within the host cells in brain and skeletal and heart muscles. Bradyzoites can be released from cysts, transform back into tachyzoites, and cause recrudescence of infection in immunocompromised patients.

## Transmission

Human transmission can occur by the following means:

1. Ingestion of tissue cysts by handling infected meat or eating undercooked meat. In France, the infection is primarily acquired through the consumption of undercooked meat. Bradyzoites are found in 8 per cent of beef, 20 per cent of pork and 20 per cent of lamb.[4] Hence, mutton should be cooked to an internal temperature of 67°C or by freezing to below –12°C which kills bradyzoites. Generally, after acute infection the disease remains latent, except in immunocompromised individuals.
2. Ingestion of infective oocysts excreted in faeces of infected cat.
3. Rarely, infection can be caused by tachyzoites through transfusion of blood from infected patient.
4. Very rarely, transmission can occur by organ transplantation from a seropositive donor to a seronegative recipient and is a potential cause of disease in heart, heart-lung, kidney, liver, and liver pancreas transplant patients.
5. *Congenital transmission*: This occurs if the woman develops primary infection during pregnancy. The parasite enters the foetal circulation by infection of the placenta.The risk is 0-9 per cent in first trimester, upto 27 per cent in second trimester and 59 per cent in third trimester.[5]

## Clinical Presentation

Toxoplasmosis in immunocompetent adults is generally asymptomatic and remains unrecognised. Occasionally mild malaise, lethargy, and lymphadenopathy may be present. The enlarged lymph nodes are discrete, either tender or non-tender and firm, but not suppurative. Immunocompromised adults may develop hepatitis, chorioretinitis, polymyositis, dermatomyositis or myocarditis. In the United States, overall 5 to 10 per cent of human immunodeficiency infected adults will contract toxoplasmic encephalitis. The incidence of perinatal transmission is found to be 3.7 per cent in HIV- infected women.

## Effect of Toxoplasmosis on Pregnancy

Primary infection with *Toxoplasma gondii* during pregnancy is associated with increased adverse pregnancy outcomes. Previously infected subjects only rarely are reinfected once they have had an adequate immune response. Maternal infection acquired before gestation poses little or no risk to foetus except in women who become infected a few months (usually upto 3 months) before conception. The outcome depends on the period of gestation at the time of infection. The rate of congenital infection increases with advance in gestational age at the time of maternal infection. It is about 15 per cent in early pregnancy and about 60 per cent in third trimester. Severity of infection is inversely proportional to the increase in period of gestation. Neonatal infection is less likely to occur following maternal infection in the first trimester. However, if it occurs it is likely to be severe leading to spontaneous abortion, severe neurologic damage and significant neonatal sequelae. In contrast in 3rd trimester infection usually results in normally looking newborns. The overall frequency of subclinical infection with congenital toxoplasmosis is as high as 85 per cent. Hence, it may go unnoticed and if these babies are not treated they will later develop chorioretinitis or delay in growth in 2nd or 3rd decade of life.

Congenital toxoplasmosis can present in one of the four forms.[6]

1. Symptomatic neonatal disease
2. Mild to severe disease manifested within first month of life
3. Childhood or adolescent sequelae from previously undiagnosed infection
4. Subclinical infection.

Neonatal clinical manifestations of congenital toxoplasmosis vary widely and include hydrocephalus, microcephaly, intracranial calcifications, chorioretinitis, strabismus, blindness, epilepsy, psychomotor or mental retardation, petichae due to thrombocytopenia and anaemia.[7, 8] The classic triad of hydrocephalus, chorioretinitis and cerebral calcification is rather rare. Prenatal ultrasound may show intracranial calcifications, ventricular dilatation, hepatic enlargement, ascites, and increased placental thickness.[9]

## Diagnosis and Screening

Clinical diagnosis is difficult as more than 90 per cent of women are asymptomatic. Whether all pregnant women should be screened for toxoplasmosis is controversial because of the low incidence of maternal primary infection and high false positivity of IgM antibodies, which may lead to termination of uninfected foetuses.

Toxoplasmosis can be diagnosed indirectly by serological methods and directly by PCR, isolation and histology.

### *Indirect Detection*

The only sign of primary infection in asymptomatic women during pregnancy is seroconversion via detection of IgG or IgM by immunofluorescence antibody test, the enzyme-linked immune filtration assay, the immunosorbent agglutination assay (ISAGA), or other similar assays.

1. *IgG and IgM antibodies*: Absence of IgG antibodies before or early in pregnancy identifies women at risk to develop the infection. IgG antibodies arise within 1 to 2 weeks after infection and persist for the individual life time. Thus, the detection of IgG in a woman at the beginning of pregnancy indicates prior infection and thus eliminates the congenital transfer of tachyzoites. IgM antibody levels increase within days and usually remain elevated for 2 to 3 months..However, IgM antibody levels can remain positive for more than 2 years in upto 27 per cent of women.[10] Only new seroconversions (IgG or IgM) place a developing foetus at risk of congenital toxoplasmosis.
2. *Avidity of IgG antibodies*: This helps in discriminating recently acquired infection from the past. Presence of low avidity antibodies indicate recent infection but they can persist beyond 3 months of infection.[11] Presence of high avidity antibodies essentially rules out infection acquired in the recent 3 to 4 months.
3. The double-sandwich IgM ELISA and IgM immunosorbent agglutination assay (ISAGA) can be used to detect IgM antibodies that arise within the first week of infection and thereafter decline and disappear at highly variable rates.

False positive results and persistence of positive titres even years after initial infection hamper correct interpretation of results obtained in IgM antibody tests. A negative IgM has more value and it essentially rules out recently acquired infection. However, results of IgM antibodies in non-reference laboratories are sometimes unreliable with high false positive rates as high as 60 per cent.[12]

### Direct Detection

1. *Polymerase chain reaction (PCR):* It helps in early prenatal diagnosis of congenital toxoplasmosis. Sensitivity of PCR results can be affected by the appropriateness of sample handling, transport, storage conditions, technique used for amplification and detection of PCR products and by previous use of anti-*T. gondii* specific drugs. If all these things are taken care of specificity and positive predictive value of PCR results approach 100 per cent.[13] In a study conducted by Romand et al on amniotic fluid PCR showed sensitivity of 64 per cent, negative predictive value of 87.8 per cent and specificity and positive predictive value of 100 per cent.[13] Sensitivity varied greatly according to gestational age and was significantly higher for maternal infections that arose between 17 and 21 weeks of gestation. The overall sensitivity is reported to be 64 to 98.8 per cent. In the newborn suspected to have congenital toxoplasmosis PCR of the peripheral blood, cerebrospinal fluid, and urine should be performed.
2. *T gondii* can be isolated from blood or body fluids by inoculation of mice or cell cultures of human tissue. However, the test takes 3 to 6 weeks and is not available at all places.

## Management

Management of maternal infection varies considerably in different centres. There are no randomised controlled trials to assess the effect of prenatal antimicrobial therapy with either spiramycin or pyrimethamine-sulphadiazine. A large prospective cohort trial of 1208 pregnant women in Europe with primary *T. gondii* infection failed to reveal any difference in the risk of congenital infection with treatment (spiramycin or pyrimethamine-sulphadiazine) or no treatment.[14] However, these studies included very few untreated women in their analysis and most untreated women were infected during the third trimester. Other uncontrolled studies have demonstrated the benefits prenatal treatment with spiramycin or pyrimethamine-sulphadiazine. One study of 5288 susceptible pregnancies showed the risk of congenital toxoplasmosis to be four times greater in neonates born to untreated mothers when compared to treated mothers.[15]

Thus, while there are no randomised trials yet, it is recommended by authorities that all pregnant women who have been diagnosed with primary toxoplasmosis should be treated with spiramycin in the first and early second trimester and pyrimethamine-sulphadiazine along with folinic acid in late second and third trimester. Pyrimethamine is teratogenic and contraindicated in first trimester of pregnancy. The regime usually followed is spiramycin 6-9 MIU per day for 3 weeks and repeated after 2 weeks interval until delivery or until foetal infection is documented. Since maternal infection does not necessarily result in foetal infection, prenatal PCR of amniotic fluid ideally should be performed. In case of a negative PCR result, pregnant women should receive spiramycin prophylaxis until the 17th week of pregnancy and have monthly ultrasound examinations for the entire pregnancy. The presence of hydrocephalus is an indication for termination.

In France and USA spiramycin is continued through pregnancy. In Austria and Germany, spiramycin prophylaxis is followed by a 4 week course of pyrimethamine plus sulphadiazine at 17 weeks of gestation. In some countries pyrimethamine-sulphadiazine is given if PCR of amniotic fluid is positive or acquisition of maternal infection in late second or third trimester. Pyrimethamine is given as a loading dose of 100 mg once daily in two divided doses for 2 days and then 50 mg once daily. Sulphadiazine is given as 75 mg/kg daily in two divided doses for 2 days, followed by 100 mg/kg daily in two divided doses (maximum 4 gm daily).

Neonatal therapy for both symptomatic and subclinical infants has been reported to improve long-term outcomes.[16]

## Recommendations for Primary Prevention or Lowering the Risk of Primary Toxoplasmosis Infection Among Pregnant Women

1. Avoid consumption of undercooked meat. Cook all meat until its no longer pink and the juices run clear.
2. Always use gloves while, and wash hands thoroughly after, handling raw meat.
3. Thoroughly wash all utensils that are in contact with undercooked meat.
4. Wash all uncooked vegetables thoroughly.
5. Wear gloves when gardening or working in soil. Wash hand immediately after contact with soil.
6. If possible, keep cats indoors throughout pregnancy and do not feed cats undercooked meat.
7. Use gloves while, and wash hands immediately after, changing cat litter.

## Outline of Management of Toxoplasmosis with Pregnancy

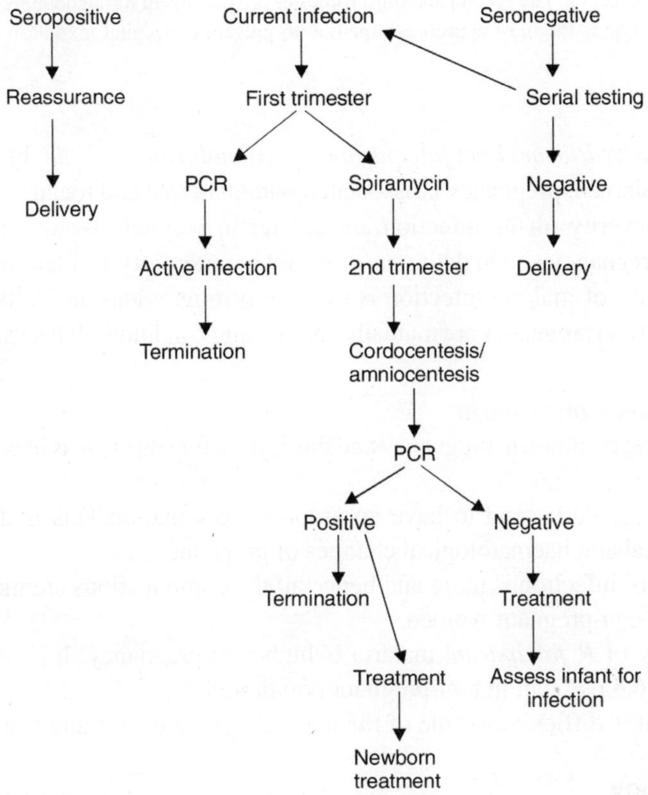


## Conclusion

Acute maternal toxoplasmosis is associated with increased risk of spontaneous abortion and can have serious effects on the developing foetus. Since most primary infections are asymptomatic and screening is problematic, primary prevention is the most appropriate method to prevent congenital toxoplasmosis.

## Key Points

- Congenital toxoplasmosis occurs if the pregnant woman acquires primary infection during pregnancy.
- The rate of congenital infection increases with advance in gestational age at the time of maternal infection. Severity is inversely proportional to the increase in period of gestation.
- IgG antibodies arise within 1 to 2 weeks after infection and persist for the individual lifetime. Thus, detection of IgG antibodies in early pregnancy indicates prior infection.
- IgM antibody levels increase within days and usually remain elevated for 2 to 3 months. Hence, they are markers of recent infection.
- PCR of the amniotic fluid or foetal blood helps in prenatal diagnosis.

- Prenatal ultrasound may show intracranial calcifications, ventricular dialatation, hepatic enlargement, ascites and increased placental thickness.
- Treatment includes spiramycin in first and early second trimester and pyrimethamine-sulphadiazine alongwith folinic acid in late second and third trimester or spiramycin throughout pregnancy.
- Primary prevention is the most appropriate method to prevent congenital toxoplasmosis.

## MALARIA

Malaria is caused by *Plasmodium falciparum*, *vivax*, *malariae* or *ovale*. In areas of endemic transmission, malaria in pregnancy is associated with maternal and foetal complications. The frequency and severity of the infection are greater in pregnant women than in the same women before pregnancy and in their non-pregnant counterparts. Epidemiological data have shown that the risk of malaria infection is more in primigravidas and falls with increasing gravidity. Malaria and pregnancy are mutually aggravating conditions. It needs multidisciplinary management.

*Effect of pregnancy on malaria*:

1. Malaria is more common in pregnancy and this is probably due to loss of acquired immunity to malaria.
2. In pregnancy, malaria tend to have an atypical presentation.This is due to hormonal, immunological and haematological changes of pregnancy.
3. The severity of infection is more and hence all the complications are more in pregnancy compared to non-pregnant women.
4. The mortality of *P. falciparum* malaria is higher in pregnancy. It is about 13 per cent compared to 6.5 per cent in non-pregnant population.
5. The treatment is difficult as some of the antimalarials are contraindicated in pregnancy.

### Pathophysiology

The pathophysiology of malaria in pregnancy is due to the physiological immunosuppression mediated by pregnancy associated hormones and involvement of the placenta. The parasites sequester along the surface of the placental membrane especially the trophoblastic villi, extravillous trophoblasts, and syncitial bridges. Intervillous spaces are filled with parasites and macrophages, interfering with oxygen and nutrient transport to the foetus.Villous hypertrophy and fibrinoid necrosis have been observed.

### Clinical Features

1. Fever – It may be continuous or intermittent, low grade or high grade.
2. Anaemia – Anaemia may be the presenting feature and hence all cases of anaemia should be investigated for malaria.
3. Splenomegaly
4. Complications – Acute pulmonary oedema and hypoglycaemia are more common in pregnancy and both carries a very high mortality. Pulmonary oedema is aggravated by

the pre-existing anaemia. Hypoglycaemia is due to the increased demands hypercatabolic state and infecting parasites.

## Risks for the Foetus

Malaria in pregnancy is detrimental to the foetus. Infection with *P. falciparum* can cause more serious complications to the foetus. The prenatal and neonatal mortality ranges from 15 to 70 per cent.

The various complications are:

1. Spontaneous abortion.
2. Prematurity
3. Stillbirth
4. Placental insufficiency and low birth weight
5. Foetal distress
6. *Congenital malaria*: It is very rare and occurs in less than 5 per cent of affected pregnancies. IgG antibodies which cross the placenta and the placental barrier may protect the foetus to some extent. It occurs with all four species of malaria but is more common with *P. malariae*. The incidence goes up during epidemics and is common in non-immune population. The chloroquine levels in the foetus are about one-third of maternal levels and are subtherapeutic. The presenting symptoms in the newborn child are fever, irritability, feeding problems, anaemia, hepatosplenomegaly, and jaundice. The diagnosis is confirmed by a smear for malaria parasite from cord blood or after birth.

## Management

A. Treatment of malaria
   1. All cases of *P falciparum* should be admitted.
   2. Severity of infection and general condition of the patient should be assessed and monitored.
   3. Foetal well-being should be closely monitored.
   4. Fluid balance and calorie intake should be maintained.
   5. Anti-malarial therapy should be started.
      - Chloroquine, Quinine and Artesunate can be given in all trimesters
      - Mefloquine can be used in 2nd and 3rd trimesters.
      - Primaquine, Tetracycline, Doxycycline and Halofantrine are contraindicated in pregnancy.

B. Management of complications like pulmonary oedema and hypoglycaemia. Anaemia should be corrected by packed cell transfusions. Renal failure if occurs should be treated by careful fluid management, diuretics and dialysis if needed.

C. *Management of labour*: Malaria can induce preterm labour. Foetal distress is commonly seen. Temperature should be brought down by paracetamol, cold sponging, etc. In cases of high parasitaemia some advocate blood transfusion.

## Chemoprophylaxis in Pregnancy

Malaria being fatal to both mother and the foetus, all pregnant women who live in malarious area during their pregnancy, should be protected with chemotherapy prophylaxis. Chloroquine being the safest drug in pregnancy is the first choice. 500 mg of chloroquine should be administered once a week.

Although a general malaria vaccine is a distant hope, a vaccine against placental malaria is possible in the near future.

## Key Points

- Malaria and pregnancy are mutually aggravating conditions.
- It is more common in pregnancy, probably due to loss of acquired immunity to malaria.
- The parasites sequester along the surface of the placental membrane especially trophoblastic with, extra hillous trophoblasts and syncitial bridges.
- Presenting complaints are fever, anaemia and splenomegaly.
- Associated complications are pulmonary oedema, hypoglycaemia and renal failure.
- Prenatal and neonatal mortality ranges from 15 to 17 per cent.

## REFERENCES


1. Robert Gangneus F, Gavinet M-F, Anelle T. Raymond J,Tourte-Schaferer CT, Dupouy-camet J. Value of prenatal diagnosis of congenital toxoplasmosis; retrospective study of 110 cases. J Clin Microbiol 1999;37:2893-98.
2. Saxena K, Bano I, Aggarwal K. Incidence of toxoplasmosis in cases of bad obstetric history. J Obst Gynae India 1993;43:703-06.
3. Wilson CB, Remington JC, Stagno S, Reynold DW. Development of adverse sequelae in children born with subclinical congenital toxoplasma infection. Paediatrics 1980;66:767-74.
4. Beazley DM. Egerman RS. Toxoplasmosis. Semin Perinatal 1998;22:332-38.
5. Desmonts G, Naot Y, Remington JS. Immunoglobulin M, immunosorbent agglutination assay for diagnosis of infectious diseases: diagnosis of acute congenital and acquired toxoplasma infection. F Clin Microbiol 1981;14:486-91.
6. Remington JS, Mcleod R, Desmonts G, Toxoplasmosis. Remington JS, Klein JO, (Eds). Infectious Diseases of the Fetus and Newborn Infant. Philadelphia: W.B, Saunders Co 1995;140-267.
7. McAuley J, Boyer KM, Patel D, et al. Early and longitudinal evaluation of treated infants and children and untreated historical patients with congenital toxoplasmosis: the Chicago collaborative treatment trial. Clin Infect Dis 1994; 18:38-72.
8. Swisher CN, Boyer K, McLeod R. Congenital toxoplasmosis. Semin Pediatr Neurol 1994;1:4-25.
9. Gay-Andrieu F, Marty P, Pialat J, Sournies G, Drier de laforte T, Peyron F. Fetal Toxoplasmosis and negative amniocentesis: necessity of and ultrasound follow up. Prenat Diagn 2003;23:558-60.
10. Gras L, Gilbert RE, Wallon M, et al. Duration of the IgM response in women acquiring *Toxoplasma gondii* during pregnancy: implication for clinical practice and cross-sectional incidence studies. Epidemiol infect 2004;132:541-48.
11. Montoya JG, Liesenfeld O, Kinney S, Press C, Remington JS. VIDAS test for avidity of toxoplasma-specific immunoglobulin G for confirmatory testing of pregnant women. J Clin Microbiol 2002;40:2504-08.
12. Liesenfeld O, Press C, Montoya JG, et al. False positive results in immunoglobulin M (IgM) toxoplasma antibody tests and importance of confirmatory testing;the Platelia toxo IgM test. F Clin microbial 1997;35:174-78.
13. Romand S,Wallon M, Franck J, Thulliez P, Peyron F, Dumon H. Prenatal diagnosis using polymerase chain reaction on amniotic fluid for congenital toxoplasmosis. Obstet Gynecol 2001;97:296-300.

14. Gilbert R, Gras L. European multicentre study on congenital toxoplasmosis. Effect of timing and type of treatment on the risk of mother to child transmission of Toxoplasma gondii. BJOG 2003;110:112-20.
15. Ricci M, Pentimalli H, Thaller R, et al. Screening and prevention of congenital toxoplasmosis : an effectiveness study in a population with a high infection rate. J Matern Fetal Med 2003;14:398-403.
16. Guerina NG, Hsu HW, Meissner HC, et al. Neonatal serologic screening and early treatment for congenital toxoplasma gondii infection. N Engl J Med 1994;330:1858-63.
17. Gilles HM, Lawson JB, Sibelas M, Voller A, Alan N. Malaria and pregnancy. Am J Trop Med Hyg 1984;33(4):517-25.
18. McGregor IA, Smith DA. A health, nutrition and parasitological survey in a rural village (Keneba) in west Kiang, the Gambia. Trans R Soc, Trop Med Hyg 1952;46:403-27.

CHAPTER 5

# Chlamydial Infection in Obstetrics and Gynaecology

*Sudha Prasad, C Jassal, Aparna Sharma*

## INTRODUCTION

Chlamydial genital tract infections are reproductive tract infections. While gonorrhoea has decreased in many parts of the developed world, but chlamydial genital tract infections remain a refractory problem worldwide. Chlamydial infection is one of the most widespread bacterial STDs in the United States. The US Centers for Disease Control and Prevention (CDC) estimates that more than 4 million people are infected each year and 2 million people are currently affected (CDC). Studies from India have reported a prevalence of Chlamydial antigen in cervical smears of upto15 per cent in young women undergoing routine gynaecological checks.[1]

### Species of Chlamydia

The genus Chlamydia contains three species that infect humans:

1. *C. psittaci*
2. *C. trachomatis*
3. *C. pneumoniae* (formerly the TWAR agent).

### Pathogenesis

Chlamydiae are obligate intracellular bacteria that are classified in their own order (chlamydiales). They possess both DNA and RNA, have a cell wall and ribosomes similar to those of gram-negative bacteria, and are inhibited by antibiotics such as tetracycline.

All Chlamydia possess a complex reproductive cycle. There are two forms of the microorganism, which participate in this cycle—the extracellular elementary body and intracellular reticulate body. The elementary body is the infective form, which is transmitted from one person to another and is required for its extracellular survival. Within 8 hour of cell entry, the elementary bodies reorganise into reticulate bodies and adapt to intracellular survival and multiplication. After 24 hour, the reticulate bodies condense and keep elementary bodies within the inclusion. The inclusion then ruptures releasing elementary bodies from the cell to initiate infection of adjacent cells or transmission to another person.

## Spectrum of *C. trachomatis* Genital Infection

As the majority of women with *C. trachomatis* infection are asymptomatic, therefore, they do not promptly seek medical care.[2] Consequently, screening is necessary to identify and treat this infection. Untreated, *C. trachomatis* infections can lead to serious complications. In certain studies, < 40 per cent of women with untreated *C. trachomatis* infections experience pelvic inflammatory disease (PID).[3,4] Of these, the majority has symptoms that are too mild or nonspecific for them to seek medical treatment. Regardless of symptom severity, the consequences of PID are severe. Of those with PID, 20 per cent will become infertile; 18 per cent will experience debilitating, chronic pelvic pain; and 9 per cent will have a life-threatening tubal pregnancy.[5]

Chlamydia trachomatis (CT) and Human papillomavirus (HPV) infections are the two commonest sexually transmitted infections. Combined screening for CT cervicitis and precancerous cervical lesions – squamous intraepithelial lesions (SIL) may be done in a high-risk population.[6]

*C. trachomatis* infection during pregnancy leads to infant conjunctivitis and pneumonia and maternal postpartum endometritis.

# CLINICAL PRESENTATION

## Mucopurulent Cervicitis

Many cases of mucopurulent cervicitis are idiopathic. However, many patients are asymptomatic, attending clinics as the partners of men with urethritis. Chlamydial infection in the lower genital tract of women affects the columnar epithelial cell lining the endocervical canal. The classic signs of cervicitis include: pain in passing urine, frequency, soreness, and a cervical discharge which, on Gram staining and microscopy, shows the presence of ten or more polymorphonuclear leukocytes per high-power field. The colour and opacity of these

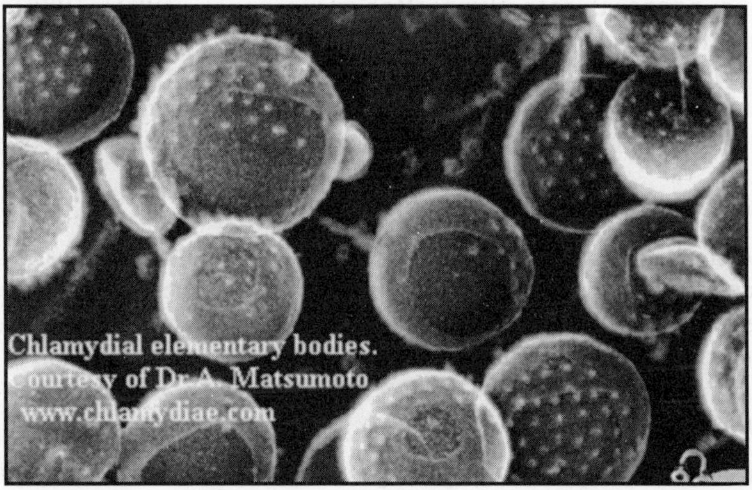


**Fig. 5.1:** Chlamydial elementary bodies. Courtesy of Dr A Matsumoto www.chlamydiae.com

exudates is very characteristics. The cervix itself may be edematous and erythematous, and may bleed easily when a sample is collected with a swab. Occasionally lymphoid follicles may be observed on the cervix.

## Pelvic Inflammatory Disease

Pelvic inflammatory disease (PID) occurs via ascending intraluminal spread of *C. trachomatis* from the lower genital tract. Mucopurulent cervicitis is thus followed by endometritis, endosalpingitis and finally pelvic peritonitis. Chlamydial endometritis can also occur in the absence of clinical evidence of salpingitis. However, chlamydial salpingitis produces milder symptoms than does gonococcal salpingitis and may be associated with less marked adnexal tenderness. *C. trachomatis* has been identified in the fallopian tubes or endometrium of upto 50 per cent of women with PID. Using enzyme immunoassay (EIA) test, *C. trachomatis* antigen was detected in 13 per cent of cases of PID.[7]

## Infertility

*C. trachomatis* produces fallopian tube scarring leading to infertility. Many infertile women will present tubal block on tubal patency test with antichlamydial antibody without the history of PID. The subclinical tubal infection (silent salpingitis) may also produce tubal blockade. Sharma et al, found that the presence of Chlamydia specific IgG antibody was significantly higher (70%) in women with infertility of tubal origin as compared to 35 per cent seropositivity in healthy fertile women and 55 per cent seropositivity in infertile women with cause of infertility other than tubal factor.[8]

## Ectopic Pregnancy

As Chlamydia produces tubal blockade in many cases, many studies suggest that, in the UK, pelvic inflammatory disease and ectopic pregnancy are primarily associated with chlamydial rather than gonococcal infections (Robertson et al, 1987, 1988). Mehanna et al, found that the geometric mean titres for *Chlamydia trachomatis* were higher among patients with tubal factor infertility and ectopic pregnancy, and they were more likely to have high antichlamydial titres (> or = 1:128 immunoglobulin G). Serum titre was significantly correlated with histologic evidence of salpingitis among the patients with an ectopic pregnancy.[9]

## Perihepatitis (Fitz-Hugh-Curtis Syndrome)

A cultural and/or serologic evidence of *C. trachomatis* is found in three quarters of women with this syndrome. This syndrome should be suspected whenever a young, sexually active woman presents with an illness resembling cholecystitis (fever and right-upper-quadrant pain of subacute or acute onset). It may be associated with symptoms and signs of salpingitis.

## Urethral Syndrome

In the absence of infection with uropathogens such as coliforms or *Staphylococcus saprophyticus*, *C trachomatis* is the pathogen most commonly isolated from women with dysuria, frequency and pyuria. Up to 25 per cent of female STD clinic patients with chlamydial urogenital infection have cultures positive for *C. trachomatis* from the urethra only. *C. trachomatis* may be isolated from the urethra of women without symptoms of urethritis.

## Infection in Pregnancy

*C. trachomatis* during pregnancy has been associated with premature delivery and postpartum endometritis. Whether these complications are in part attributable to *C. trachomatis* is not clear.

The reported prevalence of Chlamydia infections in pregnancy range from 5-30 per cent depending on age and other risk factors.[10] Pregnant women infected with Chlamydia, like non-pregnant women, are at risk for cervicitis, urethritis and pelvic inflammatory disease.

Chlamydia infections during pregnancy can also cause chorioamnionitis and post-partum endometritis and may be associated with gestational bleeding, premature rupture of membranes and preterm labour and delivery? Perinatal transmission and neonatal complications of chlamydia occur in up to 50 per cent of newborns whose mothers were infected with Chlamydia at delivery. Exposed infants are at risk for conjunctivitis (20-50% of exposed) and neonatal pneumonia (10-20% of exposed).[11]

## Perinatal Infections

- *Inclusion conjunctivitis*. Five to twenty-five per cent of pregnant women have *C. trachomatis* infections of the cervix.[10] One-half to two-thirds of children exposed during birth acquire *C. trachomatis* infection. Roughly half of the infected infants develop clinical evidence of inclusion conjunctivitis.
- Infant pneumonia *C. trachomatis* causes a distinctive pneumonia syndrome in infants.

## DIAGNOSIS

Four types of laboratory procedures are available to confirm *C. trachomatis* infection:

1. Direct microscopic examination of tissue scrapings for typical intracytoplasmic inclusions or elementary bodies.
2. Isolation of the organism in cell cultures.
3. Detection of Chlamydial antigens or nucleic acid by immunologic or hybridisation methods.
4. Detection of antibody in serum or in local secretions.

## Investigations

1. *Direct microscopic examination*: Giemsa stained cell scrapings for typical inclusions has low degree of sensitivity and false-positive interpretations by inexperienced hands.
2. *C. trachomatis culture*: Cell culture techniques for isolation of *C. trachomatis* have a low and variable sensitivity (60–80%); require rigorous transport conditions, and its high cost and technically demanding nature.

Cell culture for *C. trachomatis* involves inoculating a confluent monolayer of susceptible cells with an appropriately collected and transported specimen. After 48-72 hours of growth, infected cells develop characteristic intracytoplasmic inclusions that contain substantial numbers of *C. trachomatis* elementary and reticulate bodies. These unique inclusions are detected by staining with a fluorescein-conjugated monoclonal antibody that is specific for the major outer membrane protein (MOMP) of *C. trachomatis.*

3. *Antigen detection*:
   a. *Direct immunofluorescent antibody test*: In the (DFA) slide test, potentially infected genital or ocular secretions are smeared onto a slide, fixed and stained with fluorescein-conjugated monoclonal antibody specific for Chlamydia antigens. The antigen that is detected by the antibody in the *C. trachomatis* (DFA) procedure is either the MOMP or LPS molecule. The observation of fluorescing elementary bodies confirms the diagnosis. Compared with culture, this test is 70 to 85 percent sensitive
   b. *EIA Tests*: EIA tests detect Chlamydia LPS with a monoclonal or polyclonal antibody that has been labelled with an enzyme. The enzyme converts a colourless substrate into a coloured product, which is detected by a spectro-photometer. Specimens can be stored and transported without refrigeration and should be processed within the time indicated by the manufacturer. One disadvantage of the EIA methods that detect LPS is the potential for false-positive results caused by cross-reaction with LPS of other microorganisms, including other Chlamydia species.
4. *Nucleic acid amplification tests (NAATs)*: These tests are now the most sensitive Chlamydial diagnostic tests available being the first non-culture assays.

   The ability of NAATs to detect *C. trachomatis* and *N. gonorrhoeae* without a pelvic examination or by testing urine is a key advantage of NAATs, and this non-invasive screening facilitates increase compliance in screening other than traditional screening venues (e.g.STD and family planning clinics). Testing simply urine sample could diagnose 85 per cent of Chlamydial infection compared with 91 per cent diagnosed by genital swab testing. Therefore, NAATs are found to be highly sensitive and specific methods for the detection of *C. trachomatis* in urine specimens and can be recommended for noninvasive screening of *C. trachomatis* in urine.[12,13] The only disadvantage of NAATs is that specimens can contain amplification inhibitors that result in false-negative results.
5. *Nucleic acid hybridisation (nucleic acid probe) tests*: A DNA probe that is complementary to a specific sequence of *C. trachomatis* or *N. gonorrhoeae* rRNA hybridises with any complementary rRNA that is present in the specimen. Technical requirements and expertise necessary for performing nucleic acid hybridisation tests are similar to those for the EIAs. One of the advantages of the nucleic acid hybridisation tests is the ability to store and transport specimens for <7 days without refrigeration before receipt and testing by the laboratory.
6. *Serology tests*: Serology has limited value in testing for uncomplicated genital *C. trachomatis* infection and should not be used for screening because previous chlamydial infection frequently elicits long-lasting antibodies that cannot be easily distinguished from the antibodies produced in a current infection.

## Recommendations of the American College of Preventive Medicine for Screening for *Chlamydia trachomatis*[14]

- Assessment of risk factors for infection with *Chlamydia trachomatis* should be performed during every routine health care contact of sexually active women.
- Sexually active women with risk factors should be screened annually by any well-validated, laboratory-based amplification or antigen method, using cervical or urine specimens. Risk factors include age <25 years, a new male sex partner or two or more partners during the preceding year, inconsistent use of barrier contraception, history of a prior STD, African-American race, and cervical ectopy. All partners of women with positive tests should be tested for *Chlamydia trachomatis*. Women with mucopurulent discharge, suggestive of cervicitis, should be tested immediately.
- Pregnant women should be screened during their first trimester or at their first prenatal visit. Those with risk factors should be re-screened during their third trimester.

The CDC recommends screening sexually active women aged <20 years for chlamydial infection during routine annual examinations.[15] The CDC also recommends annual screening of women aged <20 who use barrier contraceptive measures inconsistently and who have new or multiple sex partners during the previous 3 months.

The US Preventive Services Task Force recommends routine screening for all sexually active women aged <25 years, all asymptomatic pregnant women aged <25 and/or at high-risk for infection, as well as other asymptomatic women at high-risk for infection.[16] High-risk characteristics include being unmarried or African-American, having a prior history of STD, having new or multiple sexual partners, having cervical ectopy using barrier contraceptives inconsistently. Data on the optimal interval for screening are not available. Several groups, however, recommend annual screening intervals. Re-screening at 6 to 12 months may be considered in previously infected women due to high rates of re-infection.

## Tests used for Screening Women for *Chlamydia trachomatis* (CDC Guidelines)[17]

Screening is the cornerstone of Chlamydial control for adolescents and adults.

- A non-invasive screening can be done by a nucleic acid amplification test (NAAT). It is performed by an endocervical swab specimen, if a pelvic examination is acceptable; otherwise, a NAAT performed on urine.
- An unamplified nucleic acid hybridisation test, an enzyme immunoassay, or direct fluorescent antibody test performed on an endocervical swab specimen.
- Culture performed on an endocervical swab specimen.

## Specimen-Collection Guidelines (CDC GUIDELINES)[17]

### *Endocervical Specimens*

- By established practice, specimens for *C. trachomatis* tests are obtained after specimens for Gram-stained smear or *N. gonorrhoeae* culture. When a Papanicolaou smear is to be collected, whether specimens for *C. trachomatis* or *N. gonorrhoeae* should be collected first or last is unknown. Bleeding can occur when a Papanicolaou smear is obtained first, and gross blood interferes with certain tests for *C. trachomatis* and *N. gonorrhoeae*.

- Before obtaining a specimen, a sponge or large swab should be used to remove all secretions and discharge from the cervical os.
- For non-culture tests, the swab supplied or specified by the test manufacturer should be used.
- The appropriate swab or endocervical brush should be inserted 1-2 cm into the endocervical canal (i.e. past the squamo-columnar junction). The swab should be rotated against the wall of the endocervical canal >2 times. The swabs should be withdrawn without touching any vaginal surfaces and placed in the appropriate transport medium.

### *Urethral Specimens*

- If possible, obtaining specimens should be delayed until >1 hour after the patient has voided.
- Specimens should be obtained for *C. trachomatis* tests after obtaining specimens for a Gram-stained smear or *N. gonorrhoeae* culture.
- The urogenital swab should be inserted gently 1-2 cm into the female urethra. The swab should be rotated in one direction for >1 revolutions and withdrawn. The urethral discharge, exudate collected from the urethral meatus is sufficient for *N. gonorrhoeae* culture. An intraurethral specimen is required for *C. trachomatis* testing, regardless of the presence of exudate at the meatus.

### *Urine Specimens*

- If possible, specimen collection should be delayed until >1 hour after the patient has voided.
- First-catch urine (e.g. the first 10-30 cc voided after initiating the stream) should be used.

## Treatment

The results of sensitive tests for *C. trachomatis* or *N. gonorrhoeae* (e.g. culture or nucleic acid amplification tests) should determine the need for treatment, unless the likelihood of infection with either organism is high or the patient is unlikely to return for treatment. Empiric treatment should be considered for a patient who is suspected of having gonorrhoea and/or chlamydia if:

a. The prevalence of these infections is high in the patient population.
b. The patient might be difficult to locate for treatment.
c. Patients who have chlamydial infection and also are infected with HIV should receive the same treatment regimen as those who are HIV-negative.

The CDC-STD Guidelines, 2002[18] recommend that empiric treatment should be instituted if either uterine/adnexal or cervical motion tenderness is present, and that therapy should include coverage of possible anaerobic bacterial agents. Criteria for considering inpatient as opposed to outpatient treatment were where:

- Surgical emergencies such as appendicitis could not be ruled out;
- The patient is pregnant;
- The patient has not responded to or cannot tolerate outpatient oral antibiotic regimes;
- The patient has severe illness, nausea and vomiting or fever;
- The patient has a tubo-ovarian abscess.

### Recommended Regimens: (The CDC- STD Guidelines, 2002)

Azithromycin; 1 g orally in a single dose
OR
Doxycycline; 100 mg orally twice a day for 7 days.

#### *Alternative Regimens*

Erythromycin base 500 mg orally four times a day for 7 days,
OR
Erythromycin ethylsuccinate; 800 mg orally four times a day for 7 days,
OR
Ofloxacin; 300 mg orally twice a day for 7 days,
OR
Levofloxacin; 500 mg orally for 7 days.

#### *Follow-up*

Patients do not need to be retested for Chlamydia after completing treatment with doxycycline or azithromycin unless symptoms persist or reinfection is suspected. Repeat infection confers an elevated risk of PID and other complications when compared with initial infection. Therefore, recently infected women are a high priority for repeat testing for *C. trachomatis*. All high-risk women and adolescents with chlamydial infection should to be re-screened 3-4 months after treatment. All women treated for chlamydial infection should be screened whenever they next present to hospital within the following 12 months, regardless of whether the patient believes that her sex partners were treated. Rescreening is distinct from early retesting to detect therapeutic failure (test-of-cure) (preferably by culture).

### Management of Sex Partners

Patients should be instructed to send their sex partners for evaluation, testing, and treatment. The following recommendations on exposure intervals are based on limited evaluation. Sex partners should be evaluated, tested, and treated if they had sexual contact with the patient during the 60 days preceding onset of symptoms in the patient or diagnosis of Chlamydia. Patients should be instructed to abstain from sexual intercourse until they and their sex partners have completed treatment. Abstinence should be continued until 7 days after a single-dose regimen or after completion of a 7-day regimen.

Timely treatment of sex partners is essential for decreasing the risk for reinfecting the index patient.

## Special Considerations

### *Pregnancy*

Doxycycline and ofloxacin are contraindicated in pregnant women. However, clinical experience and preliminary data suggest that azithromycin is safe and effective. Repeat testing (preferably by culture) 3 weeks after completion of therapy with the following regimens is recommended for all pregnant women, because these regimens may not be highly efficacious.

### *Recommended Regimens*

*Erythromycin base*: 500 mg orally four times a day for 7 days

OR

*Amoxicillin*: 500 mg orally three times daily for 7 days.

### *Alternative Regimens*

Erythromycin base 250 mg orally four times a day for14 days.

OR

Erythromycin ethylsuccinate: 800 mg orally four times a day for 7 days.

OR

Erythromycin ethylsuccinate: 400 mg orally four times a day for 14 days.

OR

*Azithromycin*: 1 g orally, single dose.

## Newborn

Newborns of suspected mothers may receive ocular prophylaxis and antibiotics to treat Chlamydial conjunctivitis. Ineffectiveness of the treatment, oral antibiotics should be given to these infants.

Neonates presenting with cough, tachypnoea, rales and bilateral infiltrates and hyperventilation on CXR should be immediately taken care.

Prenatal and neonatal nurses should be posted to screen the infected pregnant mothers in first and third trimesters.

Attentiveness to routine screening and perinatal complications and implications will improve health care for both mothers and their infants.

## Key Points

- Chlamydial infection is one of the most widespread bacterial STDs. Chlamydiae are obligate intracellular bacteria that are classified in their own order (chlamydiales).
- As the majority of women with *C. trachomatis* infection are asymptomatic, they do not promptly seek medical care. Consequently, screening is necessary to identify and treat this infection.

- The spectrum of genital infection includes: Mucopurulent cervicitis, pelvic inflammatory disease, infertility, ectopic pregnancy, perihepatitis (Fitz- Hugh-Curtis syndrome) and urethral syndrome.
- Infection in pregnancy can lead to premature delivery and postpartum endometritis. Perinatal transmission and neonatal complications of chlamydia occur in up to 50 per cent of newborns whose mothers were infected with chlamydia at delivery. Perinatal infections include inclusion conjunctivitis and infant pneumonia.
- Four types of laboratory procedures are available to confirm *C. trachomatis* infection: direct microscopic examination of tissue scrapings for typical intracytoplasmic inclusions or elementary bodies, isolation of the organism in cell cultures, detection of Chlamydial antigens or nucleic acid by immunologic or hybridisation methods (DFA, EIA, NAATs and Nucleic Acid Hybridisation (Nucleic Acid Probe) Tests) and detection of antibody in serum or in local secretions.
- NAATs are found to be highly sensitive and specific methods for the detection of *C. trachomatis* in urine specimens and can be recommended for noninvasive screening of *C. trachomatis* in urine.
- Sexually active women with risk factors should be screened annually by any well-validated, laboratory based amplification or antigen method, using cervical or urine specimens. Risk factors include age <25 years, a new male sex partner or two or more partners during the preceding year, inconsistent use of barrier contraception, history of a prior STD, African-American race, and cervical ectopy. All partners of women with positive tests should be tested for Chlamydia trachomatis. Women with mucopurulent discharge, suggestive of cervicitis, should be tested immediately.
- CDC recommends Azithromycin; 1 g orally in a single dose or Doxycycline; 100 mg orally twice a day for 7 days as the first line management. Patients do not need to be retested for chlamydia after completing treatment with doxycycline or azithromycin unless symptoms persist or reinfection is suspected. Azithromycin is safe and effective in pregnancy. Repeat testing (preferably by culture) 3 weeks after completion of therapy with the following regimens is recommended for all pregnant women.

## REFERENCES


1. Chowdhary A, Malhotra VL, Deb M, Rai U. Screening for chlamydial infections in women with pelvic inflammatory diseases. J Commun Dis 1998;30(3):163-66.
2. Stamm WE. Chlamydia trachomatis infections of the adult. In: Holmes KK, Sparling PF, Mardh P-A, et al (Eds): Sexually Transmitted Diseases. 3rd ed. New York, NY: McGraw-Hill, 1999:407-22.
3. Rees E. Treatment of pelvic inflammatory disease. Am J Obstet Gynecol 1980;138:1042-47.
4. Stamm WE, Guinan ME, Johnson C, Starcher T, Holmes KK, McCormack WM. Effect of treatment regimens for *Neisseria gonorrhoeae* on simultaneous infection with *Chlamydia trachomatis*, N Engl J Med 1984;310:545-49.
5. Westrom L, Joesoef R, Reynolds G, Hadgu A, Thompson SE. Pelvic inflammatory disease and fertility: a cohort study of 1,844 women with laparoscopically verified disease and 657 control women with normal laparoscopy results. Sex Transm Dis 1992;19:185-92.
6. JL Anguenot, F de Marval, P Vassilakos, R Auckenthaler, V Ibéchéoleand A Campana. Combined screening for *Chlamydia trachomatis* and squamous intra-epithelial lesions using a single liquid-based cervical sample. Human Reproduction 2001;16:10:2206-10.
7. Chowdhary A, Malhotra VL, Deb M, Rai U. Screening for chlamydial infections in women with pelvic inflammatory diseases. J Commun Dis 1998;30(3):163-66.
8. Sharma M, Sethi S, Daftari S, Malhotra S. Evidence of chlamydial infection in infertile women with fallopian tube obstruction. Indian J Pathol Microbiol 2003;46(4):680-83.
9. Mehanna MT, Rizk MA; Eweiss NY, et al. Chlamydial serology among patients with tubal factor infertility and ectopic pregnancy in Alexandria, Egypt. Sex Transm Dis 1995;22(5):317-21.
10. Watts D, Brunham R. Sexually transmitted diseases, including HIV infection, in pregnancy. In Homes KK, Mardh PA, Sparling PF, et al (Eds): Sexually Transmitted Diseases. 3rd edition. New York: McGraw-Hill, 1999;1104-1105.
11. Hammerschlag M. Chlamydial infections in infants and children. In Homes KK, Mardh PA, Sparling PF, et al (Eds): Sexually Transmitted Diseases. 3rd edition. New York:McGraw-Hill, 1999:1155-57.

12. Gaydos CA, Theodore M, Dalesio N, Wood BJ, Quinn TC. Comparison of three nucleic acid amplification tests for detection of Chlamydia trachomatis in urine specimens. J Clin Microbiol 2004July; 42(7): 3041-45.
13. Berger, Richard E. Comparison of Three Nucleic Acid Amplification Tests for Detection of Chlamydia Trachomatis in Urine Specimens. Journal of Urology 173(6):1989, June 2005.
14. Hollblad-Fadiman K,Goldman SM. American College of Preventive Medicine Practice Policy Statement. Screening for Chlamydia trachomatis. Am J Prev Med 2003;24(3):287-92.
15. CDC recommendations for the prevention and management of *Chlamydia trachomatis* infections. MMWR Recomm Rep 1993;42:1-39.
16. CDC recommendations for Screening Tests To Detect *Chlamydia trachomatis* and *Neisseria gonorrhoeae* Infections 2002. MMWR Recomm Rep 2002; 51:RR-15:1-48.
17. US Preventive Services Task Force. Screening for chlamydial infection. Am J Prev Med 2001;20:90-93.
18. Sexually Transmitted Diseases Treatment Guidelines 2002. MMWR Recomm Rep 2002;51:RR-6:1-84.

CHAPTER 6

# Genital Tuberculosis

*Usha Manaktala, S. Chandra, Rimpi Singla*

Tuberculosis, a major public health problem in India, is the most common cause of death due to a single infectious agent in adults.

## EPIDEMIOLOGY

Actual incidence of genital tuberculosis is difficult to determine as many of these patients are asymptomatic and the disease is diagnosed incidently.[1] Autopsy studies by various authors show that 4 to 12 per cent women who died of pulmonary tuberculosis had genital tuberculosis.[2] There has been a dramatic reduction of female genital tuberculosis in the developed world in 20th century. However, similar trend has not been observed in developing countries. Earlier studies reported a high incidence from India, Scotland and Scandinavia.[3] More recently, most reports on genital tuberculosis have come from India, South Africa, Russia and Turkey. Incidence of genital tuberculosis has been estimated to range from 1 to 19 per cent in various studies in India.[4-6] Worldwide incidence of genital tuberculosis in infertile women is estimated to be 5 to 10 per cent[7] although this incidence varies greatly, being less than 1 per cent in USA to nearly 13 per cent in India.[7,8]

## FACTORS AFFECTING THE INCIDENCE OF THE DISEASE

### Age

Classically, female genital tuberculosis has been described as a disease of young women, with 80 to 90 per cent patients first diagnosed between the age of 20 and 40 years.[7]

### *Socio-economic Conditions*

- Malnutrition
- Debilitating diseases affecting the caloric intake and absorption
- Overcrowding and homelessness.

### *Occupation*

Women with silicosis have an increased risk of developing pulmonary tuberculosis due to impaired function of macrophages.

### *Alcoholism and Smoking*

- Immunosuppression
- Steroid intake and immunosuppression in patients with chronic renal failure or lymphoproliferative disease.
- Other diseases with impaired cell mediated immunity such as leukaemias, lymphoma, disseminated malignancy, diabetes, hypothyroidism.

### HIV

Tuberculosis is one of the most common opportunistic infections in patients with AIDS.

### *Genetic Predisposition*

Some people are genetically predisposed to develop the disease as reflected from the racial differences in resistance to mycobacterial disease and also from twin studies.

## PATHOGENESIS

The human strain of *Mycobacterium tuberculosis* is responsible for majority of the cases of tuberculosis. The mode of infection is droplets or the dust of dried sputum from an open case of pulmonary tuberculosis. Congenital tuberculosis is very rare and is due to infection acquired *in utero*.

*Mycobacterium tuberculosis* is a slender, non-motile and non-sporing bacillus and is an obligate aerobe. Its waxy content makes it impermeable to the usual stains. It grows very slowly on very complex artificial media that should contain egg yolk and glycerol.

The following sequence of events occurs when tubercle bacilli are introduced into the tissues.

- A transient acute inflammatory reaction with an infiltration of polymorphs.
- An infiltration of macrophages derived from local histiocytes and monocytes.
- The macrophages phagocytose the bacilli and change into epithelioid cells.
- Some macrophages form typical Langhans' giant cells with many peripherally arranged nuclei.
- Within 10-14 days coagulative necrosis begins in the centre of the mass.

*The typical tubercle follicle consists of a central mass of caseation surrounded by epitheloid cells and giant cells, which in turn are surrounded by a diffuse zone of small round cells.*

## ROUTES OF INFECTION

Genital tuberculosis is almost always secondary to tuberculosis elsewhere.

The tubercle bacilli reach the genital tract by one of the following mechanisms:

### *Bloodstream*

This mechanism accounts for at least 90 per cent of cases, the primary focus being most often situated in lungs, lymph nodes, urinary tract, bones and joints in that order.[3]

### *Descending*

The infection may also reach the pelvic organs by direct or lymphatic spread from infected adjacent organs such as peritoneum, bowel and mesenteric nodes.[7]

### *Ascending*

A few cases of tuberculosis of vulva and vagina and of primary disease of cervix are explained by children sitting unclothed where others have spat or coughed, and in adults having coitus with a male suffering from urogenital tuberculosis.[9]

## PATHOLOGY

### Fallopian Tubes

Fallopian tubes are involved in at least 90 per cent of cases[7,10] and genital disease possibly starts there. Tuberculosis accounts for 5 per cent of all cases of salpingitis.[11] The disease tends to be bilateral. Ampullary portion is the most common site of disease. The disease begins at the outer ends of the tube and generally progress inwards.

Grossly the tubes may sometimes look completely normal or more often they appear red, oedematous and swollen when infection is active. In early cases flimsy adhesions and fine miliary tubercles on the surface of tube and other pelvic organs may be seen. In severe cases, dense plastic adhesions between fallopian tube and surrounding organs are seen. The tubal wall is thickened. Generally there are multiple obstructions. Localised closure at the outer end results in the formation of hydrosalpinx or pyosalpinx. Fallopian tubes may remain patent in many cases with everted fimbrial end and remaining tube being enlarged and distended giving rise to 'tobacco pouch appearance'.[12]

Microscopically, presence of epithelioid cell granulomas with or without caseation necrosis and Langhans' giant cells may be evident. The tubal mucosa may be totally destroyed or may have hyperplastic or adenomatous appearance that may be confused with adenocarcinoma.[11] This may actually predispose to adenocarcinoma.[13]

### *Endometrium*

Endometrium is involved in 50 to 60 per cent cases of genital tuberculosis[14] and is secondary to tubal involvement.[14]

Grossly, the endometrium initially looks normal to the naked eye although microscopically it may show inflammatory response. As the disease advances, inflammatory response increases and even tuberculous ulcer may be seen. This may be followed by scarring of the endometrium leading to atrophic endometrium or an obliterated endometrial cavity due to extensive intrauterine adhesions. In 2.5 per cent cases, there may be total destruction of endometrium leading to secondary amenorrhoea.[12]

Microscopically, diagnosis is based on the presence of chronic inflammatory cells with or without caseation, granulomas with lymphocytes, Langhans' giant cells and epitheloid cells. Presence of dilated glands, destruction of epithelium, inflammatory exudates in the lumen are also suggested to be additional criteria for diagnosis of tuberculous endometritis.[15]

### *Ovaries*

Ovarian involvement occurs in 15 to 25 per cent of cases[10] and most often results from direct extension of disease from fallopian tubes.[3] The disease may manifest as surface tubercles, adhesions and thickening of capsule, retention cyst and sometimes by caseating abscess cavities in the substance of ovary.[7,12] Often the ovaries have normal microscopic appearance.

### *Cervix*

Tuberculosis of cervix may be seen in 5 to 15 per cent cases of genital tuberculosis.[10] Cervix gets affected by the downward spread of the disease from the endometrium. However, rarely cervical disease may occur secondary to deposition of infected semen by male partner having active genitourinary infection.[9]

Grossly, cervix may look normal or ulcerative but more often appears as bright red papillary erosion that bleeds easily. Cervical lesion may be hypertrophic resembling cervical carcinoma.[16]

Microscopically, multinucleated giant cells, histiocytes or epithelioid cells arranged in clusters simulating granulomas are characteristic of Pap smear in tuberculosis of cervix.[17]

### *Vagina, Vulva and Bartholin's Gland*

They constitute less than 2 per cent of genital tract disease.[7,10] Involvement of vulva and vagina is usually secondary to the involvement of other parts of genital tract. However, transmission by a male partner due to involvement of epididymis or seminal vesicles has been reported.

Grossly, vulval lesion starts as a nodule over the labia or vestibular region and subsequently gets ulcerated with sinuses discharging caseous material. Tuberculosis of vagina may resemble carcinoma in gross appearance.

Microscopic appearance is similar to granulomatous lesions seen elsewhere.

### *Abdominal Tuberculosis*

Abdominal tuberculosis is seen in combination with female genital tract tuberculosis in approximately 45 per cent of patients and is responsible for the extensive adhesions. It may present as tender abdominal masses or with ascitis, peritonitis, fever, abdominal pain, weight loss and anorexia. Peritoneal fluid is exudative with predominance of lymphocytes. With advanced disease all organs are densely matted.

### *Tuberculosis with HIV*

TB and HIV are closely linked. Because of progressive depression of cell mediated immunity in HIV infected patients, person is increasingly vulnerable to the wide range of infections including tuberculosis. Patients are unable to limit the multiplication of *mycobacteria*. More commonly HIV infected patients with dormant tuberculosis infection have reactivation of latent infection. Tuberculosis is the earliest manifestation of AIDS in over half of all the cases in developing countries and accounts for about a third of AIDS deaths, and therefore is the leading killer of people living with HIV in the developing world.[18]

## CLINICAL FEATURES

The clinical diagnosis of genital tuberculosis requires a high index of suspicion.

Tuberculosis should be suspected in following circumstances:

- Family history of tuberculosis and exposure to tuberculosis. About 20 per cent of patients with the genital tuberculosis give family history of tuberculosis.
- Women from areas where tuberculosis is endemic.
- Unexplained infertility or amenorrhoea.
- Signs of chronic pelvic infection or any pelvic infection which is slow to respond to ordinary treatment or show exacerbation after curettage or tubal patency test or one which is not accompanied by polymorphonuclear leucocytosis.
- Adnexal disease with ascites in unmarried women.

### Presenting Features

Systemic symptoms tend to be mild and include weight loss, fatigue and a tendency towards evening pyrexia. Presenting symptoms of genital tuberculosis include infertility, pelvic pain, menstrual disturbances, vaginal discharge and poor general condition.

#### *Infertility*

The most common initial symptom is infertility. Reported incidence of infertility in patients with female genital tuberculosis has varied between 40 to 80 per cent even though the fallopian tube may be open.[5,15,19] The average incidence of tuberculosis in infertility clinics throughout the world is 5-10 per cent.[7]

#### *Pain*

Chronic lower abdomen or pelvic pain is the second most common symptom in patients with female genital tuberculosis. Reported incidence varies between 20 to 50 per cent.[15] Pain is non-characteristic and dull aching type. Occasionally acute pain may occur similar to that of acute pelvic inflammatory disease or a twisted pelvic organ. Acute pain may be secondary to superimposed bacterial infection and require antibiotics and may occur after diagnostic procedures.

#### *Alteration in Menstrual Pattern*

Menstrual pattern may be disturbed in 10 to 60 per cent of cases.[5,15,20,21] The change in menstrual pattern may be towards menorrhagia or metrorrhagia as in other pelvic infections but more commonly it causes oligomenorrhoea or amenorrhoea. Various Indian studies have reported the occurrence of primary and secondary amenorrhoea in 18.9 to 60 per cent cases.[20,21] Amenorrhoea is attributed to endometrial damage or rarely it is explained by suppression of ovarian function. Postmenopausal bleeding has been noted as one of the presenting features of genital tuberculosis. In series from India and abroad, postmenopausal bleeding has been reported as the presenting symptom in 1-20 per cent patients with female genital tuberculosis.[15,20]

### Vaginal Discharge

Blood stained discharge may be present due to ulceration of cervix or endometrium. Discharge is most likely to occur with endocervical or vaginal tuberculosis.

Tuberculosis of cervix may also present as post-coital bleeding or may resemble a malignant growth.

Vulvar lesions are usually painful and tender. Vaginal ulcers, unless situated at introitus are painless.

### Ectopic Pregnancy

Every woman who has had a tubal pregnancy should be suspected of having tubal tuberculosis, active or healed due to altered tubal morphology and adhesions.

### Unusual Symptoms

Abdominal swelling, uterovesical fistulae, tubointestinal and tuboparietal fistulae have also been described. Unusually, genital tuberculosis may present as Bartholin's gland swelling,[22] vesicovaginal fistula,[23] pelvic masses, uterocutaneous fistula, reten-tion of urine due to pelvic masses of tuberculous origin or as an asymptomatic pelvic masses with rising levels of serum CA-125.

## Clinical Signs

Thirty to fifty per cent cases of genital tuberculosis may have entirely normal examination.[24] Minimal induration in adnexal areas on both sides is the most commonly noted physical finding during pelvic examination. Bilateral tubo-ovarian masses, especially in nullipara or unmarried girls in the absence of fever should raise suspicion.[10] Adnexal masses may be due to thickened edematous tubes, pyosalpinx, a conglomeration of pelvic structures matted together by adhesions. Enlargement of uterus due to pyometra especially in a postmenopausal patient may be due to pelvic tuberculosis.[25]

Lower genital tract lesions may present as variety of ulcerative or proliferative lesions. Shallow superficial indolent ulcers with undermined edges are suggestive. Ulceration tends to spread slowly with healing in some area with formation of scar. Less often non-healing ulcers of vulva may be seen. It may also cause elephantiasis of vulva.

Abdominal distention may be due to involvement of peritoneum or ascites. Presence of ascites or doughy feel of the abdomen especially in a young unmarried girl with low-grade fever and alteration of menstrual pattern should raise suspicion of genital tuberculosis.

## Investigations

### Investigations Suggesting the Infection

Haematological examination show tendency towards lymphocytosis.

Chest X-ray may show the picture suggestive of active or healed tubercular lesions. A negative chest X-ray does not rule out the diagnosis of pelvic tubercular disease, since the majority of pulmonary lesions heal by the time the genital disease manifests.

Microscopic haematuria, abacteriuric pyuria suggest concomitant urinary tract involvement.

### *Mantoux or Tuberculin Test*

Tuberculin test is done to detect the TB infection. A tuberculin test does not measure the immunity or indicate the disease; it only indicates the infection with mycobacterium.[26] A skin reaction is considered to be positive if the diameter of skin induration is more than 10 mm, but it is always better to interpret the test in conjunction with other clinical features. Many healthy people may have positive test result indicating that they have been infected with TB but did not develop the disease. On the other hand, there are conditions in which patients with active disease have negative tuberculin test like HIV infection, use of immunosuppressive drugs, certain viral infections, and cancer. Positive results are found in 90 per cent of patients with genitourinary tuberculosis.[27] In one study, Mantoux test had sensitivity of only 55 per cent and a specificity of 80 per cent in women with laparoscopically diagnosed tuberculosis concluded the limited utility of Mantoux in diagnosing active genital TB during child-bearing age. In infertile women with positive Montoux test laparoscopy should be advocated early.[28]

Various methods used to diagnose genital tuberculosis:

- Histopathological examination
- Culture
- Laparoscopy
- Hysterosalpingography
- Ultrasonography
- Rapid methods like BACTEC
- Biochemical markers
- CT scan
- Immunodiagnosis.

### *Bacteriological Examination*

If tuberculosis is suspected and the lesion is accessible, the diagnosis is made by examining biopsy material both bacteriologically and histologically. The specimen is fixed and sections made for microscopic examination. Bacilli may be demonstrated by Ziehl-Neelsen staining with basic fuschin. For the bacilli to be detected on smear $10^5$ AFB/ml are required. Auramine-rhodamine staining and fluorescence microscopy are used by laboratories that process large number of specimens.

### *Histopathological Examination*

Difficulty arises in diagnosing those cases of genital tuberculosis where infection has occurred in adolescence and patient presents with the sequelae of the disease and there are no active organisms. Otherwise also genital tuberculosis is a paucibacillary disease and it is not possible to demonstrate *Mycobacterium tuberculosis* in every case. For the diagnosis of genital tuberculosis, tissue is most commonly obtained from endometrium. During laparoscopy or exploratory laparotomy if the disease is suspected, the tissue is taken for histopathology from tubes, ovaries and peritoneum.

*Endometrial biopsy for histopathological examination* remains the most commonly used procedure for the diagnosis of female genital tuberculosis. Specimen of endometrium is obtained by endometrial biopsy or by aspiration or by dilatation and curettage. Specimen should preferably be taken from the cornual regions. The most likely time in cycle to find evidence of endometrial tuberculosis is during the week preceding menstruation[10] or within 12 hours of onset of menstruation. This is because the tubercles and bacteria are mostly found in the surface layers that are shed during menstruation and have to be reformed and reinfected from the tubes downwards. Endometrial biopsy may be difficult to obtain in case of nulliparous women. Menstrual blood collected in cervical cap provides additional material for culture. This may again be difficult in cases of oligohypomenorrhoea and obviously not possible in women presenting with amenorrhoea. Histologically proven tuberculosis is present in 50 to 60 per cent of patients with genital tuberculosis. A negative endometrial biopsy does not rule out the pelvic involvement since sampling errors are common and disease may have involved other pelvic organs without tubercular endometritis.[3]

### *Culture*

Definitive diagnosis requires isolation of tuberculosis bacilli. Culture takes 4 to 8 weeks and gives positive result in 50 to 60 per cent of cases. A period of 40 days is required for 75 per cent of positive cultures to show growth. Culture can be positive even when the bacterial load is 10 bacilli/ml.

Traditionally 2 types of media are used; egg based media (e.g. Lowenstein – Jensen) and agar-based media (e.g. Middle – Brook medium). It takes 6-8 weeks for the colonies to appear. Thereafter, same length of time is required for complete identification and sensitivity testing. Species identification is done on the basis of rate of growth, temperature requirement, pigment production, photoreactivity of pigment.

Guinea pig inoculation was once a popular method but now with the improved culture techniques, it has been demonstrated that at present it does not offer any additional advantage.[29] Most studies have found a higher diagnostic yield with histopathological examination of endometrium than culture of biopsy material.[30]

### *Laparoscopy*

Laparoscopy is now a well-recognised procedure in the diagnostic work-up of patients with infertility. Laparoscopy provides the direct visualisation of the pelvic organs and peritoneal surfaces and helps in establishing tubal patency. In a clinically suspicious case, endometrial biopsy should be followed by laparoscopy.[56] Studies from India and elsewhere have reported 5 to 33.8 per cent incidence of genital tuberculosis at laparoscopy in patients with infertility.[8,31]

In subacute form there may be miliary granulations, whitish yellow and opaque plaques surrounded by hyperemic areas over the fallopian tubes and uterus. Pelvic organs may be congested red and oedematous with adhesions.

In chronic stage there may be small yellow nodes on normal looking tubes, or tubes may be short and swollen with agglutinated fimbriae. Bilateral hydrosalpinx may occur due to agglutination of fimbriae. Tubes may be filled with caseous material. Bands of adhesions covering the tubes and ovary and fixing them are occasionally seen in chronic phase of genital tuberculosis.[56]

In one Russian study laparoscopy was shown to increase the diagnostic potentialities by 19.7 per cent by morphologically verifying the diagnosis based on biopsies specimen among people with prior TB of other site or history contact with infected persons.[32] In another study out of 101 women suspected to have pelvic TB on diagnostic laparoscopy alone, definitive evidence was later found in 70 cases[31] (Figs 6.1 to 6.4 in Plate 1).

### *Hysterosalpingography*

It is done to check the tubal patency in women with infertility. On hysterosalpingographic visualisation of uterine cavity and fallopian tubes, uterine cavity is shrivelled and deformed with associated intrauterine adhesions. Tubes may show ragged outline with small lumen defects or multiple strictures giving rise to beaded appearance. Tube may also have straight rigid contour of the lumen with stem-pipe like appearance. Calcification of the tubes and ovaries may also be seen.[56]

### *Several Radiographic Signs Presumptive of Tuberculosis[33] (Figs 6.5 and 6.6)*

- Golf club appearance, when only isthmus and proximal ampulla are visualised, isthmic segment has a rigid stove pipe appearance;
- Beaded appearance due to alternate areas of tube filled with or without contrast.
- Maltase cross appearance; completely filled tube with rigid, irregular outline.
- Rosette type; distal end of tube is filled with dye giving a rosette type image.
- Numerous diverticula in isthmic area.
- Leopard skin-like speckled appearance of the ampulla due to tube being partially filled with contrast.

Hysterosalpingography is unreliable as a diagnostic tool and it can cause exacerbation of the disease. So laparoscopy should be preferred if the disease is suspected. Tubes may be patent in 37 per cent of the cases of tubercular endometritis[34] (Figs 6.5 and 6.6).

### *Ultrasonography*

Bilateral predominantly solid, adnexal masses containing scattered small calcifications is highly indicative of tuberculosis involvement.[35]

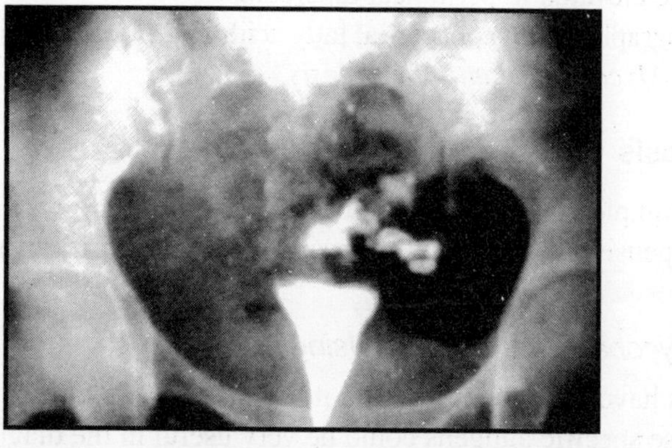

**Fig. 6.5:** Hysterosalpingogram showing beaded appearance of fallopian tube

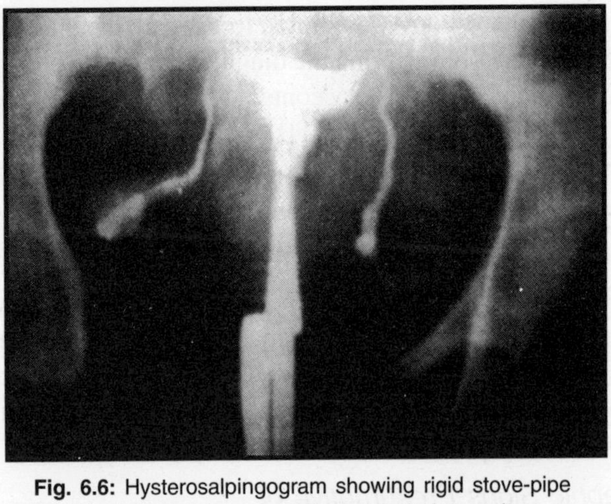

**Fig. 6.6:** Hysterosalpingogram showing rigid stove-pipe like fallopian tubes and irregular uterine cavity

### *Computed Tomography*

Findings suggestive of abdominal and pelvic tuberculosis include low density, uncommon patterns of adenopathy, presence of multiple pelvic lesions, hepatic, adrenal and splenic lesions.

### *Radiometric Methods*

BACTEC radiometric system uses fatty acid substrates like palmitic acid or formic acid labelled with radioactive carbon. As the mycobacteria metabolises these fatty acids, radioactive carbon dioxide is released which is measured as a marker of bacterial growth.

MGIT (Mycobacterial growth indicator tube) is another rapid method for detection of mycobacterial growth that is non-invasive and cheaper than BACTEC.[36]

With the help of rapid methods results are obtained within 2 weeks.

### *Biochemical Markers*

Adenosine deaminase activity is related to proliferation and differentiation of lymphocytes. Enzyme levels are elevated in peritoneal tuberculosis.[37]

Gas chromatography of mycobacterial fatty acids and alcohols has been utilised for rapid identification of *Mycobacterium tuberculosis.*

## Immunodiagnosis

These tests are complementary to other investigations and are not performed routinely as they are very expensive and are not affordable by the majority of patients in developing countries.

### *Detection of Mycobacterial Antigen Using ELISA*

Specific epitopes have been identified and it has been reported that detection of antibodies by ELISA to these specific antigens could be very useful in the diagnosis of tuberculosis.

Using a monoclonal antibody that recognises a 45 kDa protein antigen, when sandwich ELISA was applied to serum samples from patients with genital tuberculosis, the test was positive in nine of the twelve cases, while only one of the 15 non-tuberculosis controls gave a positive reaction.[38]

Using a competitive inhibition ELISA format with monoclonal antibodies to the 35 kDa *Mycobacterium tuberculosis* antigen, 73 per cent of cases of extrapulmonary tuberculosis and 70 per cent of smear-negative pulmonary tuberculosis cases could be detected.[39]

Recently, the dot-ELISA test was used to detect 55-kDa mycobacterial antigen in the serum sample of individuals with extra-pulmonary TB. The DOT-ELISA detected the target antigen in 90 percent sera of individuals with extra-pulmonary TB and in 87 per cent sera of individuals with pulmonary TB with a specificity of 97 per cent among control individuals, concluded that the detection of the 55 kDa antigen using DOT-ELISA can be routinely employed to support clinical diagnosis of extra-pulmonary TB.[40]

### *Nucleic Acid Probes*

When labelled, DNA/RNA fragment containing the appropriate sequence that is complementary to a DNA/RNA base sequence of organism are able to detect small numbers of Mycobacterial when allowed to hybridise. In one study sensitivity was shown to be 90.5 per cent and specificity 83.8 per cent.[41]

### *Polymerase Chain Reaction (PCR)*[42]

PCR for DNA is done on endometrial tissue. It may be positive even with dead bacilli and does not reflect active disease. Similarly PCR for RNA can detect small amounts of ribosomal RNA and indicate the presence of actively multiplying bacilli.

Diagnostic value—In one study PCR on endometrial curettage specimen showed 80 per cent sensitivity and high specificity in the diagnosis of genital tuberculosis.[43] In another study done to evaluate PCR, the sensitivity of the test to diagnose genital tuberculosis was shown to be 94.7 per cent.[44]

### *Comparing ELISA and PCR*[45]

In one study directly comparing DOT-ELISA and PCR for tuberculous lymphadenitis FNAC was done of enlarged lymph nodes and tested for AFB and DOT-ELISA and PCR. ELISA was more sensitive and detected 93.2 per cent of cases. PCR and fine needle aspiration cytology (FNAC) detected 82.5 per cent and 61.0 per cent cases, respectively. AFB positively was 33.1 per cent concluding that the application of DOT-ELISA was more sensitive but less specific as compared to PCR. PCR, though expensive, should be used in problem cases because of its high specificity.[56]

PCR is a very sensitive test but it can detect even fraction of bacterial DNA which are not significant. So it gives positive results in many cases that may not need treatment. So this should not form the basis of therapy.[46]

## TREATMENT

### General

It is important to improve the patient's natural resistance to the disease by attention to diet and general well-being.

### Chemotherapy[10,47,48]

The mainstay of the treatment is medical though surgery may be required in some cases mainly to treat the complications and sequelae of the disease. Any surgical procedure should be undertaken only after adequate chemotherapy.

The treatment of pelvic tuberculosis is similar to pulmonary tuberculosis. Patients are usually commenced on isoniazid(H), rifampicin (R), pyrazinamide (Z) and ethambutol(E). Maintenance therapy is usually with INH and rifampicin. Pyridoxine 10 mg should be added in the regime. Advantages of using multiple drugs are rapid bacteriological conversion, low failure rate, decreased emergence of drug resistant bacilli, shorter duration of therapy and thus better compliance.

Under Revised National Tuberculosis Control Programme, directly observed treatment short course (DOTS) is used to ensure better compliance and for prevention of multi-drug resistant tuberculosis. The principle is to give four drugs (H,R,Z,E) for initial 2 months, i.e. during intensive phase, followed by two drugs (H,R) for the remaining four months, i.e. during continuation phase.[49] DOTS is a strategy to ensure cure by providing the most effective medicine and confirming that it is taken. In DOTS, during the intensive phase of treatment a health worker or other trained person watches as the patient swallows the drug. During continuation phase, the patient is issued medicines for one week in a multiblister combipack of which the first dose is swallowed by the patient in presence of health worker. The consumption of the medicines is confirmed by the return of empty combipacks when the patient comes to collect medicines for next week. In the programme alternate day treatment regime is followed.[48]

According to a theoretical model of tuberculosis, four different populations of mycobacterium are known to exist in the lesions. First, the actively growing organisms found in the caseous material. These are particularly sensitive to isoniazid, which is a bactericidal drug and acts on fast multiplying bacilli. Second population is made up of organisms that exist in acidic pH and located intracellularly. These grow very slowly. Pyrazinamide, a highly bactericidal drug is particularly active in acidic pH and is effective against these bacilli. Third population consists of organisms located in solid caseous areas. These remain dormant or multiply very slowly and intermittently. These are killed most effectively by rifampicin that is again a bactericidal drug. Fourth population is completely dormant. Ethambutol is the only main antitubercular drug used today which is bacteriostatic. Streptomycin is also a bactericidal drug.

During antitubercular treatment, the risk of selection of resistant mutants lasts as long as bacterial load is not significantly reduced. This forms the rationale for administration of combination of several drugs in the intensive phase of chemotherapy. Further drugs like Isoniazid, Rifampicin, Streptomycin and Ethambutol prevent the emergence of resistant mutants.

### *Recommended Adult Dosage of Anti-tuberculosis Drugs*

| Drug | Daily Dosage |
|---|---|
| Isoniazid | 5-10 mg/kg, usually 300 mg |
| Rifampicin | 10 mg/kg, up to 600 mg |
| Pyrazinamide | 20-40 mg/kg up to 1500-2000 mg |
| Ethambutol | 15-25 mg/kg usually 800 or 1200 mg |
| Streptomycin | 15 mg/kg usually 750 mg |

### *Major Adverse Effects of Anti-tubercular Drugs*

| Drug | Adverse reaction |
|---|---|
| Isoniazid | Hepatitis, rash, peripheral neuropathy, neurological disturbance |
| Rifampicin | Gastrointestinal side-effects, rash, flu-like syndrome, elevation of liver enzymes, renal failure, thrombocytopenia, haemolytic anaemia |
| Pyrazinamide | Hepatitis, rash, hyperuricaemia, arthralgia, gout |
| Ethambutol | Retrobulbar neuritis |
| Streptomycin | Vestibular and auditory toxicity, nephrotoxicity |

Patients with tuberculosis resistant to first-line drugs are treated with second line drugs. These have lower efficacy and higher toxicity. These include kanamycin, amikacin, capreomycin, ethionamide, cycloserine, para-aminosalicylic acid, ofloxacin, clofazimine, thiacetazone and amoxycillin/clavulanic acid.

In case of endometrial tuberculosis, the patient is subjected to endometrial aspiration after 6 months for test of cure. If it is negative, then chemotherapy is continued for another 3 months. Repeat endometrial aspiration is done after 6 months of cessation of antibiotics. Sometimes after an initial apparent cure, positive endometrial cultures are obtained again 12 or more months later. Thus, patients should be followed up annually.

## Surgery

There is a place for excision of the affected area when the disease can be remarkably localised and is accessible. A hypertrophic lesion of the vulva that fails to respond to antibiotics may require excision. Removal of uterus and adnexa for tuberculous salpingitis and endometritis in well-chosen cases is safe when the surgery is covered by antibiotics.[50]

### *Indications of Surgery*[10]

- Progression or persistence of active disease despite adequate medical treatment
- Presence of large inflammatory masses, pyosalpinx, ovarian abscess and pyometra
- Persistence of symptoms like menorrhagia or pelvic pain
- Post menopausal woman with recurrent pyometra due to tuberculosis
- Recurrence of positive endometrial culture or histology after six months of chemotherapy.

### *Contraindications to Surgery*

- Active tuberculosis elsewhere in the body
- Presence of plastic peritonitis and dense adhesions around the pelvic organs for the fear of injury to bowel and bladder.

Any sort of surgery should be preceded by 3 to 6 weeks treatment with antitubercular drugs, in full dosage. When tuberculosis affects the upper genital tract the appropriate surgical procedure is usually total hysterectomy and bilateral salpingectomy. If the ovaries are involved or the age of the woman is more than 45 years, they are usually removed.

## PREGNANCY

Full term pregnancy is uncommon after treatment of histopathologically proven genital tuberculosis.[51] If the tubes are open, pregnancy is possible but because of residual infection or of scarring and distortion of endosalpinx, tubal implantation is likely. Ectopic pregnancy following antibiotic therapy for pelvic tuberculosis is now a recognised clinical syndrome.[52] Abortion of intrauterine pregnancies is also common.

Of all the women treated, only 8 per cent conceive. Of the pregnancies, 50 per cent are tubal and 20 to 30 per cent end in abortion. Only 20-30 per cent result in live births.[53]

If the tubes are closed at the outset, permanent sterility is likely and attempts at tuboplasty after suppression of active disease may be followed by reclosure. Reactivation of silent pelvic tuberculosis may also occur.[54]

### In Vitro Fertilisation

This is a possible alternative for the patients with treated genital tuberculosis. However lower pregnancy rate per cycle and higher spontaneous abortion rates have been reported.[55] Basal FSH levels are higher and peak estradiol levels following exogenous gonadotropin therapy are lower. When the results are compared with other patients with tubal factor responsible for infertility, fewer oocytes and embryos are obtained in women with genital tuberculosis.

## REFERENCES

1. Goldin AG, Baker WT. Tuberculosis of female genital tract. J Ky Med Assoc 1985;83:75.
2. Schaefer G. Tuberculosis of the female genital tract. Clin Obstet Gynecol 1970;13:965-98.
3. Anderson JR.Genital tuberculosis.In:Jones HW, Wentz AC, Burnett LS (Eds). Novak's text book of gynaecology.11th edition.Baltimore:Williams and Wilkins;1988:557-69.
4. Gupta S.Pelvic tuberculosis in women. J Obstet Gynaecol India 1956;7:181-98.
5. Bobnate SK, Kadar GP, Khan A, Grover S. Female genital tuberculosis. A pathological appraisal. J Obstet Gynaecol India 1986;36:676-80.
6. Malkani PK, Rajani CK. Endometrial tuberculosis. Indian J Med Sci 1954;8:684-97.
7. Schaefer G. Female genital tuberculosis. Clin Obstet Gynecol 1976;19:223-29.
8. Krishna VR, Sathe AV, Mehta H. Tubal factors in sterility. J Obstet Gynecol India 1979;29:663-67.
9. Sutherland AM,Glean ES, MacFarlane JR. Transmission of genitourinary tuberculosis. Health Bull 1982;40: 87-91.

10. Schaefer G.Female genital tuberculosis. In:Zuspan FP,Quilligan EJ, Eds.Current therapy in obstetrics and gynecology.4th edition.Philadelphia:WB Saunders Company;1994:.51-55.
11. Novak ER, Woodruff JD. Novak's Gynaecologic and Obstetric Pathology, 8th edn: 328 WB Saunders, Philadelphia, PA, 1979.
12. Nogales Ortiz F, Tarancon I, Nogales FF Jr.The pathology of female genital tuberculosis—a 31-year-study of 1436 cases.Obstet Gynecol 1979;53:422-28.
13. Vinall PS, Buxtox N. Primary carcinoma of fallopian tubes with tubercular salpingitis.Br J Obst Gynae 1979;53:422-28.
14. Schaefer G.Tuberculosis of the genital organs.Am J Obstet Gynaecol 1965;91:714-20.
15. Bazaz-Malik G, Maheshwari B, Lal N.Tuberculous endometritis:A clinicopathological study of 1000 cases.Br J Obstet Gynaecol 1983;90:84-86.
16. Chahtane A, Rhrab B, Jirari A, Ferhati D, Kharbach A, Chaoui A. Hypertrophic tuberculosis of the cervix.Three cases.J Gynecol Obstet Biol Reprod Paris 1992;21:424-27.
17. Angrish K, Verma K.Cytologic detection of tuberculosis of uterine cervix.Acta Cytol 1981;25:160-62.
18. UNAIDS. AIDS epidemic update, December 2001. UNAIDS Geneva 2001.
19. Klein TA, Richmond JA, Mishell DR. Pelvic Tuberculosis.Obstet Gynecol 1976;48:99-104.
20. Chhabra S. Genital tuberculosis—A baffling disease.J Obstet Gynecol India 1990;40:569-73.
21. Mukherjee K, Wagh KV, Aggarwal S.Tubercular endometritis in primary infertility. J Obstet Gynecol India1967;17:619-24.
22. Dhall K, Das SS, Dey P. Tuberculosis of Bartholin's gland (letter).Int J Gynecol Obstet 1992;37:127-30.
23. Ba-Thike K, Than-Aye, Nan OO.Tuberculous vesicovaginal fistula. Int J Gynecol Obstet 1992;37:127-30.
24. Simon HG. Genito-urinary tuberculosis.Clinical features in a general hospital.Am J Med 1977;68:410-20.
25. Schaefer G, Marcus RS, Kramer EE.Postmenopausal endometrial tuberculosis.Am J Obstet Gynecol 1972;112:681-87.
26. Crofton J, Horne N, Miller F. Clinical Tuberculosis. 2nd edition. 1999;43:200-203.
27. Alversez S. Mccabe Medicine 1984;63:25-55.
28. Raut VS, Mahashur AA, Sheth SS. The Mantoux test in the diagnosis of genital tuberculosis in women.Int J Gynaecol Obstet 2001 Feb;72(2):165-69.
29. Roy A, Mukherjee S, Bhattacharya S, Adhya S, Chakraborty P. Tuberculous endometritis in hills of Darjelling: A clinicopathological and bacteriological study. Indian J Pathol Microbiol 1993;36:361-69.
30. Falk V, Ludviksson K, Agren G.Genital tuberculosis in women.Analysis of 187 newly developed cases from 47 Swedish hospitals during the ten-year- period., 1968 to 1977.Am J Obstet Gynecol 1980;138:974-77.
31. Merchant R. Endoscopy in the diagnosis of genital tuberculosis. J Reprod Med 1989;34:468-74.
32. Semenovskii AV, Barinov VS, Kochorova MN, et al. Laparoscopy in the complex diagnosis abdominal and genital tuberculosis. Probl Tuberk.1999;(3)36-39.
33. Rozin S. The X-ray diagnosis of genital tuberculosis. J Obstet Gynecol Br Empire 1952;59:59-63.
34. Sharman A. Genital tuberculosis in the female. J Obstet Gynecol Br Empire 1952;59:740-42.
35. Walzer A, Koenigsberg M. Ultrasonographic demonstration of pelvic tuberculosis.J Ultrasound Med 1983;2: 139-40.
36. Hanna BA, Walters SB,et al. Detection of Mycobacterium tuberculosis directly from patient specimens with the Mycobacterium Growth Indicator Tube; A new rapid method. Abstr. C 112, 93rd Ann Meet Am Soc Microbiol. Las Vegas, USA,1994.
37. Bhargava DK, Gupta M, et al. Adenosine deaminase (ADA) in peritoneal tuberculosis: Diagnostic value in ascitic fluid and serum. Tubercle 1990;2:121-26.
38. Rattan A, Gupta SK, Singh S, Takkar D, Kumar S, Bai P, et al. Detection of antigens of *Mycobacterium tuberculosis* in patients of infertility by monoclonal antibody based sandwiched ELISA .Tuber Lung Dis 1993;74:200-03.
39. Wilkins EGL, Ivanyi J. Potential value of serology for diagnosis of extrapulmonary tuberculosis. Lancet 1990;36:641-44.
40. Attalah AM, Osman S, et al. Application of a circulating antigen detection immunoassay for laboratory diagnosis of extrapulmonary and pulmonary tuberculosis. Clin Chim Acta 2005;356 (1-2):58-66.

41. Pao CC, Lin SS, et al. The detection of mycobacterial DNA sequences in uncultured clinical specimens with cloned *Mycobacterium tuberculosis* DNA as probes. Tubercle 1988;69:27-36.
42. Manjunath N, Shankar P, Rajan L, Bhargava A, Sahuja S, Shriniwas. Evaluation of a polymerase chain reaction for diagnosis of tuberculosis.Tubercle 1991;72:22-27.
43. Mirlina ED, Lantsov VA, et al. Diagnostic value of polymerase chain reaction test in females with genital tuberculosis. Probl Tuberk 1998;1:46-48.
44. Vishnevskaia EB, Marttila NJ, et al. Polymerase chain reaction and ligase chain reaction in the diagnosis of gynecological tuberculosis. Probl Tuberk 2002;1:49-51.
45. Jain A, Verma RK, Tiwari V et al. Dot-ELISA vs. PCR of fine needle aspirates of tuberculous lymphadenitis;a prospective study in India. Acta Cytol 2005;49(1):17-21.
46. Grosset J, Mouton Y. Is PCR a useful tool for the diagnosis of tuberculosis in 1995? Tubercle Lung Dis 1995;76:183-84.
47. Richard J, Wallace Jr, David E. Griffith. Antimicrobial agents: In Kasper DL, Fauci AS, Longo DL, Braunwald E, et al. Eds. Harrisons principles of internal medicine 16th Edn. McGraw Hill, 946-51.
48. K Park.Tuberculosis. In: K Park Ed. Park's textbook of preventive and social medicine.17th edition.Banarsi Das Bhanot pbl 2002:138-53.
49. Govt. of India, RNTCP at a Glance, Revised National TB Control Programme, Central TB division, Ministry of Health and Family Welfare, New Delhi.
50. Sutherland AM.Surgical treatment of tuberculosis of female genital tract. Br J Obstet Gynaecol 1980;87: 310-12.
51. Schaefer G. Full term pregnancy following genital tuberculosis(review).Obstet Gynecol Surv 1964;29:81-124.
52. Varma TR. Genital tuberculosis and future fertility. Int J Gynecol Obstet 1991;35:1-11.
53. Infections. In: Bhatla N, Eds. Jeffcoate's Principles of Gynaecology. 6th edition Arnold;2001: 298-324.
54. Ballon SC, Clewell WH, Lamb EJ. Reactivation of silent pelvic tuberculosis by reconstructive tubal surgery. Am J Obstet Gynecol 1975;122:991.
55. Gurgan T, Urman B, Yarali H. Results of *in vitro* fertilization and embryo transfer in women with infertility due to genital tuberculosis. Fertil Steril 1996;65:367-70.
56. Manaktala U, Srivastava N. 'Role of ELISA in genital tuberculosis' International Journal of Gynecology and Obstetrics; 1997;57:205-06.

## CHAPTER 7

# Urinary Tract Infections in Pregnancy

*Anjali Tempe, Leena Wadhwa*

Although some diseases of urinary tract may be pre-existing or associated with pregnancy by chance, pregnancy often predisposes to development of urinary tract disorders, an example being acute pyelonephritis.[1]

### Changes in Pregnancy

There are significant changes in the urinary tract during pregnancy. They are as follows:

- There is a marked dilatation of renal calyces and ureter more on the right side than left, due to dextro-rotation of the uterus and direct pressure.
- There is increased renal parenchymal volume due to intra-renal fluid accumulation hence sometimes massive dilatation of renal pelvis or ureter occurs. This is seen even at the gestational age of 14 weeks and is attributed to hormonal influences in pregnancy which is relieved by 2 to 4 days of postpartum period normally.[2]
- By second trimester, there is increased renal blood flow upto 70 to 80 per cent and also glomerular filtration rate by 45 to 50 per cent.
- There is increased creatinine clearance and serum creatinine level falls during pregnancy, but rises gradually till third trimester, concentration of many other constituents change.
- The excretion of glucose is raised to 10 times as much as normal non-pregnant women, i.e. 20 to 100 mg/day. Therefore glycosuria is not a reliable indicator of carbohydrate metabolism during pregnancy.
- There is a change in the osmoregulatory mechanism of body which tolerates the decrease in osmolality of plasma by 10 mosmol/L.
- There is a vesicoureteral reflux seen in pregnancy.

The pregnancy associated urinary stasis, glycosuria, vesicoureteric reflux are predisposing factors for development of urinary tract infections.

### Urinary Tract Infections

They are the most common bacterial infections encountered during pregnancy. Asymptomatic bacteriuria is usual, symptomatic infection may involve the lower urinary tract to cause cystitis and upper urinary tract to cause pyelonephritis.

## Pathogenesis

Various bacteria which are responsible for infection are *E.coli* (75-90%), *Klebsiella* (10-15%) and *Proteus* (5%) species. Pseudomonas streptococci and staphylococci are present infrequently.[3] The infection can be due to transperineal route of spread to urinary tract of these bacteria. The stasis during pregnancy, the perineal discomfort in postpartum period due to tears or episiotomy or injury, the bladder insensitivity to increased urinary tension in immediate postpartum period, the need for catheterisation due to over distension are the factors leading to urinary tract infection in pregnancy and postpartum period.

## Asymptomatic Bacteriuria (ASB)

It is defined as presence of 100,000 organisms of the same species/ml of urine in an otherwise asymptomatic woman; present in 2 consecutive specimens. The incidence varies and is about 5 per cent in general population. About 5 per cent women are positive for the first time when screened. Subsequently 1.5 per cent are added to increase the incidence to (6.5%). After treatment about 80 per cent are found to be negative for growth of organisms. Out of a cohort of 1000 women, 990 were negative after they were given the antibiotic treatment twice, still 10 women remained positive.[3] This indicates the recurrent nature of infection in some patients, or underlying pathology.

## Significance of ASB

1. 11.8 per cent of bacteriuric women subsequently developed signs and symptoms of urinary tract infections against 3.2 per cent of those pregnant women who had sterile urine.[4]
2. About 20 per cent of patients having bacteriuria may have underlying renal abnormality. This is particularly so, if the infection is recurrent, resistant to treatment or there is postpartum recurrence.[5] Postpartum urography is reserved for these symptomatic and chronic women.
3. There is a significant controversy regarding the cost effectiveness of routine screening in pregnancy for ASB. It is said to be cost effective if the pregnant population is showing an incidence of >10 per cent, i.e. high risk. In low risk, i.e. < 5 per cent incidence it's not cost effective.[2]
4. The gold standard for diagnosis of asymptomatic bacteriuria is urine culture, other methods like dipstick method or uri screen based on (LEN)-leucocyte esterase nitrite strip test which is easier to do, are not found effective.[6,7]
5. Untreated ASB can lead to acute pyelonephritis (25-40%),[3] maternal hypertension, pre-eclampsia and anaemia in mother and preterm and low birth weight infant and foetal loss.[8-10] There is a beneficial effect of antibiotic therapy in reducing pyelonephritis and in apparent reduction in preterm births, but the association of preterm and low birth weight infants with ASB needs to be interpreted with caution.[11]

   Gilstrap and colleagues have found no association of ASB with anaemia, hypertension or low birth weight infants.[12]

## Predisposing Factors

Incidence depends on parity, race, socio-economic status. Highest incidence is found in Afro-American multipara with sickle cell trait and the lowest incidence was found in affluent white women of low parity.
Although definition wise ASB is > 100,000 bacterial/ml of urine, lower colony counts of 20 to 40,000/ml of single pathogen can cause pyelonephritis and should not be ignored.

## Management

Most commonly used antibiotics are ampicillin, cephalosporin, nitrofurantoins and sulfonamides. Single dose of antimicrobials are also used with success.

### *Single Dose*

Amoxycillin 2 gm or ampicillin 2 gm. Cephalosporins 2 gm or nitrofurantoin 200 mg, etc. can be used. Recurrence rate with single dose is around 30 per cent.

### *Three Days Course*

Amoxycillin 500 mg three times a day, Ampicillin 250 mg 4 times a day, cephalosporin 250 mg 4 times a day or nitrofurantoin 50 to 100 mg 4 times a day, sulfonamides 500 mg 4 times a day can be given.

### *Protracted Therapy*

For recurrent infections, 100 mg of nitrofurantoin at bed time daily for 10 to 21 days may be required, or it may be continued throughout the pregnancy to prevent further infections.[13]

## Cystitis and Urethritis

Symptomatic bacteriuria without flank pain or fever is caused by this infection. Urinary urgency, frequency, dysuria are the common symptoms and treatment does not differ from asymptomatic bacteriuria. Haematuria or pyuria and bacteriuria are present. If the symptoms are present with sterile urine, the infecting agent could be *Chlamydia trachomatis* and will respond to erythromycin therapy. About 90 per cent of women have infection limited to bladder only. Mucopurulent cervicits usually co-exists. Before treatment, concomitant pyelonephritis must be confidently excluded.

## Acute Pyelonephritis

This is a potentially life-threatening condition occurring in pregnancy. In contrast to non-pregnant women, in pregnancy acute pyelonephritis leads to acute renal failure if not treated. Complications such as septic shock, renal abscess and renal vein thrombosis may develop. When symptomatic kidney infection does occur the underlying defects like unrecognized diabetes, congenital anomalies of kidney, analgesic abuse nephropathy, reflux nephropathy, calculi etc. may be present.

### *Pathology*

Incidence is 1 to 2 per cent in pregnancy. It presents as a febrile illness with loin pain, vomiting. Dysuria pyuria, bacteriuria are present. Most cases are bilateral or right sided. If only limited to left side, it may indicate presence of anomalous kidney or ureter.

Between 75 to 90 per cent or renal infections are caused by bacteria that have p-fimbriae adhesins.[14] About 15 percent of the women with acute pyelonephritis also have bacteraemia. Almost all clinical findings are because of endotoxaemia. The changes are mediated by cytokines and TNF release.

### *Differential Diagnosis*

Labour, chorioamnionitis, appendicitis, placental abruption, infarcted myoma and in puerperium, metritis with pelvic cellulitis.

### *Complications*

Premature rupture of membranes, IUGR or foetal death. Severe complications can be perinephric cellulitis or abscess, septicaemia, septic shock, ARDS and death.

### *Treatment*

It is as follows:

1. Initially at least hospitalisation is necessary.
2. IV antibiotics with IV fluids to maintain adequate urine output are started. Ampicillin is not recommended as *E. coli* are resistant to it. Second or third generation cephalosporins are preferred instead with or without aminoglycosides according to sensitivity of the organisms. If within 24 hours, the patient is afebrile, oral cephalosporins may be started and administered for a total of 7 to 10 days.
3. Plasma creatinine should be measured early.
4. β-agonist tocolysis may precipitate respiratory insufficiency, so cautious use of these to avoid preterm labour is advocated.
5. Haemolysis and anaemia is present, so haemogram, electrolytes and KFT is to be performed.
6. Blood pressure, temperature, urine output are monitored closely.
7. Chest X-ray is indicated if patient is breathless.
8. Urine and blood cultures are to be sent and treated accordingly.
9. Intravenous antibiotics therapy, as already discussed, is started.
10. Patient is preferably only managed by hospitalisation as full compliance is poor in outdoor patients.
11. If the patient does not respond within 48 to 72 hours, further investigations for urinary tract obstruction or other pathology is indicated like ultrasonography or single shot pyelography, etc. Plain X-ray abdomen may also help in ruling out calculi in 50 per cent of patients.
12. Passing of double ureteral stent may relieve the obstruction in most cases.
13. For renal stones which cause obstruction of the outflow tract, invasive procedures like stenting, percutaneous nephrostomy, laser lithotripsy, basket extraction of calculus or occasionally surgical exploration may be needed.

### *Follow-up*

Recurrence of infection is common in 30 to 40 per cent women. Therefore 100 mg nitrofurantoin at bed time is recommended to prevent relapse. Recurrence also suggests underlying pathology, therefore further investigations are needed in the postpartum period if the urine culture is still not sterile.

## Chronic Pyelonephritis

The disease is chronic interstitial nephritis, thought to be caused by bacterial infection.

### *Clinical Picture*

Fewer than half of the women have any preceding symptoms of cystitis or acute pyelonephritis or obstructive disease. The origin of this disease is therefore obscure and probably not due to only bacterial infection. Mostly there is radiological scarring of the kidney with reflux uropathy. Chronic infection is not symptomatic and symptoms are that of renal insufficiency and not of infection. If superimposed acute pyelonephritis develops, there may be further deterioration. The maternal and foetal prognosis depends on the extent of renal destruction. The maternal and foetal prognosis is good if hypertension is minimal or absent and renal pavenchyma is at the most moderately compromised. If severely diseased kidney is present, the chances of good pregnancy outcome are rare and therefore in severe disease of kidney, patients should not undertake pregnancy as they may go into end stage disease and pregnancy may be planned after kidney is transplanted in such unfortunate patients.

## Key Points

- There are significant changes in the urinary tract during pregnancy. The urinary stasis, glycosuria, vesicouretric reflux are predisposing factors for development of urinary tract infections.
- Asymptomatic bacteriuria (ASB) is present in about 5 to 6.5 per cent pregnant women. Untreated ASB can lead to acute pyelonephritis in 25 to 40 per cent patients. Association of ASB with preterm and low-birth weight infants and maternal hypertension, anaemia needs to be interpreted with caution.
- Asymptomatic bacteriuria is treated by administering antibiotics such as ampicillin, cephalosporins, nitrofurantoins and sulphonamides in pregnancy.
- Acute pyelonephritis is a potentially life-threatening condition in pregnancy. Incidence is 1 to 2 per cent in pregnant patients. Hospitalisation is advisable, at least in the initial phase. The preferred antibiotics in the treatment of acute pyelonephritis are second or third generation cephalosporins with or without aminoglycosides according to the sensitivity of the organisms cultured.

## REFERENCES

1. William's, Obstetrics. "Renal and urinary tract disorders": 21st edition edited by Cunningham FG, Ganl NF, Leveno KJ, Gilstrap III LC, Hauth JC, Wenstrom KP. Mcgraw-Hill Medical Publishing Division, 2001; Chapter 47:1251-59.
2. Turnbull's, Obstetrics. "Urinary tract in pregnancy": 3rd edition, edited by Chamberlain G, Steer P, Churchill Livingstone, 2001,Chapter 23:383-402.
3. Danforth's. Obstetrics and Gynecology. "Medical and surgical complications of pregnancy: Edited by Scott JR, Gibbs RS, Karlon BY, Haney AF, Publisher Lippincott Williams and Wilkins, 9th edition 2003, chapter 17:292-94.

4. Chng PK, Hall MH. 'Antenatal prediction of urinary tract infection in pregnancy': Brit J Obst Gynecol 1982;89:8-11.
5. Schwartz MA, Wang CC, Eckert L, et al. 'Risk factors for urinary tract infection in the postpartum period': Am J Obstwet Gynecol 1999;181:547-53.
6. Mcissac W, Carroll JC, Biringer A, Benstein P, Lynos FE, Low DE, Permaul JA. 'Screening for asymptomatic bacteriuria in pregnancy': J of Obstet. Gynecol Can. 2005;27(1):20-4.
7. Teppa RJ, Roberts JM. "The uri-screen test to detect significant asymptomatic bacteriuria during pregnancy": J Soc Gynecol Investig 2005;12(1):50-3.
8. Romero R, Oyazun E, Mazar M, et al. 'Meta-analysis of the relationship between asymptomatic bacteriuria and preterm delivery/low birth weight': Obstet Gynecol 1989;73:576-82.
9. Locksmith G, Duff P. "Infection, antibiotics and preterm delivery": Semin Perinatal 2001;25(5):295-309.
10. Le J, Briggs GG, Mckeown A, Bustillo G. "Urinary tract infections during pregnancy":Ann Pharmaca other 2004;38(10):1692-701 Epub 2004 Aug 31.
11. Smaill F. 'Antibiotics for asymptomatic bacteriuria in pregnancy': Cochrane database Syst Rev 2001(2) CD000-490 Review PMID 11405965.
12. Gilstrap LC III, Leveno KJ, Cunningham FG, Whalley PJ, Roark ML. 'Renal infection and pregnancy outcome': Am J Obstet Gynecol 1981b;141:708.
13. Lucas MJ, Cunningham FG, William's. 'Urinary tract infections complicating pregnancy'. William's Obstetrics 19th edition (Suppl. 5) Norwalk CT Appleton and Lange, Feb/march 1994.
14. Stenquist K, Sandberg T, Lidin-Janson G, Orskov F, Orskav I, Svanborg-Eden C. "Virulence factors in *Escherichia coli* in urinary isolates from pregnant women":J Infect Dis 1987;156:870.

**CHAPTER 8**

# Preterm Labour, Prelabour Rupture of Membranes and Chorioamnionitis

***Asmita Muthal Rathore***

This chapter will focus mainly on role of infections in preterm labour, premature rupture of membranes (PROM) and chorioamnionitis and thus use of antibiotics in their prevention and management.

## PRETERM LABOUR

Preterm birth is an important cause of perinatal morbidity and mortality. The aetiology of preterm labour is multifactorial with increasing evidence that infection plays a major role in its causation and is thought to be responsible for preterm birth in up to 40 per cent of cases.[1] The earlier in pregnancy that labour occurs, the more likely this results from a pathological signal as infection. The mechanisms by which infection results in preterm labour are many. Endo-and exotoxins released from invading bacteria activate the decidua and foetal membranes to produce cytokines thereby activating local inflammatory reaction or the host response to infection may directly stimulate monocytes and macrophages resulting in phospholipase and PG production. PG release from foetal membranes and decidua stimulates uterine contractions. It is likely that both maternal and foetal signals in response to infection are what initiate preterm labour after silent chorioamnionitis.[2] The infections implicated in aetiology of preterm labour include vaginal infections, urinary tract infections (UTIs) and recently periodontal infections.

### Vaginal Infections in Preterm Labour

The ascending infection from cervix and vagina is most common pathway of intrauterine infection and resulting amniotic infection. Infection may occur early in pregnancy or even before pregnancy and remain asymptomatic and undetected for months until preterm labour or prerupture of membranes (PROM) occurs. Almost all vaginal infections are studied as a potential contributor to preterm labour.

#### *Group B Streptococcus*

Up to 30 per cent pregnant women are colonised with Group B *Streptococcus* (GBS). In mother, it can cause clinical chorioamnionitis, UTI or asymptomatic bacteriuria in pregnancy and endometritis and wound infection after delivery. In neonate, vertical transmission can result in pneumonia, septicaemia and meningitis. However, the association between preterm birth and colonisation is less clear. Klebanoff et al,[3] in placebo-controlled double blind randomized controlled trials (RCT), treated pregnant women with GBS colonisation with erythromycin or placebo for up to 10 weeks. There was no statistically significant benefit for birth weight < 2.5 kg, delivery < 37 weeks or preterm PROM. According to current recommendations (Grade C) issued by RCOG,[4] there is no evidence to support the antenatal treatment of asymptomatic women colonised with GBS.

### *Bacterial Vaginosis*

Bacterial vaginosis (BV) is a syndrome characterised by reduction or elimination of normal lactobacilli and overgrowth of other endogenous organisms. BV has been consistently associated with an increased risk of preterm birth, but it is not known whether it actually causes preterm birth or is only a marker for intrauterine colonisation. BV is associated with increased concentration of elastase, mucinase and sialidase in vagina and certvix and may be a marker for microbial colonization of upper genital tract.[2] In a meta-analysis by Riggs et al,[5] there were 11 studies which evaluated the association between treatment of BV and gestational age < 37 weeks. Eight of these found no significant association and combined odds ratio (OR) of 0.89 [95% confidence interval (CI) 0.66–1.20] was not statistically significant. However, there was significant heterogenecity between studies. In a subgroup analysis, six studies evaluated association between treatment of BV with any antibiotic and preterm birth when the mother had a prior preterm birth. Three of these studies found a significant benefit, one found significant harm, and two found no difference with treatment. The combined OR was 0.61 (95% CI 0.28–1.34), but the results were extremely variable. The antibiotics used in these studies were metronidazole, metronidazole + erythromycin, vaginal clindamycin, oral clindamycin. The US Preventive Task Force[6] notes that current evidence does not support screening and treatment of BV in general population and heterogeneity between studies preclude making definitive recommendation on screening and treating women with a prior preterm birth. Study group recommendations of RCOG[4] state that clinical trials of screening for and treatment of bacterial vaginosis have yielded conflicting results, but treatment may reduce the risk of preterm birth in women with a previous preterm delivery (Grade C recommendation).

### *Other Vaginal Infections*

Genital infections with *Chlamydia trachomatis*, *Ureaplasma urealyticum* and *Trichomonas vaginalis* are also studied for their impact on preterm labour.

*Chlamydia trachomatis* prevalence varies widely in different populations from 5 to 15 percent and has been associated with adverse pregnancy outcomes in several reports. Martin et al[7] studied the effect of treatment of *Chlamydia* on prevention of preterm labour and noted that there was no significant reduction in low birth weight (LBW) (OR 0.74, 95% CI 0.38–1.45) or preterm birth (OR 0.89, 95% CI 0.49–1.62). Although treatment of *Chlamydia* may not prevent preterm birth, there are other reasons to screen and treat this organism. Firstly, there is public health benefit of detection and treatment of this sexually transmitted disease (STD), and treatment during pregnancy may prevent maternal postpartum morbidity as well as transmission to infant at delivery with the attendant morbidity. The RCOG study group[4] recommends adequate chemotherapy and counselling for women with genital chlamydial infection, followed by a test of cure not less than three weeks after end of therapy along with contact tracing and appropriate management of their partners in a genitourinary medicine clinic (Grade C recommendation).

Eschenbach et al[8] treated women colonised with *Ureaplasma urealyticum* and found no significant improvement in LBW (OR 1.36, 95% CI 0.85–2.17) or preterm birth (OR 1.02, 95% CI 0.67-1.54).

Infection with *Trichomonas vaginalis* during pregnancy has been associated with preterm delivery. In Vaginal Infections and Prematurity Study (VIP study),[9] pregnant women colonised with *T. vaginalis* had a 30 per cent higher risk of delivering an infant with LBW or preterm and 40 per cent higher risk of giving birth to an infant who was both preterm and LBW. Two RCTs studied effect of treatment of trichomoniasis to prevent preterm labour. The drugs used for treatment were metronidazole, azithromycin and cefixime. Both studies found an elevated risk of preterm labour in treated group which was significant in one. The combined OR in the 2 trials was 1.71 (95% CI 1.19–2.46).[5] There was no significant heterogenecity in the studies. There is no obvious explanation for this surprising finding, although it has been reported that many isolates of *T. vaginalis* are infected with *M. hominis* which might be released when the parasite is killed. With these results, it is a difficult question to whether treat the infection or not? It would perhaps be reasonable for the physician to explain the evidence to woman, offer the option of treating or delaying treatment until after pregnancy unless symptoms develop and advise condom use.

## Urinary Tract Infections

Asymptomatic bacteriuria and UTI are risk factors for foetal and maternal morbidity including development of pyelonephritis, preterm labour and impaired intrauterine development. The pathophysiology and effect of UTI on pregnancy is dealt with in detail in a separate chapter.

## Periodontal Infections

Periodontal disease appears to be a new potential risk factor for preterm labour. Moderate-to-severe periodontal disease is highly prevalent among pregnant women (much more common than genitourinary infections) with about 15 per cent affected during the first trimester and overall about 25 per cent showing worsening periodontal progression during pregnancy.[10] Periodontal disease creates a significant systemic inflammatory and microbial assault to the host. This is a chronic infection and presents a potential infectious and inflammatory cytokines reservoir and its characteristic haematogenous dissemination may become threat to foetoplacental unit.[10]

Jeffcoate et al[11] conducted prospective study on 1,313 women and found that antenatal maternal periodontitis is an independent risk factor for preterm birth (OR 5.28, 95% CI 2.05–13.6) and very preterm birth (OR 7.07, 95% CI 1.7–27.4). Radnal et al[12] have reported odds ratio of 5.5 at the 95 per cent confidence interval. On multivariate logistic regression analysis, only bleeding on probing and a probing depth of 4 mm or more significantly predicted preterm birth.

Dartbudak O et al[13] conducted a periodontal examination and collection of amniotic fluid at 15 to 20 weeks of pregnancy in 36 women at risk for pregnancy complications. Amniotic fluid bacteria and cytokine levels, vaginal smears and intraoral plaque samples were studied. The odds ratio of preterm delivery and having periodontitis was 20.0 (95% CI: 2.0–201.7, $p < 0.01$). The odds of > 60 colony-forming units (CFU) in subgingival plaque and preterm birth was 32.5:1 (95% CI: 3.0–335.1, $p < 01$). Amniotic interleukin-6 (IL-6) ($r = 0.56$, $p < 0.01$) and prostaglandins $E_2$ ($PGE_2$) ($r = 0.50$, $p < 0.01$) cytokine levels were correlated with CFU from subgingival plaque samples ($r = 0.44$) thus implying that periodontitis can induce a primary host response in the chorioamnion leading to preterm birth.

However, Moore S,[14] in a case-control study to investigate an association between adverse pregnancy outcome and periodontal disease, found no association between the severity of periodontal disease and pregnancy outcome in the UK population.

Though current literature supports a connection between periodontal infection in pregnant women and preterm birth, more studies are needed to determine whether the association is a causal and also if the risk varies in different populations.

## Role of Antibiotics

Antibiotics may be of benefit in management of preterm labour with intact membranes in the following situations:

1. For prevention of preterm labour in women with abnormal genital tract colonisation.
2. To delay delivery in patients who present with preterm labour.
3. Intrapartum prophylaxis for prevention of early onset GBS infection in neonate.

### *For Prevention of Preterm Birth*

As already discussed, studies of prophylactic antibiotics in women with abnormal genital tract colonisation have used different methodologies to diagnose abnormal genital tract colonisation and various antibiotic regimens with conflicting results.

In spite of consistent association between a variety of lower genital tract infections and adverse pregnancy outcome, latest meta-analysis by Riggs et al[5] shows that screening and treatment of vaginal infections in general population of asymptomatic pregnant women does not reduce the rate of preterm birth or LBW. The only exception may be the treatment of BV in those with prior preterm delivery, but definite conclusion is not possible due to heterogeneity in studies.

Kiss H et al[15] conducted multicentre, prospective randomised controlled trial of an infection screening programme to reduce the rate of preterm delivery, to evaluate whether a screening strategy in pregnancy lowers the rate of preterm delivery in a general population of pregnant women. A total of 4,429 pregnant women presenting for their routine prenatal visits early in the second trimester were screened by Gram stain for asymptomatic vaginal infection and women received standard treatment in the intervention group. In the intervention group, the number of preterm births was significantly lower than in the control group (3.0% v 5.3%,

95% CI 1.2–3.6; p = 0.0001). They concluded that integrating a simple infection screening programme into routine antenatal care leads to a significant reduction in preterm births and reduces the rate of late miscarriage in a general population of pregnant women. A latest Cochrane Systematic Review[16] included six randomised controlled trials which recruited 2,184 women to detect the effect of prophylactic antibiotic administration on pregnancy outcomes in the second or third trimester. Antibiotic prophylaxis in unselected pregnant women reduced the risk of PROM (OR 0.32, 95% CI 0.14–0.73). In women with a previous preterm birth, there was a risk reduction in LBW (OR 0.48, 95% CI 0.27–0.84) and postpartum endometritis (OR 0.46, 95% CI 0.24–0.89). There was a risk reduction in preterm delivery (OR 0.48, 95% CI 0.28–0.81) in pregnant women with a previous preterm birth associated with BV during the current pregnancy, but there was no risk reduction in pregnant women with previous preterm birth without BV during pregnancy (OR 1.06, 95% CI 0.68–1.64). However, vaginal antibiotic prophylaxis during pregnancy did not prevent infectious pregnancy outcomes and there is a possibility of adverse effects such as neonatal sepsis (OR 8.07, 95% CI 1.36–47.77).

Debate continues as to the best antibiotics, optimum route of administration, and stage of gestation. Antibiotics like amoxycillin, ampicillin, erythromycin, clindamycin, azithromycin, cefixime, and metronidazole have been studied.[17] Regarding the route of administration, vaginal route seems logical due to 1000-fold increase in intravaginal organisms in BV, but this route may not be effective against organisms already in decidua which may need systemic administration.

The optimal timing and duration of antibiotic therapy is another controversial area. Very early spontaneous preterm labour and preterm birth is more likely to be of infectious aetiology than preterm birth just before term. The earlier in pregnancy at which abnormal genital tract flora is detected, the greater is the risk of an adverse outcome suggesting that whatever damage abnormal flora induces, this is at an early gestation, even if the flora subsequently reverts to normal. It follows, therefore, that if antibiotics are to be of help in preventing spontaneous preterm labour and preterm birth of infectious aetiology, these must be administered early in pregnancy. Antibiotics used prophylactically for the prevention of preterm birth are more likely to be successful, if they are used in women with abnormal genital tract flora [rather than other risk factors for preterm birth, e.g. low body mass index (BMI), twins, previous preterm birth]; they are used early in pregnancy prior to infection (tissue penetration/ inflammation and tissue damage); they are used in women with the greatest degree of abnormal genital tract flora.[18]

### *For Treatment of Preterm Labour*

Subclinical and clinical infection have been implicated in the aetiology of preterm labour. This has led to the suggestion that women with preterm labour should be treated with antibiotics in order to reduce the incidence of preterm birth. Despite the evidence linking intrauterine infection and preterm labour, no consistent benefit has been found between antibiotic treatment and pregnancy prolongation or reduction of perinatal mortality or morbidity in patients with established preterm labour. In a large NICHD-funded multicentre trial in the USA,[19] which compared ampicillin or erythromycin with placebo in women in preterm labour with intact membranes, there was no improvement in latency or maternal or neonatal morbidity with antibiotic treatment. Thus, currently, there is no evidence to support use of antibiotic in women who are in preterm labour without PROM. The latest Cochrane review[20] found that antibiotic treatment in women with preterm labour with intact membranes reduces maternal infection defined as chorioamnionitis or endometritis [Relative risk (RR): 0.74; 95% CI: 0.64–0.87) but has no effect on reduction of preterm birth or adverse neonatal outcomes. The role of antibiotics in women in preterm labour with PROM is discussed later in this chapter.

### *As Intrapartum Chemoprophylaxis for Early Onset GBS Infection in Neonate*

Though the relationship between maternal GBS colonisation and initiation of preterm labour remains uncertain, GBS infection is a leading cause of neonatal sepsis and substantial fraction of neonatal GBS occurs among preterm infants and intrapartum prophylaxis significantly reduces the incidence of early onset GBS infection. The CDC in consultation with the ACOG published revised guidelines[21] which support either risk-based or screening-based approach to select women for intrapartum prophylaxis. According to the risk-based approach, women presenting with preterm labour, who had intrapartum fever > 38°C or had prolonged ROM > 18 hours should receive GBS prophylaxis. The screening-based approach recommended screening of all pregnant women between 35 and 37 weeks of gestation for GBS colonisation and prophylaxis for women who were positive and risk approach for those whose status was not known. All women with invasive GBS disease in past pregnancies must receive prophylaxis irrespective of risk status The screening-based protocol showed 88 per cent reduction in early onset GBS sepsis.[22] The RCOG[4] recommends that all women with a history of having delivered an infant with GBS infection or of PROM, and all women found incidentally to have GBS in the urine or vagina during the current pregnancy should be offered intrapartum chemoprophylaxis.

Intrapartum penicillin 4 hourly given intravenously till delivery is recommended for GBS prophylaxis. For those women who are allergic to penicillin, a combination of clindamycin and erythromycin should be used.

## PRELABOUR RUPTURE OF MEMBRANES

Prelabour rupture of membranes (PROM) is a significant obstetric problem responsible for about one-third of all preterm births and causes important maternal morbidity. It is defined as rupture of membranes (ROM) one or more hours before onset of labour[23] and can be grouped as term PROM and preterm PROM (PPROM). PPROM can be further subdivided into near term (34–36 weeks), remote from term (26–34 weeks) and previable PROM (less than 26 weeks) according to gestational age at ROM which is the most important determinant of neonatal outcome.

## Aetiology

The aetiology of PROM is multifactorial[24] involving infectious, inflammatory and mechanical processes and factors like maternal enzymes, maturational and mechanical forces, chorioamniotic membrane, phospholipids content, etc. and probably foetal signals.

Choriodecidual infections appear to play an important role in aetiology of PROM, especially at early gestational ages; and of all the reasons PROM occurs, bacterial infection is the most likely to result in termination of pregnancy (TOP).[25] The role of infection in PROM is supported by an association with BV and asymptomatic bacteriuria. The mechanical forces like cervical incompetence, polyhydramnios work by exposing membranes to vaginal flora. The probable mechanism includes collagen disruption by bacterial endotoxins and enzymes like bacterial phospholipase, proteases and collagenase. The inflammatory processes may lead to activation of prostaglandin (PG) pathway with direct destruction of foetal membranes. Foetal signals induced by some messenger system is also supposed to contribute to preterm labour mainly by release of amniotic cell cytokines.

Clinical risk factors associated with PROM include low socioeconomic status, cigarette smoking, sexually transmitted infections, prior cervical colonisation, prior preterm delivery, prior preterm labour in current pregnancy, overdistension of uterus, cervical cerclage, amniocentesis, and vaginal bleeding in pregnancy.[26] In many cases, the ultimate cause of PROM is not known.

## Diagnosis

The approach to diagnosis of membrane rupture is clinical. The presence of suspicious history or USG findings followed by demonstration of fluid passage from cervix suggest the diagnosis. Sterile speculum examination can confirm the diagnosis and provide the opportunity to inspect for cervicitis, cervical dilatation and effacement, cord prolapse and to perform appropriate cultures. Demonstration of ferning or nitrazine positivity (due to alkaline pH of amniotic fluid) on pool of fluid is also useful. If initial testing is negative, but clinical suspicion remains, then the patient should be retested after prolonged recumbency. The confirmation of diagnosis in doubtful cases by invasive techniques like USG-guided infusion of indigocarmine, followed by observation for passage of blue fluid per vaginum or amnioscopy is generally not required. Other plausible causes of vaginal discharge like urinary incontinence, vaginitis, cervicitis, mucoid show, semen, and vaginal douches should be excluded.

Until diagnosis of ROM is excluded, digital cervical examination, which is shown to decrease latency and increase infectious morbidity, should be avoided. A single examination also increases the risk substantially.

## Complications of PROM

### *Maternal*

Maternal risks associated with prolonged PROM include mainly the risks due to sepsis. Clinical chorioamnionitis complicates 15 to 20 per cent cases and postpartum infection occurs in up to 12 per cent cases of PPROM.[27] With appropriate antibiotic therapy and expeditious delivery serious maternal complications are rare. The higher risk of refractory labour or abruption also contributes to the morbidity mainly due to interventions needed.

### *Perinatal*

Main foetal concern in PROM is the chorioamnionitis and foetal infection which occurs in a substantial subset of patients. Infection significantly affects latency and thus perinatal outcome. In patients with PROM, median latency with a positive foetal blood culture was 2 days, with a positive amniotic fluid culture was 9 days and with no signs of infection was 41 days.[28] The risk of sepsis is inversely related to gestational age. Prolonged PROM can result in oligohydramnios which if untreated results in oligohydramnios tetrad comprised of pulmonary hypoplasia, peculiar facies, deformities of extremities and growth delay in foetus.

Neonatal implications include risks of prematurity [like respiratory distress syndrome (RDS), intraventricular haemorrhage (IVH), necrotising enterocolitis (NEC)], neonatal sepsis and pulmonary hypoplasia. Long-term complications include cerebral palsy, developmental delay and chronic lung diseases.

## Management of PROM

Appropriate management can be done by gestational age-based approach as gestational age at rupture of membranes and delivery determines the risk of perinatal complications. A central tenet of care of patient with PROM is that pregnancy prolongation should be considered only when significant foetal benefit can be expected, in the absence of significant maternal risk. The risks of conservative management should be considered against the risk of prematurity with immediate delivery after individual assessment of patients for maternal, foetal and neonatal complications. It is important that the patients be well informed regarding the potential for subsequent maternal, foetal and neonatal complications regardless of the management approach.

### *Preterm Prelabour Rupture of Membranes (PPROMs)*

Although practice varies and there is considerable controversy regarding the optimal management of PPROM, there is general consensus regarding some issues. Firstly, gestational age should be established based on clinical history and prior USG assessment where available. Secondly, the woman with PPROM should be evaluated for evidence of advanced labour, chorioamnionitis, abruptio placentae, and foetal compromise and those with these problems are best delivered regardless of gestational age. The women with genital herpes infection and HIV infection should generally not be managed conservatively.

### *PPROM Near Term*

When PPROM occurs at 34 to 36 weeks of gestation, the risk of acute severe morbidity and mortality in neonate is low with expeditious delivery. Conversely, conservative management at 34 to 36 weeks is associated with an increased risk of amnionitis (16% vs 2%, $p = 0.01$), prolonged maternal hospitalisation (5.2 vs 2.6 days, $p = 0.06$) and a lower mean umbilical cord pH at delivery (7.25 vs 7.35, $p = 0.09$) without the benefit of a significant reduction in perinatal complications related to prematurity.[29] Thus, these women are generally best served by expeditious delivery. Corticosteroids and concurrent antibiotics are not necessary if immediate delivery is planned.

### *PPROM Remote from Term (26–34 weeks)*

Delivery before 34 weeks is associated with significant risk of neonatal morbidity and mortality. Hence, when PROM is diagnosed before 34 weeks of pregnancy, expectant management is indicated, if mother and foetus are stable, in the hope of prolonging pregnancy and reduce gestational age-dependent neonatal morbidity. If conservative management is to be persued, the patient should be admitted to the facility capable of providing emergency delivery and undertake intensive maternal and foetal monitoring.

## Adjunctive Therapy in Expectant Management

### *Antibiotics*

The goal of adjunctive antibiotic therapy during conservative management is to treat or prevent ascending decidual infection in order to prolong pregnancy and offer opportunity for reducing neonatal infectious and gestational age-dependent morbidity. The administration of antibiotics after PROM is associated with a delay in delivery and reduction in maternal and neonatal morbidity. Many prospective randomised controlled trials (RCTs) are conducted to evaluate benefit of antibiotics in conservative management of PPROM; and Kenyon et al,[30] in a recent meta-analysis, found that antibiotics were associated with a statistically significant reduction in maternal infection and chorioamnionitis. There also was reduction in number of infants born within 48 hours and 7 days with following morbidities:neonatal infection (RR 0.67. 95% CI 0.52–0.85), positive blood culture (RR 0.75, 95% CI 0.60–0.93), use of surfactant (RR 0.83. 95% CI 0.72–0.96), oxygen therapy (RR 0.88, 95% CI 0.81–0.96), and abnormal cerebral ultrasound scan before discharge from hospital (RR 0.88, 95% CI 0.62–0.99). Perinatal mortality was not significantly reduced (RR 0.91, 95% CI 0.75–1.11). Despite the discontinuation of antibiotics after 7 days, treated women continue to remain pregnant for at up to 3 weeks. The benefit was present both in trials where penicillin and erythromycin were used. Amoxycllin/clauvulanate was associated with a highly significant risk of necrotising enterocolitis (RR 4.60, 95% CI 1.98–10.72) in this study and should be avoided. Antibiotics can used for 5 to 7 days.

### *Antenatal Corticosteroids*

Administration of antenatal corticosteroids to women with preterm labour is the most effective obstetric intervention directed to reduce perinatal morbidity and mortality. In most recent meta-analysis on this issue, Harding et al[31] found corticosteroid administration in setting of PPROM to substantially reduce the risk of RDS (20% vs 35.4%, OR 0.56; CI0.46–0.70), IVH (7.5% vs 15.9%, OR 0.47; CI 0.31–0.70) and NEC (0.8% vs 4.6 %, OR 0.21; CI 0.05–0.82) without significantly increasing the risk of maternal (9.2% vs 5.1%, OR 1.95; CI 0.83-4.59), or neonatal infection (7% vs 6.6%, OR 1.05; CI 0.66-1.68). It is recommended to patients with PPROM in the dose of betamethasone 12 mg intramuscularly (IM) two doses every 24 hours or dexamethasone 6 mg intramuscularly-4 doses every 12 hours along with a course of concurrent antibiotics.

### *Tocolytic Therapy*

There is inadequate data regarding tocolytic therapy in setting of PPROM. Results are at present conflicting with regard to pregnancy prolongation but no benefit is conferred in neonatal outcome. Further research is needed in this area before any recommendations can be made.

## Monitoring in Expectant Management

Intensive maternal and foetal monitoring is necessary for early detection of complications in patients on expectant treatment. Chorioamniotic infection occurs frequently in patients with PROM and a significant part of patient's surveillance is directed at the early recognition of infection.

### *Maternal*

Sepsis is rare but a serious complication of PROM and the woman should be monitored daily for any evidence of sepsis by clinical parameters like pulse rate or uterine tenderness or foul-smelling liquor. Since clinical signs of infection appear late, laboratory parameters like total leucocyte count (TLC) or C-reactive proteins can be useful though they are nonspecific. Cultures should be performed whenever necessary.

### *Foetal*

In PPROM, foetus is at risk of cord compression, abruption and intrauterine infection and early signs of these problem needs to be looked for.

*Clinical monitoring:* It should include recording of foetal movements and foetal heart rate (FHR) daily.

*Biophysical testing* The changes in foetal behaviour during intrauterine infection is thought to be due to different mechanisms like increased concentration of PGs, vasoconstriction of chorionic and umbilical vessels. The simple noninvasive tests of foetal behaviour are found to be useful in monitoring patients of PPROM for infection.

*Non-Stress Test (NST)* The presence of foetal tachycardia has always been used as a marker of intrauterine infection. Intrauterine infection is significantly associated with nonreactive (NR) NST or foetal tachycardia, but the predictive value decreases significantly when the test is performed more than 24 hours from delivery. The NST alone has similar negative predictive value as complete biophysical profile (BPP) in identifying patients at risk for developing maternal or neonatal infection within 24 hours.

### *USG*

1. *Amniotic fluid (AF) volume*: Very low volume of AF volume after PPROM is good predictor of poor outcome.
2. *Foetal BPP:* In patients with intrauterine infection NST is the first test to be affected followed by a decrease in foetal breathing. As more biophysical parameters become compromised, the higher the frequency of infection. There is consistent association between an abnormal NST, absent foetal breathing activity and a low BPP score and

maternal and neonatal infection. To be predictive of intrauterine infection, NST/BPP must be performed on daily basis and predicted value is optimal when the test is conducted within 24 hours of delivery.

### *Previable PROM (less than 26 weeks)*

When PROM occurs before 26 weeks of gestation, the prognosis is guarded. Perinatal mortality is 60 to 90 per cent and 16 per cent of surviving newborns have long-term sequelae. Approximately 50 per cent mothers will have chorioamnionitis, 50 per cent will be delivered by caesarean section and 6.8 per cent will have abruptio.[32] It is associated with higher incidence of maternal infectious morbidity like chorioamnionitis, endometritis and abruptio than in PROM near term and can rarely result in maternal death. The incidence of neonatal complications is also high with higher incidence of stillbirth, pulmonary hypoplasia and skeletal deformities seen. On long-term, it is associated with developmental delay, delayed motor development, cerebral palsy, chronic lung disease, hydrocephalus and mental retardation. The risks and benefits of expectant management with antibiotic therapy compared to TOP should be discussed with the patient including a realistic appraisal of neonatal outcomes and need for obstetric monitoring and neonatal intensive care. Many patients will elect TOP because of significant risk of adverse maternal and neonatal sequelae, which should be performed by suitable methods. Those who opt for, should be treated expectantly in tertiary care hospital. Most of the survivors are patients who extend their latent period for 2 or more weeks. The benefit of amnioinfusion or cervical cerclage in such patients is not established.

### Term PROM

In patients with term PROM, there is no benefit to the foetus by conservative management and general idea should be to deliver the patient as early as safely possible. Two important points should be assessed after confirming the diagnosis—condition of cervix and any evidence of infection. For patients with infection, immediate induction should be done along with therapeutic antibiotics. For patients who do not have any signs of infection, induction or expectant management can be considered. In patients with favourable cervix, labour should be induced with oxytocin. For patients with unfavourable cervix, management plan is less straightforward. Hannah et al[33] conducted a large prospective RCT, comparing intervention versus expectant management and oxytocin versus prostaglandin for induction of labour in term patients with PROM. A total of 5,000 women were assigned to four groups—immediate induction with oxytocin or $PGE_2$ gel, or expectant management followed by induction with oxytocin or $PGE_2$ gel if labour did not ensue within 4 days. The frequency of caesarean section did not differ significantly among these four groups. Women in expectant management-oxytocin group had higher rate of infection than women in induction-oxytocin group. Neonatal infection rates were overall low in all groups, but neonates in induction-oxytocin group were less likely to need antibiotics suspected sepsis than other groups. Women in this study expressed significantly greater preference for induction. Immediate induction of labour with oxytocin was less expensive than either immediate induction with $PGE_2$ gel or expectant management followed by induction after 4 days.[34]

## Management of Labour in PROM

Labour in patients with PROM is at increased risk of prolonged labour, chorioamnionitis, abruptio and foetal distress and thus need careful monitoring with partogram and preferably continuous CTG monitoring. The number of vaginal examinations should be minimised, especially, in latent phase of labour and patients should be observed for earliest warning signs of chorioamnionitis.

GBS prophylaxis is recommended as per local protocol if risk factors are present. Therapeutic broad-spectrum antibiotics (BSA) should be given in case of overt infection. When required, the combination of antibiotics should cover gram-positive, negative and anaerobic organisms.

Newborn baby should be observed for any evidence of sepsis.

*Induction of labour*: Recently, many studies have described the use of prostaglandin preparation in the treatment of patients with PROM and an unfavourable cervix and found all agents to be safe and effective in this clinical setting. However, oxytocin alone seems to be equally effective in PROM. In the RCT by Hannah et al,[33] women in induction-oxytocin group had shorter labours, shorter interval between ROM and delivery than induction-PG group. Thus, induction in patients with PROM is generally done by oxytocin; and if PGs are used, patients should be carfully monitored for hyperstimulation.

## CHORIOAMNIONITIS OR INTRA-AMNIOTIC INFECTION

Chorioamnionitis is an infection of amniotic cavity and foetal membranes. Despite advances in antibiotic therapy, it is associated with increased maternal and neonatal mortality and morbidity. The likely mechanism is by ascending vaginal infection. Though associated with many conditions, most often it is a complication of PPROM. According to the available studies, chorioamnionitis occurs in 3 to 25 per cent[35] of women who have ruptured membranes for more than 24 hours. Preterm and PROM predict 5 to 10-fold increase in incidence of chorioamnionitis as compared to term gestation (20% vs 2%).[36]

### Aetiology

Organisms commonly associated with chorioamnionitis are:

- *Aerobic*
  - Gram-negative: *Escherichia coli*, other gram-negative bacilli
  - Gram-positive: *Streptococcus agalactiae*, *Enterococcus faecalis*, *Staphylococcus aureus*
- *Anaerobic*
  - *Gram-negative*: *Bacteroides fragilis*, *Fusobacterium* species, *Gardnerella vaginalis*
  - *Gram-positive*: *Peptostreptococcus* species, *Peptococcus* species, *Clostridium* species
- Others: *Mycoplasma hominis*, *Ureaplasma urealyticum*.

## Predisposing Factors

The factors increasing the risk of chorioamnionitis are obstetric manipulations, PROM, genital tract colonisation (GBS, BV), meconium-stained amniotic fluid, lowered host resistance like nutritional disorders, drug abuse, HIV infection, drugs like corticosteroids or cancer chemotherapy.

## Complications

### *Maternal*

Immediate complications include death, septic shock (resulting in acute renal failure, coagulopathy, ARDS), septic pelvic thrombo-phlebitis, dystocia, wound infection, puerperal infections, though serious complications are rare with advances in medical treatment. Long-term complications include chronic pelvic infection resulting in increased risk of infertility, ectopic pregnancy and chronic pelvic pain.

### *Foetal*

Perinatal mortality and morbidity like neonatal sepsis, pneumonia, and respiratory distress. Intra-amniotic infection in preterm neonates is associated with higher mortality and morbidity.

## Clinical Features

According to severity, they can be grouped in three groups—those without signs of infection, those with signs of intra-amniotic infections, those with foetal infection. Since the clinical signs of infection appear late, it is important to have a high index of suspicion and make early diagnosis and treatment to improve outcome.

### *Clinical Features of Chorioamnionitis*

Include fever more than 100.4°F or 38°C in the absence of any other obvious cause, maternal and/or foetal tachycardia, uterine tenderness, foul-smelling liquor. Clinical signs of chorioamnionitis are present in only 25 per cent of patients who have histologic chorioamnionitis at delivery.[35]

### *Investigations*

Various laboratory tests can be used for diagnosis.

### *Blood Tests*

*ESR* It is a nonspecific test for systemic inflammation and levels are also elevated during normal pregnancy. The lack of sensitivity limits the clinical usefulness.

*Maternal WBC count* It is a clinical gold standard for systemic infection but is nonspecific. In PPROM, PPV ranged from 40 to 75 per cent and NPV from 52 to 89 per cent. No single cut-off level is determined and though sensitive lacks specificity. Generally, leucocytosis > 15,000 cells/mm$^3$ is considered significant.

*Maternal C-reactive protein* It is a product of hepatic acute phase reaction to infection and is mediated by inflammatory cytokine IL-6. An elevated maternal CRP is associated with infection and neonatal morbidity, but diagnostic performance is poor in most of the studies and not sensitive for clinical use.

### *Amniotic Fluid (AF) Tests*

*AF Gram stain* It is the oldest and most widely used method because of low cost and ready availability. It is used to evaluate for the presence of leucocytes and bacteria. It will not identify *Mycoplasma*. The test has poor sensitivity but good NPV is of value in ruling out infection.

*Cytokines* Placental tissue has been found to produce many inflammatory cytokines in intrauterine infection. Increased levels of AF IL-6 is associated with short latency and neonatal morbidity and mortality. Restricted availability and cost are limiting factors in developing countries.

*Culture* It is the current gold standard for intrauterine infection. The major drawback is prolonged time for culture results. It also does not identify localised infections of decidua, and difficulty in descrimination between true infection and contamination. Repeatedly, it has been found that patients with positive AF culture have short latency and increased risk of maternal and neonatal infection.

Currently, combined use of gram stain and culture is the best method for diagnosis of subclinical chorioamnionitis.[35]

## Management

Once the diagnosis of chorioamnionitis is made, parenteral antibiotics should be started followed by early delivery.

*Antibiotics* Two essential qualities of antibiotic regimen are: the ability to cover organisms associated with intra-amniotic and early neonatal infection and the ability to cross the placenta in quantities sufficient to begin foetal/neonatal therapy. Many different regimes are proposed, but ampicillin along with aminoglycoside like gentamycin is proved to be safe and effective. Anaerobic coverage can be given in cases of suspicion by clindamycin or metronidazole.

[Broad-spectrum antibiotics are to be given by parenteral route till the patient is afebrile for 48 hours after delivery].

Antibiotic regimes for treatment of chorioamnionitis.[35]

*First choice—*

1. Ampicillin 1 gm plus sulbactam 0.5 gm im or iv 6.8 hourly
2. Amoxycillin 1 gm plus clauvulinic acid 0.2 gm im or iv 6-8 hourly
3. Cefuroxime 750 mg or 1.5 gm im or iv 8 hourly
4. Cefazoline 0.5 – 1 gm 6 hourly plus gentamicin 1.5 mg/kg 8 hourly
5. Ampicillin 0.5 – 1 gm 8 hourly plus gentamicin 1.5 1 kg 8 hourly

*Secone choice (based on placental transfer)*

1. Cefixitin 1.2 gm im or iv 6-8 hourly
2. Erythromycin 250–500 mg 6 hourly

*Penicillin allergic—*
1. Cefuroxime 750 mg or 1.5 gm im or iv 6-8 hourly
2. Cefazoline plus gentamicin 1.5 mg/kg hourly
3. Vancomycin 0.5–1 gm 6-12 hourly plus gentamicin 1.5 mg/kg hourly.

*Contraindicated—*
1. Quinilones
2. Chloramphenicol
3. Tetracyclines

Duration of therapy – Broad spectrum antibiotics are to be given by parenteral route till patient is afebrile for 48 hours after delivery.

Though current consensus is for the intrapartum administration of antibiotics when the diagnosis of intra-amniotic infection is made; the results of latest Cochrane review[37] neither support nor refute this, although there was a trend towards improved neonatal outcomes when antibiotics were administered intrapartum. No recommendations can be made on the most appropriate antimicrobial regimen to choose to treat intra-amniotic infection.

*Antenatal corticosteroids:* They are contraindicated in women with chorioamnionitis.

*Obstetric management:* Vaginal delivery is preferred with caesarean being reserved for obstetric indication. Maternal infectious morbidity increases five times when the patient is delivered by caesarean section.

Labour in these patients can be abnormal and should be carefully monitored by partogram and CTG. These patients may require large doses of oxytocin due to ineffective uterine activity. Foetal monitoring may pose problems due to pre-existing foetal tachycardia and attempts should be made to keep maternal temperature normal by antipyretics and hydrotherapy in a hope of reducing foetal tachycardia. The incidence of PPH can also be high and third stage should be managed actively. There are different opinions about the length of time that a patient with PROM and chorioamnionitis may be in labour. These studies are not conclusive and persistence in attempts to obtain a vaginal delivery in these patients may be potentially dangerous.[23]

Caesarean in these patients is associated with increased risk of septic pelvic thrombophlebitis and wound infection and should be covered by appropriate antibiotics.

All these women should be carefully observed for puerperal sepsis.

## Key Points

- Infection is a cause of spontaneous preterm labour in up to 40 per cent of cases.
- Bacterial vaginosis in early pregnancy is significantly associated with preterm labour, PPROM and preterm birth.
- Treatment of BV in women with previous preterm birth may reduce the risk of preterm labour in this pregnancy.
- The earlier in pregnancy the antibiotics are used prophylactically, more likely there is to be benefit.
- Periodontal infection appears to be risk factor for preterm labour and more studies are necessary to establish causal association and benefit of treatment.
- Use of antibiotics in women in preterm labour does not reduce incidence of preterm birth.

- GBS prophylaxis in high-risk cases reduces the incidence of early onset of neonatal disease and should be used as per local protocol.
- PROM is associated with significant maternal and perinatal morbidity.
- Antibiotics given in the second trimester can reduce the risk of PPROM in women at risk.
- Term PROM and PPROM after 34 weeks of pregnancy should be managed by expeditious delivery.
- PPROM between 26 and 34 weeks should be conservatively managed with careful monitoring if there are no contraindications. Antibiotics and corticosteroid are beneficial in these patients.
- Antibiotics given in PPROM delay delivery and may reduce foetomaternal infectious morbidity.
- PPROM before 26 weeks is associated with high maternal and perinatal morbidity and termination of pregnancy should be offered.
- Chorioamnionitis is associated with high maternal and perinatal morbidity.
- Chorioamnionitis should be treated by antibiotics and early delivery.
- For therapeutic use, intravenous antibiotics are most likely to be of most benefit.

## REFERENCES

1. Lettieri L, Vintzileos AM, Rodis JF, et al. Does idiopathic preterm labour resulting in preterm birth exists? Am J Obstet Gynaecol 1993;168:1480-85.
2. Goldenberg RL, Hauth JC, Andrews WC. Intrauterine infection and preterm delivery. N Engl J Med 2000;342:1500-07.
3. Klebanoff MA, Regan JA, Rao AV, et al. Outcome of the vaginal infections and prematurity study: Results of a clinical trial of erythromycin among pregnant women colonized with GBS. Am J Obstet Gynaecol 1995;172:1540-45.
4. RCOG-Study group recommendations. Infection and Pregnancy. June 1,2004-RCOG website-www.rcog.org.uk.
5. Riggs MA, Klebanoff MA. Treatment of vaginal infections to prevent preterm birth: A meta analysis. Clin Obstet Gynaecol 2004;47(4):796-807.
6. Guise JM, Mahon SM, Aickin M, et al. Screening for BV in pregnancy. Am J Prev Med 2001;20:62-72.
7. Martin DH, Eshenbach DA, Cotch FA, et al. Double blind placebo controlled treatment trial of *Chlamydia trachomatis* endocervical infections in pregnant women. Inf Dis Ob Gynaecol 1997;5:10-17.
8. Eshenbach DA, Nugent RP, Rao AV, et al. A randomized placebo controlled trial of erythromycin for treatment of *Ureaplasma urealyticum* to prevent premature delivery. Am J Obstet Gynaecol 1991;164: 734-42.
9. Cotch MF, Pastrek JG 2nd, Nugent RP, et al. *T vaginalis* associated with LBW and preterm delivery. Sex Trans Dis 1997;24:353-60.
10. Offenbacher S. Maternal periodontal infections, prematurity and growth restriction. Clin Obstet Gynaecol 47/ 4:808-21.
11. Jeffcoate MK, Gerus NC, Reddy MS, et al. Periodontal disease and preterm birth: Results of prospective study. J Am Dent Assoc 2001;132:875-80.
12. Radnal M, Gorzo I, Nagy E, Urban E, Novak T, Pal A. A possible association between preterm birth and early periodontitis: Pilot study. Obstet Gynecol Surv 2005 Mar;60(3):150-51.
13. Dortbudak O, Eberhardt R, Ulm M, Persson GR. Periodontitis: A marker of risk in pregnancy for preterm birth. J Clin Periodontol 2005 Jan;32(1):45-52.
14. Moore S, Randhawa M, Ide M. A case-control study to investigate an association between adverse pregnancy outcome and periodontal disease. J Clin Periodontol 2005 Jan;32(1):1-5.
15. Kiss H, Petricevic L, Husslein P. Prospective randomised controlled trial of an infection screening programme to reduce the rate of preterm delivery. BMJ 2004 Aug 14;329(7462):374.
16. Thinkhamrop J, Hofmeyr GJ, Adetoro O, Lumbiganon P. Prophylactic antibiotic administration in pregnancy to prevent infectious morbidity and mortality (Cochrane Review). In: The Reproductive Health Library, Issue 8, 2005. Oxford: Update Software Ltd. Available from http://www.rhlibrary.com. (Reprinted from The Cochrane Library, Issue 4, 2004. Chichester, UK: John Wiley and Sons, Ltd.).
17. Lamont RF, Ruth Mason M, Adinkra PE. Advances in use of antibiotics in prevention of preterm birth. Rec Adv Obstet Gynecol 2001;21:35-44.

18. Lamont RF. Can antibiotics prevent preterm birth—the pro and con debate. BJOG 2005 Mar;112 Suppl 1: 67-73.
19. Romero, Sibai B, Cartitis S, et al. Antibiotic treatment of preterm labour with intact membranes—a multicentre, randomized double blind, placebo controlled trial. Am J Obstet Gynecol 1993;169:764-74.
20. Adewole I. Antibiotics in preterm labour with intact membranes: RHL commentary (last revised: 15 November 2002). The WHO Reproductive Health Library, No 8, Update Software Ltd, Oxford, 2005.
21. American Academy of Paediatrics Committee on Infectious Diseases and Committee on foetus and newborn—Revised guidelines on prevention of early onset GBS infection. Paediatrics 1997;99:489-96.
22. Kubota T. Relationship between maternal GBS colonization and pregnancy outcome. Obstet Gynecol 1998;92:926-30.
23. Arias F. Premature rupture of membranes. In Arias F (Ed): High Risk Pregnancy and Delivery, 2nd Indian edition, Reprint 2002. New Delhi: Mosby Elsevier Publication, 2002; 100-13.
24. Berkowitz KM. Preterm premature rupture of membranes. In Mishell Jr, Goodwin TM, Brenner TF (Eds): Management of Common Problems in Obstetrics and Gynaecology. 4th edn. Oxford: Blackwell Publishing, 2002; 77-78.
25. Polzin W, Brady K. The etiology of premature rupture of membranes. Clini Obstet and Gynaecol 1998,;41(4):810-16.
26. Mercer BM. Preterm premature rupture of membranes. Obstet Gynecol 2003; 101:178-93.
27. Mercer BM. Management of premature rupture of membranes before 26 weeks of gestation. Obstet Gynecol Clinics North Am 1992;19:339-51.
28. Carroll S, Ville Y, Greenough A, et al. Preterm prelabor amniorrhexis; intrauterine infection and interval between membrane rupture and delivery. Arch Dis Child 1995;72:F43-46.
29. Naef RW, Allbert JR, Ross EL, Weber BM, Martin RW, Morrison JC. Premature rupture of membranes at 34-37 weeks of gestation; aggressive versus conservative management: Am J Obstet Gynaecol, 1998;178:126-30.
30. Kenyon S, Boulvain M, Neilson J. Antibiotics for preterm premature rupture of membranes: A systematic review. Obstet Gynecol 2004; 104:1051-57.
31. Harding JE, Pang J, Knight DB, Liggins GC. Do antenatal corticosteroid help in setting of preterm ROM? Am J Obstet Gynaecol 2001;184:131-39.
32. Bengston JM, Van marter LJ, Barss V, et al. Pregnancy outcome after PROM at or before 26 weeks. Obstet Gynecol 1980;73:921-26.
33. Hannah ME, Ohlsson A, Farine D, et al. Induction of labour compared with expectant management for prelabour rupture of membranes at term N Engl J Med 1996;334:1005-10.
34. Gafni A, Goeree R, Myth TL, et al. Induction vs expectant management for prelabour rupture of membranes at term; an economic evaluation. Can Med Assoc J 1997;157:1519-25.
35. Incerpi MH. Chorioamnionitis: Significance and management. In Mishell Jr, Goodwin TM, Brenner PF (Eds): Management of Common Problems in Obstetrics and Gynaecology, 4th edn. Oxford: Blackwell Publishing, 2002;82-84.
36. Greig PC. The diagnosis of intrauterine infection in women with preterm PROM. Clini Obstet and Gynaecol, 1998;41(4):795-808.
37. Hopkins L, Smaill F. Antibiotic régimens for management of intraamniotic infection (Cochrane Review). In: The Reproductive Health Library, Issue 8, 2005. Oxford: Update Software Ltd. Available from http://www.rhlibrary.com. (Reprinted from The Cochrane Library, Issue 4, 2004. Chichester, UK: John Wiley and Sons, Ltd.).

# CHAPTER 9

# Puerperal Sepsis

Poonam Sachdeva, Sumita Mehta, Ruchira Singh

## DEFINITION

Puerperal sepsis is defined as an infection of the genital tract which occurs as a complication of delivery. Puerperal pyrexia is considered to be due to genital tract infection unless proved otherwise.

### Predisposing Factors

1. Malnutrition and anaemia.
2. Low socioeconomic status.
3. Low host resistance.
4. Prolonged rupture of membranes > 18 hours.
5. Chronic debilitating illness.
6. Repeated vaginal examinations.
7. Traumatic operative vaginal delivery.
8. Retained bits of placental tissue and membranes.
9. Caesarean delivery without prophylactic antibiotics.
10. Haemorrhage – Antepartum or postpartum.
11. Application of internal monitoring devices.
12. Diabetes.

### Microbiology

In a great majority of instances, bacteria responsible for pelvic infections are those that normally reside in bowel and also colonize the perineum, vagina and cervix. Usually, multiple species of bacteria are isolated and although typically considered to be of low virulence, they may become pathogenic as a result of haematomas and devitalised tissue.

a. Aerobic gram-positive organisms Group A, B and D streptococcus:
   - β haemolytic streptococci of group A are unusual but cause the most serious type of infection
   - Group B streptococci have been isolated from 7 to 20 per cent of gravid patients. They are significant cause of neonatal deaths due to septicaemia
   - *Staphylococcus aureus*.

b. Aerobic gram-negative bacteria–
   - *E. coli* is the most commonly isolated organism in puerperal period.

- *Klebsciella* sps., Proteus and Enterobacteriaceae
- Gardnerell vaginalis—is found more commonly in younger women.

It is not clear whether these organism are truly pathogenic or they are simply markers of risk factors.

c. Anaerobic bacteria
   - Peptostreptococci and peptococci are the most commonly isolated anaerobes. Necrotic deciduas and retained POC's provide an ideal environment for growth of anaerobes
   - Bacteroides are important because of their role in intraperitoneal abscess formation and their resistance to antibiotics
   - Clostridia—occur in endocervical culture in about 5 per cent of asymptomatic women
   - Fusobacterium

d. Others
   - Mycoplasma (*M. hominis* and *Ureaplasma urealyticum*). Its importance in the postpartum period is supported by the observation of a rise in antibody titre to this organism in women with otherwise unexplained puerperal pyrexia
   - *Chlamydia trachomatis*—has been implicated as a cause of late onset; indolent metritis that may develop in one-third of women who had antepartum chlamydial cervical infection. It is isolated significantly more on from adolescents with postcaesarean metritis as compared with adults. It should be suspected in women whose infants have conjunctivitis or pneumonitis.

## Mode of Infection

a. *Endogenous*: It is caused by organisms present in genital tract before delivery. Anaerobic streptococcus being the predominant pathogen.
b. *Autogenous*: It is due to organism present elsewhere in body (skin, throat) which migrate to genital tract by bloodstream or direct contact.
c. *Exogenous*: The infection is contracted from sources outside the patient (hospital or attendants), group B streptococcus, staphylococcus and *E. coli* are important.

## Clinical Features

1. *Local infection*:
   a. *Wound infection*: Incidence of abdominal incisional infections following caesarean section ranges from 3 to 15 per cent. When prophylactic antibiotics are given, the incidence is less than two per cent.

      Risk factors for wound infections are:
      - Obesity
      - Diabetes
      - Anaemia
      - Poor haemostasis and haematoma formation. Signs and symptoms indude fever, usually on about fourth postoperative day associated with malaise. On local examination, the wound is red and swollen. Pus formation may lead to wound disruption.

b. *Wound dehiscence*: This refers to separation of wound involving the fascial layers which mostly manifests on fifth postoperative day with serosanguinous discharge.

c. *Necrotising fascitis*: This may involve abdominal incisions or may complicate episiotomy or perineal laceration. It is associated with significant tissue necrosis.
   - Risk factors are diabetes mellitus, obesity and hypertension
   - Infection is mainly polymicrobial
   - Clindamycin given along with a β lactam agent is the most effective spectrum.

2. *Uterine Infection*:

It is characterised by–
- Rise in temperature
- Offensive and copious lochial discharge (in severe cases lochia may be scanty or odourless)
- Uterine tenderness and sub-involution

Infection is also associated with increased incidence of secondary postpartum haemorrhage than retained products. Antibiotic therapy is the first line of management, when there is no clear evidence of retained products.

3. *Extrauterine infection*:

a. Parametritis—The onset is usually on 7-10th day of puerperium
   - If cellulitis is extensive it can form an area of induration called phlegmon within the leaves of broad ligament.
   - The spread is usually unilateral. If inflammatory reaction is more intense, cellulitis extends along the base of broad ligament with a tendency of extend to lateral pelvic wall.

Posterior extension may involve the rectovaginal septum, producing a firm mass posterior to cervix.

b. Pelvic peritonitis

May be seen with infections following caesarean delivery when there is uterine incisional necrosis and dehiscence. Rarely, late in course of pelvic cellulites, a parametrial or adnexal abscess may rupture and produce peritonitis. Patient presents with pyrexia and lower abdominal pain. Muscle guarding may be absent. Vaginal examination reveals tenderness in both fornices and with movement of cervix. If infection begins in the uterus and extends into the peritoneum, the treatment in usually medical.

Conversely, peritonitis as a consequence of a bowel lesion or uterine incisional necrosis is usually best treated surgically.

c. Pelvic abscess

A parametrial phlegmon may suppurate and form a fluctuant broad ligament mass that points above the inguinal ligament. These abscess dissect anteriorly and may be amenable to needle drainage. If they dissect posteriorly to rectovaginal septum, surgical drainage is easily done by colpotomy incision.

Patients usually present with swinging temperature, diarrhoea and bulging fluctuant mass felt through the posterior fornix.

They often develop five or more days after delivery.

d. Septic pelvic thrombophlebitis:
   Incidence – 1:3000 deliveries
   *Pathogenesis*: Bacterial infection begins in the placental implantation site or the uterine incision. These infections are associated with myometrial venous thrombosis. The ovarian veins, which drain the upper uterus get involved. Septic phlebitis of left ovarian vein may extend to renal vein. In one-fourth of patients with pelvic thrombosis, clot extends into inferior vena cava.

   Women with septic thrombophlebitis usually experience clinical improvement of pelvic infection following antimicrobial therapy. However, they continue to have hectic fever spikes. They usually don't appear clinically ill and may be asymptomatic except chills. It is also called enigmatic fever. Symptoms include spiking fever with or without pain despite antibiotic therapy. The patient may have tender palpable mass. The diagnosis is by ultrasonography, CT scan or MRI. If there is doubt about diagnosis, a trial of heparin therapy is given. Rapid improvement of symptoms after heparin administration is diagnostic.
e. *Adnexal infections*: Fallopian tubes are involved only with perisalpingitis without subsequent tubal occlusion. Ovarian abscess develops from bacterial invasion through a rent in ovarian capsule. It is usually unilateral and presents 1 to 2 weeks after delivery. Rupture leads to peritonitis which requires surgical exploration.
f. Bacteraemia, Toxic shock syndrome
   - It is an acute febrile illness with severe multisystem derangement. Fatality rate is 10 to 15 per cent.
   - Characterised by fever, headache, mental confusion, diffuse erythematous rash, nausea, vomiting and watery diarrhoea.
   - If may lead to renal failure followed by hepatic failure, DIC and circulatory collapse. This clinical picture is called toxic shock syndrome.
   - *Staphylococcus aureus* has been recovered from almost all affected patients and is due to exotoxin which causes profound endothelial injury.
   - Principal therapy is supportive allowing reversal of capillary endothelial injury. Treatment is similar to that for septic shock.

## Diagnosis

Clinical features of puerperal sepsis will depend on:
- Nature of infecting organisms
- The site of primary infection
- The rapidity and extent of spread.

### *History*

- History of antecedent pregnancy and course of labour should be carefully received.
- Possible risk factor to be noted
- Nature of any prior antibiotics

*Examination*: Examination is done to detect source and location of infection, also to rule out any other cause of pyrexia.

It should include the following:

- Head, neck and spine—look for evidence of anaemia, jaundice and throat infection. Neck stiffness especially if spinal or epidural anaesthesia has been given.
- Breasts—engorgement and inflammation suggestive of any abscess.
- Heart and lungs—valvular disease, Rule out pneumonia or collapse especially if patient has been given inhalational anaesthesia.
- Abdomen—Look for free fluid, liver or spleen enlargement or any other organomegaly
  - Uterine size and tenderness
  - Renal angle tenderness
  - Presence of bowel sounds
  - Signs of peritonitis
- Pelvis—Lochia—colour and unpleasant odour
  - External genitalia—lacerations
  - Bimanual examination of uterus and parametrial tissues to look for
    - > Size of the uterus
    - > Any pelvic abscess
- Limbs—Check for evidence of thrombosis or thrombophlebitis

## Investigations

1. Blood: Haemoglobin estimation total and differential leucocyte count to estimate the efficacy of immune response. Serial counts will map progress of infection.
   Platlet count—low count indicates septicaemia or DIC.
   Thick blood film—for malarial parasite.
   Blood urea and electrolytes—Initial measurement required as renal failure may ensue later.
2. Urine culture—A clean catch midstream urine sample for microscopy and culture sensitivity.
3. High vaginal swabs and endocervical swabs for culture and sensitivity.
   Appropriate culture according to site of infection.
4. Chest radiography:
   - To detect infection or collapse
   - Lung complications may be a result of septic or non-septic embolism
   - Early signs of ARDS in septicaemia can be detected
5. Pelvic ultrasonography
   - To detect any retained bits of POC's and to locate any abscess within pelvis.
   - For collecting samples (pus or fluid) from pelvis for culture and sensitivity.
6. Colour flow Doppler: To diagnose and localize venous thrombosis.
7. CT scan and MRI—To confirm pelvic vein thrombosis or when diagnosis is in doubts.

### *Differential Diagnosis*

1. Breast engorgement—About 15 per cent of delivered women develop fever due to breast engorgement.
   - i. Fever rarely exceeds 39ºC
   - ii. Characteristically lasts no longer than 24 hours
   - iii. Responds to milk expression, hot fomentation and simple analgesics.
2. Respiratory tract infections
   - i. Most often seen within first 24 hours following delivery and almost invariably in women following caesarean delivery.
   - ii. If complicated can lead to atelectasis, aspiration pneumonia and occasionally bacterial pneumonia.
   - iii. Airway obstruction from thick secretions and diminished cough reflex increases the possibility of atelectasis and superimposed infection.
   - iv. Atelectasis is best prevented by routine coughing and deep breathing on a fixed schedule usually every four hours for at least 24 hours following operative delivery.
3. Pyelonephritis (UTI)
   - Bacteriuria, pyuria, costovertebral angle tenderness and spiking temperature indicate renal infection.
   - Risk factors are occult bacteriuria, bladder trauma and catheterisation.
   - Around 1 to 5 per cent of patients with single short-term catheterisation develop bacteriuria, this rises to 50 per cent with repeated catheterisation.
4. Thrombophlebitis
   - Superfical or deep vein thrombosis of legs may cause peurperal pyrexia.
   - Painful swollen leg accompanied by calf tenderness is a pointer towards disease.
   - Doppler confirms the diagnosis.

## Prophylaxis

### *Antenatal*

- Improvement of nutritional status
- Eradication of any septic focus (skin, throat, etc)

### *Intranatal*

- Full surgical asepsis during delivery
- Screening for group B streptococcus in high-risk patients
- Prophylactic use of antibiotics before LSCS.
- Delivery of placenta by controlled cord traction even during
- Caesarean section.

### *Postpartum*

- Aseptic precautions for at least one week following delivery
- Restriction of the number of visitors
- Use of sterilised sanitary pads
- Isolation of infected mother and babies.

## Treatment

1. *General Care*:
   - Adequate fluid and caloric intake must be ensured by intravenous infusion if necessary.
   - Anaemia should be corrected
   - Pain relief with adequate dosage of analgesics
   - An indwelling catheter may be required to relieve any urine retention due to pelvic abscess. It is also helpful in recording the urine output.
   - Record of pulse, respiration, temperature, lochial discharge and fluid intake and output to be maintained.
2. *Antibiotics*:
   a. For endometritis after vaginal delivery – Antibiotics should include good anaerobic coverage (either single agent such as broad spectrum antibiotic coverage such as cephalosporin or a penicillin and β-lactamase inhibitor combinations).
   b. For patients with endometritis after caesarean section
   The response to antibiotics is poorer. Initial therapy should consist of broad spectrum antibiotic with activity against all anaerobes, gram-positive and gram-negative organisms. Most widely used regimen which has 90 to 97 per cent efficacy is clindamycin 900 mg every 8 hours and gentamicin injections 1.5 mg/kg intravenous 12 hourly. Ampicillin is added in sepsis syndrome or suspected enterococcal infection.

   β-lactam antibiotics also have activity against many anaerobic pathogens and their main advantage lies in fewer side effect. The ones commonly used are cephalosporins–cefoxitin, cefatetan and cefotaxime.

   Metronidazole plus ampicillin and aminoglycoside provides coverage against most organisms causing severe pelvic infections.

   Imipenem plus cilastin (which inhibits renal metabolism of imipenem) is reserved for more serious infections.

## Causes of Failure to Response within 48 to 72 Hours of Antibiotic Therapy

a. An infected mass such as abscess or haematoma of the wound or pelvis, extensive pelvic cellulitis, septic pelvic thrombophlebitis.
b. Retained products of conception.
c. A nongenital source of infection such as pyelonephritis, pneumonia or intravenous catheter phlebitis.
d. A non-infectious fever such as drug fever.
e. A resistant organism such as enterococcus in patients treated with cephalosporin like antibiotics.
f. Inadequate route of otherwise correct antibiotic.

It is recommended that parenteral therapy should be continued for 24 to 48 hours after the patient becomes completely afebrile and asymptomatic. Intravenous antibiotics then may be discontinued and the patient discharged without oral antibiotics unless the patient has had staphylococcal bacteriuria.

3. *Surgical Therapy*:

Perineal and abdominal wound

Stitches of perineal wound will have to be removed to facilitate drainage of pus and relieve pain.

After infection is controlled, secondary sutures are applied later.

Antibiotics may need to be changed according to pus culture sensitivity.

Retained uterine products should be evacuated after 24 hours of antibiotic therapy as instrumentation in the presence of active sepsis can cause septicaemia.

Pelvic abscess—drained by colpotomy or percutaneous drainage under ultrasound guidance.

Laparotomy—In unresponsive peritonitis not controlled by conservative means, laparotomy is indicated. Even if no palpable pathology is found, drainage of pus may be effective.

Indications for hysterectomy are:

- Uterine rupture or perforation
- Gangrenous uterus
- Multiple abscess
- Gas gangrene uterus

## Key Points

- Puerperal pyrexia is considered to be due to genital infection until proved otherwise.
- Puerperal sepsis is still a significant cause of maternal morbidity and mortality. The risk factors are malnutrition and anaemia, low Socioeconomic status, low host resistance, prolonged rupture of membranes >18 hr, chronic debilitating illness, repeated vaginal examinations, traumatic operative vaginal delivery, retained bits of placental tissue and membranes, caesarean delivery without prophylactic antibiotics, haemorrhage – Antepartum or postpartum, Application of internal monitoring devices, diabetes.
- Beta haemolytic streptococcus group A is the main cause of Puerperal sepsis and it must be treated vigorously and the patients isolated.
- Prophylactic antibiotics reduces the risk of wound infection in caesarean sections from 3- 15% to < 2 percent so its use is strongly recommended.[4]
- Failure to respond within 48 to 72 hr could be due to pelvic abscess, pelvic thrombophlebitis, retained products of conception, non-genital sources of infections, resistant organisms so timely evaluation will decrease morbidity and mortality of the patients.
- Indications for hysterectomy are infected uterine tissue, multiple abscess or gangrene.
- Metronidazole plus ampicillin and aminoglycoside provides coverage against most organisms causing severe pelvic infections.

## REFERENCES

1. Daftary SN, Chakravarti S. The Puerperium: Holland and Brews manual of obstetrics 15 ed.507–33.
2. Anteby Ey, Yagel S, Hanoch, et al. Puerperal and intrapartum streptococcal infection. Infect Dis Obstet and Gynae 1999;7:276.
3. Blanco JD, Gibbs RS, Malherbe H, et al. A controlled study of genital mycoplasmas in amniotic fluid from patients with intra-amniotic infection. J Infect Diseases 1983;147:650.
4. Steer JP. Puerperal sepsis. Turnbul Obstetrics: 3rd ed. 2001;662-70.
5. Brown CandL, Stettler RW, Twickler D, et al. Puerperal septic thrombophlebitis: Incidence and response to heparin therapy. Am J Obst Gynecol 1991;181:143.

6. Duff P, Gibbs RS. Pelvic vein thrombophlebitis: Diagnostic dilemma and therapeutic challenge. Obst.and Gynecol Surv 1983;38:365.
7. Dunnihoo DR, Gallaspy JW, Wise RB, Otterson WN. Postpartum ovarian vein thrombophlebitis: A review Obst and Gynecol Surv 1991;46-415.
8. Brown CEL, Dunn DH, Harrell R, Setiawan H. Computed tomography for evaluation of Puerperal infection. Surg. Gynecol Obst 1991;172:2.
9. Guerinot GT, Gitomer SD, Sanko SR: Postpartum patients with toxic shock syndrome. Obst Gynecol 1982;72:169.
10. Gilstrap LC III, Cunninghan FG. The bacterial pathogenesis of infections following cesarean section. Obstet Gynecol 1979;53:545.
11. Dinsmoor MJ, Newton ER, Gibbs RS. A randomized double blind placebo controlled trial of oral antibiotic therapy following HIV antibiotic therapy for postpartum endometritis: Obstet Gynecol 1979;134:238.

**CHAPTER 10**

# Septic Abortion and Septic Shock

*Leena Wadhwa, Anjali Tempe*

## SEPTIC ABORTION

A septic abortion is a spontaneous or therapeutic/artificial abortion complicated by a pelvic infection. The condition remains a primary cause of maternal mortality in the developing world, mostly as a result of illegal abortions.[1] Abortion related deaths contribute to 17.6 per cent of all maternal deaths in India. The risk of death from septic abortion rises with the progression of gestation.

### History

Patients with septic abortion usually present with complaints including the following:

- Fever
- Abdominal pain
- Vaginal discharge
- Vaginal bleeding
- History of recent pregnancy

### Physical Examination

- Abdominal examination look for guarding, rebound tenderness and bowel sounds.
- Pelvic examination—assess vaginal discharge, bleeding, cervical motion tenderness, uterine and adnexal tenderness and masses

### Causes

a. Retained products of conception due to incomplete spontaneous or therapeutic abortion.
b. Introduction of infection into the uterus. Pathogens causing septic abortion usually are mixed and derived from normal vaginal flora and sexually transmitted bacteria. These organisms includes the following:
   *Escherichia coli* and other aerobic, enteric, gram-negative rods, Group B beta-haemolytic *Streptococcus*, *Staphylococcus* *Bacteroides* species, *Neisseria gonorrhoeae*, *Chlamydia trachomatis*, *Clostridium perfringes*, *Mycoplasma hominis* and *Haemophilus influenzae*.

### D/D

1. Appendicitis, acute

2. Pelvic inflammatory disease
3. Pregnancy, ectopic
4. Pregnancy, trauma
5. Pregnancy, urinary tract infections
6. Shock, septic
7. Urinary tract infection
8. Vaginitis/vulvovaginitis

## Lab Testing

- Complete blood count, ESR
- Electrolytes, glucose, BUN and creatinine
- Blood type and screen
- Endocervical cultures (e.g. aerobic, anaerobic, gonorrhoeal chlamydial) and Gram stain.
- Blood cultures

## Imaging Studies

1. Ultrasound to rule out retained products of conception, adnexal masses and free fluid in the cul-de-sac.
2. Both supine and upright radiographs of the abdomen assist in detection of free air or foreign bodies.

## Management

- Monitor vital signs
- Administer IV fluids
- Administer oxygen
- Perform evacuation of retained tissues from the uterine cavity after stabilizing the patient under broad-spectrum antibiotic coverage
- Laparotomy may be needed if above measures elicit no response

### *Indications for Exploratory Laparotomy in Cases of Infected Abortion*

1. Failure to respond to curettage and appropriate medical therapy
2. Perforation and infection with suspected bowel injury
3. Pelvic or adnexal abscess
4. Poor response to vigorous medical therapy and debridement techniques
5. Gas gangrene (clostridial necrotizing myometritis)
   - Because of the likelihood of multiple organisms and bacteraemia in septic abortion, broad-spectrum antibiotic therapy is started. Once sensitivities are known the use of antibiotic monotherapy is recommended.

*Antibiotics commonly used are:*

1. Doxycycline: 100 mg IV 12 hourly with cephalosporin IV for atleast 48 hr followed by 100 mg BD × 10-14 d

Effective against gram-negative, gram-positive organisms and *Rickettsia*, *Chlamydia* and *Mycoplasma*.

2. Cephalosporins (e.g. Cefotaxime, ceftriaxone): 1-2 gm IV BD
   Effective against gram-negative, *Pseudomonas*.
3. *Gentamicin:* 1-1.5 mg/kg IV BD
   Aminoglycoside antibiotic for gram-negative coverage.
4. *Imipenem and Cilastatin (Primaxin):* 250-500 mg IV 6 hourly,
   Wide spectrum coverage.
5. *Ampicillin and sulbactam (Unasyn):* 1.5 to 3 gm IV 6-8 hourly
   Covers skin, enteric flora and anaerobes.
6. *Metronidazole:* 15 mg/kg IV over 1 hr followed by 7.5 mg/kg IV over 1 hr 6-8 hourly.

*For anaerobic coverage.*

7. Ciprofloxacin: 400 mg IV 12 hourly
   Activity against streptococci, and *S. epidermidis* and against gram-negative organisms.
8. Piperacillin and Tazobactam Sodium (zosyn) (Antipseudomonal penicillin plus beta-lactamase inhibitor): 12 gm piperacillin/1.5 gm tazobactam × 7-10 days IV in divided doses.
9. Ticarcillin and clavualanate (Timentin) (Antipseudomonal penicillin plus beta-lactamase inhibitor): 3.1 gm IV (4-6) hourly.

Coverage against most gram-positive and gram-negative organisms and most anaerobes. The agents selected should be based on following considerations.

a. The likely pathogens at the probable site of infection.
b. Recent antibiotic use.
c. The patterns of antimicrobial resistance within the hospital and community.

- When the uterus is too large for an operator to undertake suction curettage, high dose oxytocin administration often is successful.
- Use of prostaglandin E2 suppositories is contraindicated in the presence of sepsis because it causes fever. 15-methyl prostaglandin F2-alpha (carboprost tromethamine) 250 microgram intramuscularly can be used every 3 to 4 hours. A large Foley catheter (50 ml balloon) may be placed in the lower uterus as an alternative method.[2]

## Prevention

- Contraception to prevent unwanted pregnancies
- Safe and legal abortion
- Early access to prenatal care
- Prompt diagnosis of septic abortion
- Timely treatment with IV antibiotics
- Prompt evacuation of retained tissues from the uterus

## Complications

- Pelvic inflammatory disease

- Reproductive potential after an infected abortion may be compromised by Asherman's syndrome, pelvic adhesions or incompetent cervix
- Peritonitis
- Haemorrhage
- Sepsis
- Septic shock
- Inferior vena cava thrombosis.

## Medical/Legal Pitfalls

- Failure to obtain information about recent termination of pregnancy may lead to a wrong diagnosis or delayed/inappropriate treatment
- Failure to promptly administer broad-spectrum antibiotic therapy may result in complications including sepsis and septic shock
- Failure to evaluate retained products of conception from the uterus leads to treatment failure and possible complications.
- Failure to diagnose uterus perforation may lead to litigation
- Failure to diagnose bowel injury may lead to litigation.

## SEPTIC SHOCK

Septic shock is the most common cause of mortality in the intensive care unit. Despite aggressive treatment mortality ranges from 15 per cent in patients with sepsis to 40-60 per cent in patients with septic shock. Infections that most commonly cause bacteraemia and septicaemic shock in obstetrical patients are antepartum pyelonephritis, chorioamnionitis and puerperal sepsis, septic abortion and necrotising fasciitis.[3] Most commonly bacteria that cause shock are from members of the endotoxin producing enterobacteriaceae family especially *E.coli*. Pathogens that less often cause shock are aerobic and anaerobic streptococci and *Bacteroides* and *Clostridium* species. Group A beta-haemolytic streptococci as well as *Staphylococcus aureus* produce virulent exotoxins that cause all features of the sepsis syndrome. In pyelonephritis, *E.coli* and *Klebsiella* species most likely cause bacteraemia or septicaemia.[4]

## CLINICAL FEATURES

There is a continuum of clinical manifestations from systemic inflammatory response syndrome (SIRS) to sepsis to severe sepsis to septic shock to multiple organ dysfunction syndrome (MODS).

## CONSENSUS CONFERENCE DEFINITIONS

Data from the American college of chest physicians:Society of critical care medicine consensus conference.[5]

**A: Systemic inflammatory response syndrome (SIRS):**
Two or more of the following clinical signs of systemic response to endothelial inflammation:

Temperature > 38°C or < 36°C

Elevated heart rate > 90 beats/min

Tachypnoea R/R > 20 breaths/min or hyperventilation ($PaCO_2$ < 32 mmHg)

Altered white blood cell count > 12.0 cells × $10^9$/L or < 4.0 cells × $10^9$/L or

Presence of > 10 per cent immature neutrophils (Bands)

**B: Sepsis:** SIRS plus a documented infection site (documented by positive culture for organisms from that site). Blood cultures do NOT need to be positive.

**C: Severe sepsis:** Sepsis associated with organ dysfunction, hypoperfusion abnormalities, or hypotension. Hypoperfusion abnormalities include but are not limited to:
1. Lactic acidosis
2. Oliguria
3. Or an acute alteration in mental status.

**D: Septic shock:** Sepsis induced hypotension despite fluid resuscitation plus hypoperfusion abnormalities.

Organ dysfunctions associated with severe sepsis and septic shock:

*Lungs:* A common and serious consequence of sepsis is adult respiratory distress syndrome (ARDS). Early fall in arterial $PO_2$, tachypnoea, hyperpnoea.

*Kidneys:* (Acute renal failure): oliguria, anuria, azotaemia, proteinuria

*Liver:* Elevated levels of serum bilirubin, alkaline phosphatase, cholestatic jaundice

*Digestive tract:* Nausea, vomiting, diarrhoea and ileus

*Skin:* Moist, cold, or clammy

*Heart:* The key target organ in sepsis is the heart; mediated through myocardial depressant factor, cardiac output is initially normal or elevated. As shock worsens, cardiac output decreases and severe vasoconstriction ensues leading to hypotension and further cardiac dysfunction.

*Brain:* Confusion,coma

*Hypothalamus:* Fever, hypothermia

*Haematological:*Thrombocytopenia, leucocytosis, consumptive coagulopathy

*Multiple organ dysfunction syndrome (MODS):* Presence of altered organ function in an acutely ill patient such that homeostasis cannot be maintained without intervention.

**Pathophysiologic events in septic shock:**
- Infection becomes established
- Organisms proliferate
- Toxins are released
- Toxins activate monocytes or macrophages

- Cytokines are released (tumor necrosis factor (TNF) and Interluekin-1 (IL-1)
- System activation occurs
- Organ dysfunction develops
- Shock develops
- Refractory hypotension, multiorgan system failure, and death or recovery evolve

## PATHOGENESIS OF SEPTIC SHOCK

Sepsis is caused by an inflammatory response to a trigger—most often microbial endotoxins (released upon lysis of cell wall of gram-negative bacteria) and exotoxins. (e.g. *Pseudomonas aeruginosa*, toxic shock syndrome—*Staphylococcus aureus*). These and other toxins stimulate inflammatory cytokine production by vascular endothelium (Fig. 10.1).

Cytokines play key mediating role in sepsis, with tumor necrosis factor alpha (TNF-alpha) and interleukin-1-(IL-1) and 8 being central mediators in the cascade. Cytokines also

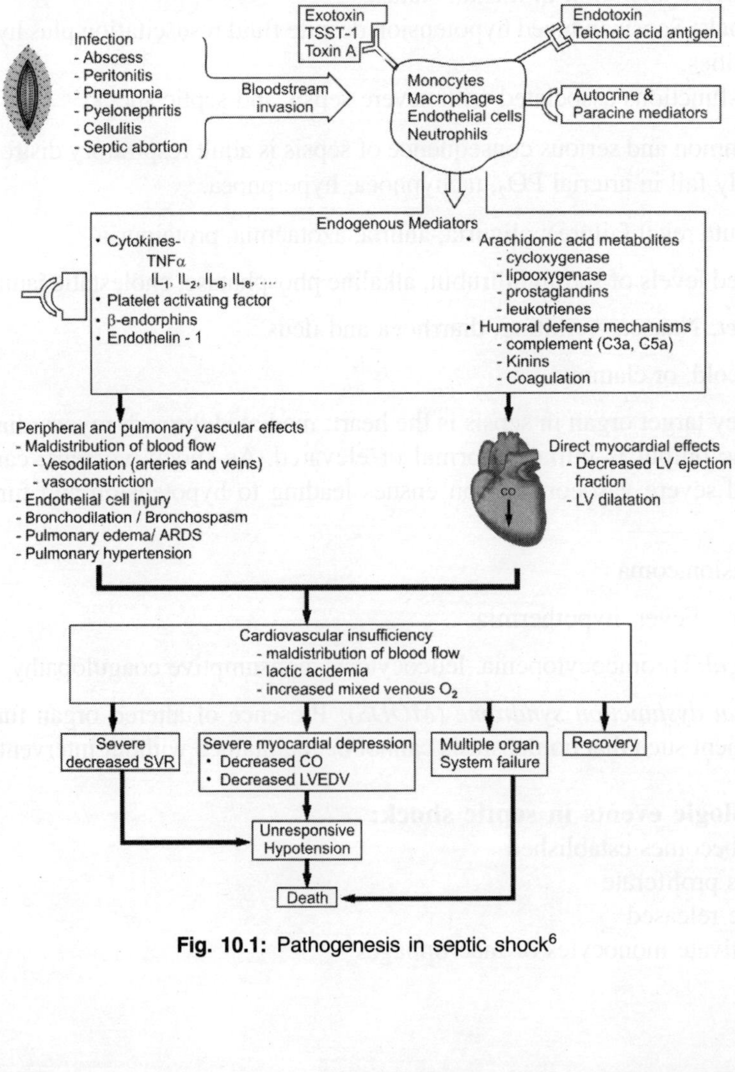


**Fig. 10.1:** Pathogenesis in septic shock[6]

play an essential role in the defense against infection, such as by up-regulating the cytolytic activity of lymphocytes and the expression of complement receptors; activating macrophages, enhancing the oxidative burst of leucocytes and stimulating B-cell and T-cell proliferation.

## Haemodynamic Changes in Septic Shock

If circulating volume is initially restored, then septic shock can be characterised as a high cardiac output, low systemic vascular resistance condition (warm phase of septic shock). If hypotension is not corrected following vigorous fluid infusion, prognosis is guarded. Oliguria and continued peripheral vasoconstriction characterise a secondary, cold phase of septic shock, from which survival is uncommon.

Differential Diagnosis

- Hypovolaemic shock
- Less common are—
  - Acute pulmonary embolus
  - Amniotic fluid embolus
  - Cardiogenic shock
  - Cardiac tamponade
  - Dissection of aorta
  - Haemorrhagic pancreatitis
  - Diabetic ketoacidosis

## Laboratory Data

Respiratory alkalosis signals impending shock that is reversible with fluid resuscitation. Metabolic acidosis can develop just prior to hypotension or can occur at the same time. Treatment should be instituted before metabolic acidosis beings.

Lab tests include CBC with differential count, C-reactive protein, urine analysis, coagulation profile, glucose, blood urea nitrogen, creatinine, electrolyes, liver function tests, lactic acid level, arterial blood gas, electrocardiogram, and a chest X-ray.

Cultures of blood, sputum, urine and other obviously infected sites should be performed.

Atleast 2 sets of blood cultures should be obtained over a 24-hour period. Depending on the patient's clinical status and associated risk, other studies could include abdominal X-ray, CAT scans, MRI, 2D echocardiograms, and/or lumbar puncture.

At the onset of septic shock, the leucocyte count may be significantly reduced, and the polymorphonuclear leucocytes (PMNs) may be as low as 20 per cent. This is associated with a sharp decrease in platelet count to <= 50,000/µL. However, this situation rapidly reverses within 1 to 4 h, and a significant increase in both the total WBC count and PMNs (to > 80% with a predominance of juvenile forms) usually occurs. Urinalysis may disclose that the urinary tract is the source of infection, particularly in patients who have indwelling catheters.

In early stage of septic shock, the patient may have a transient respiratory alkalosis due to endotoxin-induced hyperventilation, but it is quickly superseded by severe metabolic acidosis manifested by decreased arterial pH, serum bicarbonate and arterial $PO_2$, and increased arterial $PCO_2$.[7] Early respiratory failure leads to hypoxaemia with $PO_2 < 70$ mm Hg. The ECG may show depressed ST segments with T-wave inversions and occasionally atrial and ventricular arrhythmias. The BUN and creatinine concentrations usually increase progressively as a result of renal failure with decreased creatinine clearance.

## Management of Overt Shock

*Restore ORDER*

**O:** Provide adequate oxygen delivery
**R:** Restore circulating volume (crystalloid and blood volume replacement)
**D:** Drug therapy (Pharmacologic support of blood pressure, antibiotics, miscellaneous agents)
**E:** Evaluate response to therapy
**R:** Remedy the underlying cause.

## General Guidelines for Managing Shock[6]

The goals to be achieved are:

| | |
|---|---|
| Cardiovascular/haemodynamic | |
| Blood pressure | Systemic blood pressure > 90 mmHg; mean arterial pressure ≥ 60 mmHg |
| Pulmonary capillary wedge pressure | 14-18 mmHg |
| Central venous pressure (CVP) | 12-15 cm $H_2O$ |
| Oxygen delivery | Haemoglobin > 10 gm/dl<br>Oxygen saturation > 92%<br>Cardiac index<br>> 4.0L/min/$m^2$ (septic shock)<br>> 2.2L/min/$m^2$ (other shock states) |
| Pulmonary blood gases | Normalise alveolar- arterial gradient |
| Blood gases | Maintain<br>$PaO_2$ 80-100 mmHg<br>$PaCO_2$ 30-35 mmHg<br>PH>7.35 |
| Renal | Urine output > 20-30 ml/hr<br>Normalise blood urea nitrogen, creatinine |
| Hepatic | Bilirubin < 3 mg/dl |
| Mental status | Orientation |
| Coagulation studies | Normalise |
| Serum lactate level | < 2.32 micro mol/g |

## THERAPY

### Three Priorities

1. Immediate stabilisation of the patient. The immediate concern for patient with severe sepsis is reversal of life-threatening abnormalities (ABC: airway, breathing, circulation). Altered mental status or depressed level of consciousness secondary to sepsis may require immediate protection of the patient's airway. Intubation may also be necessary to deliver higher oxygen concentrations. Circulation may be compromised and significant decreases in blood pressure may require aggressive combined empiric therapy with fluids (with crystalloids or colloids)[8] and ionotropes/vasopressors (dopamine, dobutamine, phenylephrine, epinephrine or norepinephrine). Usual dose range of dopamine and dobutamine is 2-10 microgram/kg/min.[9] In severe sepsis monitoring of circulation is necessary (refer to guidelines for managing shock). Patients with severe sepsis should be in ICU. Their vitals signs (blood pressure, heart rate, respiratory rate and temperature) should be monitored. Maintain adequate cardiac output and ventilation with drugs. Consider dialysis to assist kidney function. Maintain arterial blood pressure in hypotensive patients with vasoactive drugs.
2. The blood must be rapidly cleared of microorganisms. Certain antimicrobial agents may cause the patients to get worse. It is believed that certain antimicrobials cause more lipopolysaccharide (LPS) to be released causing more problems for the patient. Antimicrobials that are beneficial are: Carbapenems, ceftriaxone, cefepime, glycopeptides, aminoglycosides, and quinolones. Prompt institution of empiric treatment with antimicrobials is essential. The early institution of antimicrobials has been shown to decrease the development of shock and to lower the mortality rate. After the appropriate samples are obtained from the patient a regimen of antimicrobials with broad spectrum of activity is needed.

The drugs used depend on source of sepsis (Dosages already mentioned in section of septic abortion):

1. *Community acquired pneumonia:* A 2-drug regimen is usually utilized. Usually a third (ceftriaxone) or fourth (cefepime) generation cephalosporin is given with an aminoglycoside (usually gentamicin).
2. *Nosocomial pneumonia:* Cefipime or Imipenem-cilastatin and an aminoglycoside.
3. *Abdominal infection:* Imipenem-cilastatin or pipercillin-tazobactam and aminoglycoside.
4. *Nosocomial abdominal infection:* Imipenem—cilastatin and aminoglycoside or pepercillin-tazobactam and Amphotericin-B.
5. *Skin/soft tissue:* Vancomycin and imipenem-cilastatin or piperacillin-tazobactam.
6. Nosocomial skin/soft tissue: vancomycin and cefipime.
7. *Urinary tract infection:* Ciprofloxacin and aminoglycoside.
8. *Nosocomial urinary tract infection:* Vanocomycin and cefipime.
9. *CNS infection:* Vancomycin and third generation cephalosporin or Meropenem.
10. *Nosocomial CNS infection:* Meropenem and vancomycin

(Drugs will change with time) Empiric broad-spectrum antibiotic should be replaced with specific therapy as soon as possible because of the significant adverse effects associated with long-term, broad-spectrum therapy, including disruption of normal gut mucosal barrier that increases the risk for opportunistic infection and pseudomembranous colitis.

## Other Therapy

- Use of antacid or $H_2$-blockers to prevent stress induced bleeding
- *Streroid use:* Limited, no improvemet demonstrated in overall survival of patients with severe septic shock.[10]
- *Intralipid therapy:* Judicious use in neutropenic and immunosuppressed patients because of its depressive effects on mononuclear and polymorphonuclear monocytes.
- *Amino acid therapy:* 1-1.5 g/kg is sufficient.
- *Oral, enteric or parenteral nutritional support:* Should be based on lab assessment of pre-existing nutritional status (albumin, transferrin, thyroxine-binding pre-albumin, somatomedin-C). The usual rule is to provide 25-35 kcal/kg/day fairly equally distributed between fat and carbohydrate.

3. The original focus of infection must be treated. Remove foreign bodies. Drain purulent exudates, particularly for anaerobic infections. Remove infected organs; debride or amputate gangrenous tissue. Hysterectomy is seldom indicated unless the uterus has been lacerated or is obviously intensely infected.

   (Any woman with a puerperal infection who is suspected of developing peritonitis should be carefully evaluated for uterine incisional necrosis and separation or for bowel perforation).

## New Drug in Treating Severe Sepsis

Recombinant human activated protein C (Xigris) is the first agent approved by the FDA effective in the treatment of severe sepsis proven to reduce mortality. It is a potent agent for the:

1. Suppression of inflammation
2. Prevention of microvascular coagulation
3. Reversal of impaired fibrinolysis

## S/E

Patients treated with this protein are at an increased risk of bleeding. The risk is highest during infusion of the protein.

## Complications of Septic Shock

1. Adult respiratory distress syndrome (ARDS)
2. Disseminated intravascular coagulation (DIC)
3. Acute renal failure (ARF)
4. Intestinal bleeding
5. Liver failure

6. Central nervous system dysfunction
7. Heart failure
8. Death

The management of patients with septic shock remains a challenge. However, with early recognition, prompt intervention, and continued aggressive surveillance, a satisfactory outcome can be achieved.

## Key Points

- Gram-negative microbes are by for the greatest offending organisms in obstetrics and gynaecology accounting for 75-80 per cent of all septic episodes of these *E. coli* is responsible for approximately 50 per cent of all cases.
- Progression from SIRS to septic shock can be slowed or prevented with aggressive fluid therapy, antibiotic administration and surgical drainage or excision of infected tissue.
- In septic shock, antibiotic agents should be given at maximum doses with dose modification for impaired renal function.
- Acceptable regimens include an extended spectrum penicillin or third generation cephalosporin combined with on aminoglycoside.
- End organ failure is a major contributor to mortality in sepsis and septic shock. The major complications are ARDS, DIC and ARF.

## REFERENCES


1. Rana A, Pradhan N, Gurung H, Singh M. Induced Septic abortion: A major factor in maternal mortality and morbidity. J Obstet Gynaecol Res 2004; 30(1):3-8.
2. Stubblefield PG, Grimes DA. Septic abortion. N Engl J Med 1994; 331(5):310-14.
3. Mabic WC, Barton JR, Sibai B. Septic shock in pregnancy. Obstetrics and Gynecology 1997;90:553-61.
4. Williams's Obstetrics, 21st edition Critical care and trauma: pg.1167-71.
5. ACCP. American college of chest physicians/society of critical care medicine consensus confer definitions for sepsis and organ failure and guidelines for the use and innovative therapies in sepsis. Int Care Med 1992;8:64-74.
6. Harriet O'Smith, Audrey A Romero. Shock in the gynecologic patient. Telinde's operative gynecology 9th edition: 209-32.
7. Richard L. Sweet, Ronald S.Gibbs. Post abortion infection, bacteremia and septic shock. Infectious diseases of the female genital tract 4th edition: 355-67.
8. Schierhout G, Roberts I. Fluid resuscitation with colloid or crystalloid solutions in critically ill patients: A systematic review of randomized trials. BMJ 1998; 316(7136):961-64.
9. Arthur P. Wheeler, Gordon R. Bernard. Treating patients with severe sepsis. N Engl J Med 1999;340(3):207-14.
10. Cronin L, Cook DJ, Carlet J, et al. Corticosteroid treatment for sepsis a critical appraisal and meta-analysis of the literature. Crit Care Med 1995;23(18):1430-39.

**CHAPTER 11**

# Sexually Transmitted Infections: Genital Ulcer-Adenopathy Syndrome

***Shakun Tyagi***

Most young, sexually active patients who have genital ulcers either have genital herpes, syphilis, or chancroid. The relative frequency of each differs by geographic area and client population; however, genital herpes is the most prevalent of these diseases. A high prevalence rate of 40 per cent positivity of HSV-2 antibodies in Indian patients with genital ulcers has been reported.[1] More than one of these diseases sometimes is present in a patient who has genital ulcers. Each disease has been associated with an increased risk for HIV infection. The prevalence of HIV varies from 10-65 per cent in patients with genital ulcer. Not all genital ulcers are caused by sexually transmitted infections and diagnosis based only on the patient's medical history and physical examination is often inaccurate. Therefore, evaluation of all patients who have genital ulcers should include a serologic test for syphilis and a diagnostic evaluation for genital herpes if facilities are available. In settings where chancroid, Lymphogranuloma venereum(LGV) or Granuloma inguinale is prevalent specific diagnostic tests are warranted. Health care providers often must treat patients before test results are available because early treatment decreases the possibility of ongoing transmission and because successful treatment of genital herpes depends upon prompt initiation of therapy. In this situation, the clinician should treat for the diagnosis considered most likely on the basis of clinical presentation and epidemiological circumstances. Sometimes treatment must be initiated for additional conditions because of diagnostic uncertainty.

## GENITAL HERPES SIMPLEX VIRUS INFECTION

Genital herpes is caused usually by Herpes simplex virus type-2 (HSV-2) and less commonly by type 1. The incidence of genital herpes is on the rise in most of the countries and in many countries it has become the most common cause of genital ulceration. Most persons infected with HSV-2 have mild or unrecognised infections but shed virus intermittently in the genital tract. Most genital herpes infections are transmitted by persons unaware that they have the infection or who are asymptomatic when transmission occurs.

### Clinical Features

#### *Primary Genital Herpes*

It is characterised by bilaterally distributed multiple lesions, moderate to severe local pain, dysuria, urethral or vaginal discharge, vulval irritation, perianal, or vulval fissures, sacral paraesthesia, tender inguinal lymphadenopathy and systemic symptoms. Lesions appear 3-14 days after exposure. Systemic symptoms occur early in the course of disease, they begin after a mean incubation period of 6-8 days, peak within 4 days of onset of lesions and gradually abate over the subsequent 3-4 days. About 40 per cent of men and 70 per cent of women experience constitutional symptoms during primary disease. Headache, fever, myalgias, lethargy, backache and photophobia are most frequent complaints.

The first lesions are small grouped painful vesicles or pustules on an erythematous base, which break and form ulcers in 2-4 days. New groups of lesions may appear during the second week. In the third week crust appears on the lesions and the process of re-epithelisation begins. Tender inguinal lymphadenopathy appears during the second and third week and persists for long. Inguinal and femoral lymph nodes are tender, firm and non-fluctuant. About 88 per cent of women with primary genital HSV-2 infection have cervicitis, although HSV cervicitis may be a sole manifestation of the first episode in about 8 per cent of women. The mean time from onset of lesions to complete healing is longer in women by about 20 days than in men (16.5 days). Rarely, first-episode genital herpes is manifested by severe disease that may require hospitalisation.

*First episode non-primary genital herpes*: More than 40 per cent of patients who present with the first clinical episode of Genital herpes have pre-existing antibodies to the heterologous (type-1) herpes virus. These episodes are referred to as first episode non-primary and usually are due to HSV-2 infection in an individual with HSV-1 antibodies. The patients with post primary first episode have lower frequency of systemic symptoms, shorter duration of pain, fewer lesions and shorter healing compared with the true primary infections. Constitutional symptoms are less common. Lesions are not widely distributed, the mean number of days with pain, healing time and viral shedding is about 4 days less than in true primary disease.

### *Recurrent Genital Herpes*

Genital herpes cause by HSV-2 is recurrent in 90 per cent or more of those infected and 88 per cent have at least one recurrence during 12 months after the initial episode. Emotional stress, sunlight, concurrent infection and menstruation can trigger recurrences. Lesions of recurrent genital herpes are less in number, duration of lesions is less and may be unilateral.

## Diagnosis of HSV Infection

The clinical diagnosis of genital herpes is both insensitive and nonspecific. The typical painful multiple vesicular or ulcerative lesions are absent in many infected persons. Up to 30 per cent of first-episode cases of genital herpes are caused by HSV-1, but recurrences are much less frequent for genital HSV-1 infection than genital HSV-2 infection. Therefore, the distinction between HSV serotypes influences prognosis and counselling. For these reasons, the clinical diagnosis of genital herpes should be confirmed by laboratory testing. Both virologic tests and type-specific serologic tests for HSV should be available in clinical settings that provide care for patients with STDs or those at risk for STDs.

## Virologic Tests

- Isolation of HSV in cell culture is the preferred virologic test in patients who present with genital ulcers or other mucocutaneous lesions. Tissue culture for HSV often is positive within 48 hours of inoculation. Characteristic cytopathic effect with ballooning of cells and cell death are observed, and death of the entire monolayer of cells may be rapid. Immunofluorescent staining of the tissue culture cells can quickly identify HSV and can distinguish between types 1 and 2. The sensitivity of culture declines rapidly as lesions begin to heal, usually within a few days of onset.
- Polymerase chain reaction (PCR) assays for HSV DNA are highly sensitive, but their role in the diagnosis of genital ulcer disease has not been well defined. However, PCR is available in some laboratories and is the test of choice for detecting HSV in spinal fluid for diagnosis of HSV-infection of the nervous system (CNS).
- Tzanck preparation is a time-honored procedure to assist in the diagnosis of cutaneous herpes virus infections. A positive result is the finding of multinucleate giant cells in smears prepared from the base of the ulcer and stained with Giemsa or Papanicolaou smear stain.

## Type-Specific Serologic Tests

Both type-specific and nonspecific antibodies to HSV develop during the first several weeks following infection and persist indefinitely. Because almost all HSV-2 infections are sexually acquired, type-specific HSV-2 antibody indicates anogenital infection, but the presence of HSV-1 antibody does not distinguish anogenital from orolabial infection.

## Principles of Management of Genital Herpes

Antiviral chemotherapy offers clinical benefits to most symptomatic patients and is the mainstay of management. In addition, counselling regarding the natural history of genital herpes, sexual and perinatal transmission, and methods to reduce transmission is integral to clinical management. Systemic antiviral drugs partially control the symptoms and signs of herpes episodes when used to treat first clinical episodes and recurrent episodes or when used as daily suppressive therapy. However, these drugs neither eradicate latent virus nor affect the risk, frequency, or severity of recurrences after the drug is discontinued. Randomized trials indicate that three antiviral medications provide clinical benefit for genital herpes: acyclovir, valacyclovir, and famciclovir.[2-11] Topical therapy with antiviral drugs offers minimal clinical benefit, and its use is not recommended. Many patients with first-episode herpes present with mildclinical manifestations but later develop severe or prolonged symptoms. Therefore, most patients with initial genital herpes should receive antiviral therapy.

## CDC and WHO Recommended Regimens

- *Acyclovir* 400 mg orally three times a day for 7–10 days, OR
- *Acyclovir* 200 mg orally five times a day for 7–10 days, OR
- *Famciclovir* 250 mg orally three times a day for 7–10days, OR

- *Valacyclovir* 1 g orally twice a day for 7–10 days.

  Treatment may be extended if healing is incomplete after 10 days of therapy.

## Episodic Therapy for Recurrent Genital Herpes

Effective episodic treatment of recurrent herpes requires initiation of therapy within 1 day of lesion onset, or during the prodrome that precedes some outbreaks. The drugs used are same as in primary herpes but duration of treatment is only for five days.

For episodic therapy, a randomized controlled trial indicated that a 3-day course of valacyclovir 500 mg twice daily is as effective as a 5-day course.

## Suppressive Therapy for Recurrent Genital Herpes

Suppressive therapy reduces the frequency of genital herpes recurrences by 70–80 per cent among patients who have frequent recurrences (i.e. >6 recurrences per year), and many patients report no symptomatic outbreaks. Safety and efficacy have been documented among patients receiving daily therapy with acyclovir for as long as 6 years, and with valacyclovir or famciclovir for 1 year. Quality of life often is improved in patients with frequent recurrences who receive suppressive compared with episodic treatment. The frequency of recurrent outbreaks diminishes over time in many patients, and the patient's psychological adjustment to the disease may change. Suppressive antiviral therapy reduces but does not eliminate subclinical viral shedding. Therefore, the extent to which suppressive therapy prevents HSV transmission is unknown.

## CDC and WHO Recommended Regimens for Suppressive Therapy

- *Acyclovir* 400 mg orally twice a day, OR
- *Famciclovir* 250 mg orally twice a day, OR
- *Valacyclovir* 500 mg orally once a day, OR
- *Valacyclovir* 1.0 gram orally once a day.

## Counselling

Counselling of infected persons and their sex partners is critical to management of genital herpes. Counselling has two main goals: to help patients cope with the infection and to prevent sexual and perinatal transmission. Although initial counselling can be provided at the first visit, many patients benefit from learning about the chronic aspects of the disease after the acute illness subsides. The risk for neonatal HSV infection should be explained to all patients, including men.

Asymptomatic persons diagnosed with HSV-2 infection by type-specific serologic testing should receive the same counselling messages as persons with symptomatic infection. In addition, such persons should be taught about the common manifestations of genital herpes. Antiviral therapy is not recommended for persons who do not have clinical manifestations of infection.

### Management of Sex Partners

The sex partners of patients who have genital herpes are likely to benefit from evaluation and counselling. Symptomatic sex partners should be evaluated and treated in the same manner as patients who have genital lesions. Asymptomatic sex partners of patients who have genital herpes should be questioned concerning histories of genital lesions, educated to recognize symptoms of herpes, and offered type-specific serologic testing for HSV infection.

## HIV INFECTION AND GENITAL HERPES

Immunocompromised patients may have prolonged or severe episodes of genital, perianal, or oral herpes. Lesions caused by HSV are common among HIV-infected patients and may be severe, painful, and atypical. Episodic or suppressive therapy with oral antiviral agents is often beneficial.

### *CDC and WHO Recommended Regimens for Episodic Infection in Persons Infected with HIV*

- *Acyclovir* 400 mg orally three times a day for 5–10 days, OR
- *Acyclovir* 200 mg five times a day for 5–10 days, OR
- *Famciclovir* 500 mg orally twice a day for 5–10 days, OR
- *Valacyclovir* 1.0 g orally twice a day for 5–10 days.

### *CDC and WHO Recommended Regimens for Daily Suppressive Therapy in Persons Infected with HIV*

- *Acyclovir* 400–800 mg orally twice to three times a day, OR
- *Famciclovir* 500 mg orally twice a day, OR
- *Valacyclovir* 500 mg orally twice a day.

In the doses recommended for treatment of genital herpes, acyclovir, valacyclovir, and famciclovir are safe for use in immunocompromised patients. For severe cases, initiating therapy with acyclovir 5–10 mg/kg body weight IV every 8 hours may be necessary. If lesions persist or recur in a patient receiving antiviral treatment, HSV resistance should be suspected and a viral isolate obtained for sensitivity testing. Such patients should be managed in consultation with a specialist, and alternate therapy should be administered. All acyclovir-resistant strains are resistant to valacyclovir and most are resistant to famciclovir. Foscarnet, 40 mg/kg body weight IV every 8 hours until clinical resolution is attained, is often effective for treatment of acyclovir-resistant genital herpes.

## GENITAL HERPES IN PREGNANCY

Most mothers of infants who acquire neonatal herpes lack histories of clinically evident genital herpes. The risk for transmission to the neonate from an infected mother is high (30–50%) among women who acquire genital herpes near the time of delivery and is low (<1%) among women with histories of recurrent herpes at term or who acquire genital HSV during the first half of pregnancy. However, because recurrent genital herpes is much more common than initial HSV infection during pregnancy, the proportion of neonatal HSV infections acquired from mothers with recurrent herpes remains high. Prevention of neonatal herpes depends both on preventing acquisition of genital HSV infection during late pregnancy and avoiding exposure of the infant to herpetic lesions during delivery. Women without known genital herpes should be counselled to avoid intercourse during the third trimester with partners known or suspected of having genital herpes. All pregnant women should be asked whether they have a history of genital herpes. At the onset of labour, all women should be questioned carefully about symptoms of genital herpes, including prodrome, and all women should be examined carefully for herpetic lesions. Women without symptoms or signs of genital herpes or its prodrome can deliver vaginally. Women with recurrent genital herpetic lesions at the onset of labour should be delivered by cesarean section to prevent neonatal herpes. However, abdominal delivery does not completely eliminate the risk for HSV transmission to the infant. The results of viral cultures during pregnancy in women with or without visible herpetic lesions do not predict viral shedding at the time of delivery, and therefore routine viral cultures of pregnant women with recurrent genital herpes are not recommended.

Available data do not indicate an increased risk for major birth defects compared with the general population in women treated with acyclovir during the first trimester.[11] Acyclovir suppressive therapy late in pregnancy might reduce the frequency of caesarean sections among women who have recurrent genital herpes by diminishing the frequency of recurrences at term.[12,13]

### Neonatal Herpes

Neonatal infection is caused by contact with infected genital secretions. Ninety per cent of infections are acquired perinatally, 5-8 per cent are acquired congenitally, and a few are acquired postnatally. Neonates and infants (aged <6 wk) have a very high frequency of visceral and CNS infections. Without therapy, the mortality rate is 65%, and a high degree of neurological sequelae exists. The disease may be confined to the skin, eyes, or mouth or it may manifest as encephalitis or disseminated visceral disease involving the lungs, liver, heart, adrenals, and skin. All infants who have evidence of neonatal herpes should be promptly evaluated and treated with systemic acyclovir. The recommended regimen for infants treated for known or suspected neonatal herpes is acyclovir 20 mg/kg body weight IV every 8 hours for 21 days for disseminated and CNS disease, or 14 days for disease limited to the skin and mucous membranes.

## SYPHILIS

Syphilis is a systemic disease caused by infection with a spirochaete bacterium *Treponema pallidum*, a thin helical cell approximately 0.15 mm × 6-50 mm. It a labile organism that cannot survive drying or exposure to disinfectants; thus, fomite transmission (e.g. from toilet seats) is virtually impossible. It is solely a human pathogen and does not naturally occur in other species.

Community based studies in women in various parts of India have shown a prevalence of syphilis ranging from 0.2 to 10.5 per cent.[14] In STD clinic attendees in various parts of India, the prevalence ranges from 10 to 40 per cent, while in commercial sex workers from 30 to 60 per cent.

## Clinical Features

### *Primary Syphilis*

After an incubation period of 3 to 90 days, primary chancre appears at the site of inoculation. A small red macule appears initially, which soon becomes papule and subsequently ulcerates to form a chancre, a painless indurated ulcer, with rolled borders and smooth base which may be sometimes covered with a grayish slough or a slightly haemorrhagic crust. In women, genital chancres are seen on the vulva, vagina or the cervix. It is accompanied by regional lymphadenopathy in 50 per cent of cases, which resolves spontaneously in about 4 to 6 weeks.

### *Differential Diagnosis*

Genital herpes, chancroid, granuloma inguinale, lymphogranuloma venereum, Behçet's disease, Crohn's disease, squamous cell carcinoma, fixed drug eruptions may mimic a chancre.

### *Secondary Syphilis*

The clinical manifestations of the secondary stage are protean and can involve any organ. Some patients may develop a flu-like prodrome manifestating as fever, malaise, headache, stiff neck, myalgia, arthralgia and rhinorrhoea. However, skin rash and lymphadenopathy are most common manifestations. The rash may be macular, papular, maculopapular, papulosquamous, psoriasiform, annular, pustular, or follicular. In warm and moist areas of the body such as genitals, perineum, perianal region, axilla and groin, the skin and mucosal lesions of secondary syphilis may proliferate into pale, elevated, moist sharply demarcated papules with flat surfaces. These lesions are known as condyloma lata and are highly infectious.

### *Latent Syphilis*

It is defined as reactive serology along with positive specific treponemal antigen tests in the absence clinical signs and symptoms. Latent syphilis acquired within the preceding year is referred to as early latent syphilis (this duration is taken as two years by WHO); all other cases of latent syphilis are either late latent syphilis or latent syphilis of unknown duration. The distinction is important for epidemiological reasons because patients in the early latent stage may have relapse of secondary syphilis and thus early latency is considered as infectious stage.

Patients can be diagnosed as having early latent syphilis if, within the year preceding the evaluation, they had (a) a documented seroconversion, (b) unequivocal symptoms of primary or secondary syphilis, or (c) a sex partner documented to have primary, secondary, or early latent syphilis. Patients who have latent syphilis of unknown duration should be managed as if they have late latent syphilis. All patients with latent syphilis should have careful examination of all accessible mucosal surfaces (i.e. the oral cavity, the perineum in women, and underneath the foreskin in uncircumcised men) to evaluate for internal mucosal lesions.

### *Tertiary Syphilis*

Symptomatic late syphilis is found in up to 40 per cent of individuals with late *T.pallidum* infection.[15] This consists of three major clinical manifestations, which may co-exist: neurosyphilis, cardiovascular syphilis, gummata. Tertiary syphilis refers to gumma and cardiovascular syphilis, but not to all neurosyphilis, which may occur along with primary and secondary syphilis.

- Neurological syphilis may be subdivided into two broad groups. Asymptomatic neurosyphilis is diagnosed when individuals have late syphilis with abnormal CSF examination but with no associated neurological symptoms or signs. Symptomatic neurosyphilis is a protean disease consisting of a number of neurological syndromes usually due to direct central nervous system infection by *T.pallidum* or *T.pallidum* associated endarteritis. The most common manifestations of symptomatic neurosyphilis are related to dorsal column loss (tabes dorsalis) and dementia (general paralysis of the insane/GPI) and meningovascular involvement. Although it has been suggested that in the antibiotic era more subtle and atypical presentations occur more often.[16]
- Cardiovascular syphilis is characterised by an aortitis, which usually involves the aortic root but may affect other parts of the aorta usually spreading distally from the aortic root. The most frequent clinical manifestations of aortitis associated with late syphilis are aortic regurgitation, aortic aneurysm and angina.
- Gummata are inflammatory fibrous nodules or plaques, which may be locally destructive. They can occur in any organ but most commonly affect bone and skin.

## DIAGNOSIS

- Darkfield examinations and direct fluorescent antibody tests of lesion exudate or tissue are the definitive methods for diagnosing early syphilis.
- A presumptive diagnosis is possible with the use of two types of serologic tests for syphilis:
  a. Nontreponemal tests (e.g. Venereal Disease Research Laboratory [VDRL] and Rapid Plasma Reagin [RPR]) and
  b. Treponemal tests (e.g. fluorescent treponemal antibody absorbed [FTA-ABS] and *T. pallidum* particle agglutination [TP-PA]). The use of only one type of serologic test is insufficient for diagnosis, because false-positive nontre-ponemal test results may occur secondary to various medical conditions. Nontreponemal test antibody titers usually correlate with disease activity, and results should be reported quantitatively. A four-fold change in titer, equivalent to a change of two dilutions (e.g. from 1:16 to 1:4 or from 1:8 to 1:32), is considered necessary to demonstrate a clinically significant difference between two nontreponemal test results that were obtained using the same serologic test. Sequential serologic tests in individual patients should be performed by using the same testing method (e.g. VDRL or RPR), preferably by the same laboratory. The VDRL and RPR are equally valid assays, but quantitative results from the two tests cannot be compared directly because RPR titers often are slightly higher than VDRL titers. Nontreponemal tests usually become nonreactive with time after treatment; however, in some patients, nontreponemal antibodies can persist at a low titer for a long period of time, sometimes for the life of the patient. This response is

referred to as the "serofast reaction." Most patients who have reactive treponemal tests will have reactive tests for the remainder of their lives, regardless of treatment or disease activity. However, 15–25 per cent of patients treated during the primary stage revert to being serologically non-reactive after 2–3 years. Treponemal test antibody titers correlate poorly with disease activity and should not be used to assess treatment response. Some HIV-infected patients can have atypical serologic test results (i.e. unusually high, unusually low, or fluctuating titers). For such patients, when serologic tests and clinical syndromes suggestive of early syphilis do not correspond with one another, use of other tests (e.g. biopsy and direct microscopy) should be considered. However, for most HIV-infected patients, serologic tests are accurate and reliable for the diagnosis of syphilis and for following the response to treatment.

- Patients who have syphilis and who also have symptoms or signs suggesting neurologic disease (e.g. meningitis) or ophthalmic disease (e.g. uveitis) should have an evaluation that includes CSF analysis and ocular slit-lamp examination for diagnosis of neurosyphilis. The diagnosis of neurosyphilis usually depends on various combinations of reactive serologic test results, abnormalities of cerebrospinal fluid (CSF) cell count or protein, or a reactive VDRL-CSF with or without clinical manifestations. The CSF leucocyte count usually is elevated (>5 WBCs/mm3) in patients with neurosyphilis; this count also is a sensitive measure of the effectiveness of therapy.
- All patients who have syphilis should be tested for HIV infection. In geographic areas in which the prevalence of HIV is high, patients who have primary syphilis should be retested for HIV after 3 months if the first HIV test result was negative.

## Treatment

Penicillin G, administered parenterally, is the preferred drug for treatment of all stages of syphilis. The preparation(s) used (i.e. benzathine, aqueous procaine, or aqueous crystalline), the dosage, and the length of treatment depend on the stage and clinical manifestations of disease.

The Jarisch-Herxheimer reaction is an acute febrile reaction frequently accompanied by headache, myalgia, and other symptoms that usually occurs within the first 24 hours after any therapy for syphilis. Patients should be informed about this possible adverse reaction. The Jarisch-Herxheimer reaction occurs most often among patients who have early syphilis. Antipyretics may be used, but they have not been proven to prevent this reaction.

## Treatment for Primary and Secondary Syphilis

### *CDC and WHO Recommended Regimens*

Inj. Benzathine penicillin G 2.4 million units IM in a single dose. Because of the volume involved, this dose is usually given as two injections at separate sites.

*Alternative regimen*

Procaine benzylpenicillin, 1.2 million IU by intramuscular injection, daily for 10 consecutive days

*WHO recommended alternative regimen for penicillin-allergic non-pregnant patients.*

Doxycycline, 100 mg orally, twice daily for 14 days OR
Tetracycline, 500 mg orally, 4 times daily for 14 days
Alternative regimen for penicillin-allergic pregnant patients
Erythromycin, 500 mg orally, 4 times daily for 14 days

## Treatment for Latent Syphilis

Treatment of latent syphilis usually does not affect transmission and is intended to prevent occurrence or progression of late complications.

*CDC and WHO recommended regimen*
*early latent syphilis*
Inj. Benzathine penicillin G 2.4 million units IM in a single dose.

*Late latent syphilis or latent syphilis of unknown duration*
Inj. Benzathine penicillin G 7.2 million units total, administered as three doses of 2.4 million units IM each at 1 week intervals.

## Treatment for Tertiary Syphilis

*CDC and WHO recommended regimen for adults*
Inj. Benzathine penicillin G 7.2 million units total, administered as three doses of 2.4 million units IM each at 1 week intervals.

*Alternative regimen for penicillin-allergic non-pregnant patients*
Tab. Doxycycline, 100 mg orally, twice daily for 30 days OR
Tab. Tetracycline, 500 mg orally, 4 times daily for 30 days

*WHO Recommended alternative regimen for penicillin-allergic pregnant patients.*
Tab.Erythromycin, 500 mg orally, 4 times daily for 30 days.

## Follow-up

Treatment failure can occur with any regimen. However, assessing response to treatment is often difficult, and definitive criteria for cure or failure have not been established. Nontreponemal test titers may decline more slowly for patients who previously had syphilis. Patients should be re-examined clinically and serologically 6 months and 12 months following treatment. Patients who have signs or symptoms that persist or recur or who have a sustained four-fold increase in nontreponemal test titer (i.e. compared with the maximum or baseline titer at the time of treatment) probably failed treatment or were reinfected. These patients should be re-treated and re-evaluated for HIV infection. Because treatment failure usually cannot be reliably distinguished from reinfection with *T. pallidum*, a CSF analysis also should be performed for neurosyphilis. HIV-infected patients should be evaluated more frequently (i.e. at 3 months intervals instead of 6 months intervals). If additional follow-up cannot be ensured, re-treatment is recommended.

While following up patient for latent syphilis quantitative nontreponemal serologic tests should be repeated at 6, 12, and 24 months. Patients with a normal CSF examination should be re-treated for latent syphilis if

a. Titers increase four-fold,

b. An initially high titer (>1:32) fails to decline at least four-fold (i.e. two dilutions) within 12–24 months of therapy, or signs or symptoms attributable to syphilis develop.

All patients who have latent syphilis should be evaluated clinically for evidence of tertiary disease (e.g. aortitis, gumma, and iritis). Patients who have syphilis and who demonstrate any of the following criteria should have a prompt CSF examination:

- Neurologic or ophthalmic signs or symptoms;
- Evidence of active tertiary syphilis (e.g. aortitis, gumma, and iritis);
- Treatment failure; or
- HIV infection with late latent syphilis or syphilis of unknown duration. If dictated by circumstances and patient preferences, a CSF examination may be performed for patients who do not meet these criteria.

## Management of Sex Partners

Sexual transmission of *T. pallidum* occurs only when mucocutaneous syphilitic lesions are present; such manifestations are uncommon after the first year of infection. However, persons exposed sexually to a patient who has syphilis in any stage should be evaluated clinically and serologically for syphilis.

## Syphilis Among HIV-Infected Persons

Unusual serologic responses have been observed among HIV-infected persons who have syphilis. Most reports have involved serologic titers that were higher than expected, but false-negative serologic test results and delayed appearance of seroreactivity also have been reported. However, aberrant serologic responses are uncommon, and most specialists believe that both treponemal and non-treponemal serologic tests for syphilis can be interpreted in the usual manner for most patients who are coinfected with *T. pallidum* and HIV. When clinical findings are suggestive of syphilis, but serologic tests are nonreactive or the interpretation is unclear, alternative tests (e.g. biopsy of a lesion, darkfield examination, or direct fluorescent antibody staining of lesion material) may be useful for diagnosis. Neurosyphilis should be considered in the differential diagnosis of neurologic disease in HIV infected persons.

## Primary and Secondary Syphilis Among HIV-Infected Persons

Compared with HIV-negative patients, HIV-positive patients who have early syphilis may be at increased risk for neurologic complications and may have higher rates of treatment failure with currently recommended regimens. The magnitude of these risks, although not defined precisely, is likely minimal. No treatment regimens for syphilis have been demonstrated to be more effective in preventing neurosyphilis in HIV-infected patients than the syphilis regimens recommended for HIV-negative patients. Careful follow-up after therapy is essential.

## Treatment

Inj.Benzathine penicillin G 2.4 million units IM administered at 1 week intervals for 3 weeks.

## Follow-up

HIV-infected patients should be evaluated clinically and serologically for treatment failure at 3, 6, 9, 12, and 24 months after therapy. Although of unproven benefit, some specialists recommend a CSF examination 6 months after therapy. HIV-infected patients who meet the criteria for treatment failure should be managed in the same manner as HIV-negative patients (i.e. a CSF examination and re-treatment). CSFexamination and re-treatment also should be strongly considered for patients whose nontreponemal test titers do not decrease four-fold within 6–12 months of therapy.

# SYPHILIS DURING PREGNANCY

All women should be screened serologically for syphilis at the first prenatal visit. For communities and populations in which the prevalence of syphilis is high or for patients at high risk, serologic testing should be performed during the third trimester, at 28 weeks' gestation, and at delivery in addition to routine early screening. Any woman who delivers a stillborn infant after 20 weeks' gestation should be tested for syphilis. No infant should leave the hospital if maternal serologic status has not been determined at least once during pregnancy and preferably again at delivery.

## Diagnosis

Seropositive pregnant women should be considered infected unless an adequate treatment history is documented in the medical records and sequential serologic antibody titers have declined.

## Treatment

Penicillin is effective for preventing maternal transmission to the foetus and for treating fetal infection. Treatment during pregnancy should consist of the penicillin regimen appropriate for the stage of syphilis. A second dose of benzathine penicillin 2.4 million units IM may be administered 1 week after the initial dose for women who have primary, secondary, or early latent syphilis. In the second half of pregnancy, management and counselling may be facilitated by a sonographic foetal evaluation for congenital syphilis, but this should not delay therapy. Sonographic signs of foetal syphilis (i.e. hepatomegaly, ascites, and hydrops) indicate a greater risk for foetal treatment failure. Women treated for syphilis during the second half of pregnancy are at risk for premature labour and/or foetal distress if the treatment precipitates the Jarisch-Herxheimer reaction. These women should be advised to seek obstetric attention after treatment if they notice any contractions or decrease in foetal movements. Although stillbirth is a rare complication of treatment, concern about this complication should not delay necessary treatment. All patients who have syphilis should be offered testing for HIV infection.

## Follow-up

Co-ordinated prenatal care, treatment follow-up, and syphilis case management are important in the management of pregnant women with syphilis. Serologic titers should be repeated in the third trimester and at delivery. The clinical and antibody response should be appropriate for the stage of disease. Most women will deliver before their serologic response to treatment can be assessed definitively.

## CONGENITAL SYPHILIS

Clinical evidence of early congenital syphilis is similar to that of secondary syphilis in adults. The rash has a higher probability of being atypical and can be vesicular or bullous instead of the characteristic reddish brown macular rash. Additional symptoms of early congenital syphilis are:

Haemorrhagic rhinitis, periostitis, pseudoparalysis, often from pain secondary to osteochondritis mucous patches, perioral fissures, hepatosplenomegaly, generalised lymphadenopathy, hydrops, glomerulonephritis, thrombocytopenia, neurologic, and ocular involvement.

Late congenital syphilis mainly manifests with neurologic symptoms. Cardiovascular abnormalities are rare. Symptoms include the following:

- Prominent frontal bones, depression of nasal bridge, abnormal maxilla development, anterior tibial bowing
- Clutton joints (arthritis of both knees)
- Interstitial keratitis
- Hutchinson incisors
- Mulberry molars
- Deafness
- Paroxysmal cold haemoglobinuria
- Gummatous involvement

## CHANCROID

Chancroid is an acute, sexually transmitted, autoinoculable, ulcerative disease of the genito-inguinal area caused by a gram- negative bacillus, *Haemophilus ducreyi*.

Chancroid is a cofactor for HIV transmission (high rates of HIV infection among patients who have chancroid). About 10 per cent of persons who have chancroid are coinfected with *T. pallidum* or HSV.

### Clinical Features

The typical lesion of chancroid is non-indurated (soft sore), painful ulcer with ragged or undermined edges and a necrotic base covered with a purulent discharge. It bleeds easily on touch. The ulcers are often multiple. One to two weeks after the appearance of genital ulcer, regional lymph nodes become tender and inflamed in 30 to 60 per cent of patients. It is unilateral in two-thirds of the patients.

### Diagnosis

- Gram staining of smear from ulcer base may show gram-negative streptobacilli lying in clusters either inside the leucocytes or outside in chains.

- A definitive diagnosis of chancroid requires identification of *H. ducreyi* on special culture media that is not widely available from commercial sources; even using these media, sensitivity is <80 per cent.
- PCR
- Antigen detection by Immunoflorescent test can be used.

A probable diagnosis, for both clinical and surveillance purposes, can be made if all the following criteria are met:

a. The patient has one or more painful genital ulcers;
b. The patient has no evidence of *T. pallidum* infection by darkfield examination of ulcer exudate or by a serologic test for syphilis performed at least 7 days after onset of ulcers;
c. The clinical presentation, appearance of genital ulcers and, if present, regional lymphadenopathy are typical for chancroid; and
d. A test for HSV performed on the ulcer exudate is negative. The combination of a painful ulcer and tender inguinal adenopathy, symptoms occurring in one-third of patients, suggests a diagnosis of chancroid; when accompanied by suppurative inguinal adenopathy, these signs are almost pathognomonic.

## Treatment

Successful treatment for chancroid cures the infection, resolves the clinical symptoms, and prevents transmission to others. In advanced cases, scarring can result despite successful therapy.

### *CDC and WHO Recommended Regimen for Adults*

- *Tab.Azithromycin* 1 g orally in a single dose, OR
- *Inj.Ceftriaxone* 250 mg intramuscularly (IM) in a single dose, OR
- *Tab.Ciprofloxacin* 500 mg orally twice a day for 3 days, OR
- *Tab.Erythromycin* base 500 mg orally three times a day for 7 days.

***Note*:** Ciprofloxacin is contraindicated for pregnant and lactating women. Azithromycin and ceftriaxone offer the advantage of single dose therapy. Worldwide, several isolates with intermediate resistance to either ciprofloxacin or erythromycin have been reported.

Patients should be tested for HIV infection at the time chancroid is diagnosed. Patients should be retested for syphilis and HIV 3 months after the diagnosis of chancroid if the initial test results were negative.

## Follow-up

Patients should be re-examined 3–7 days after initiation of therapy. If treatment is successful, ulcers usually improve symptomatically within 3 days and objectively within 7 days after therapy. If no clinical improvement is evident, the clinician must consider whether

a. The diagnosis is correct,
b. The patient is coinfected with another STD,
c. The patient is infected with HIV,

d. The treatment was not used as instructed, or
e. The *H. ducreyi* strain causing the infection is resistant to the prescribed antimicrobial. The time required for complete healing depends on the size of the ulcer; large ulcers may require >2 weeks. Clinical resolution of fluctuant lymphadenopathy is slower than that of ulcers and may require needle aspiration or incision and drainage, despite otherwise successful therapy. Although needle aspiration of buboes is a simpler procedure, incision and drainage may be preferred because of reduced need for subsequent drainage procedures.

## Management of Sex Partners

Sex partners of patients who have chancroid should be examined and treated, regardless of whether symptoms of the disease are present, if they had sexual contact with the patient during the 10 days preceding the patient's onset of symptoms.

## Special Considerations

### *Pregnancy*

The safety and efficacy of azithromycin for pregnant and lactating women have not been established. Ciprofloxacin is contraindicated during pregnancy and lactation. No adverse effects of chancroid on pregnancy outcome have been reported.

### *HIV Infection*

HIV-infected patients who have chancroid should be monitored closely because, as a group, these patients are more likely to experience treatment failure and to have ulcers that heal more slowly. HIV-infected patients may require longer courses of therapy than those recommended for HIV-negative patients, and treatment failures can occur with any regimen. Because data are limited concerning the therapeutic efficacy of the recommended ceftriaxone and azithromycin regimens in HIV-infected patients, these regimens should be used for such patients only if follow-up can be ensured.

# GRANULOMA INGUINALE (DONOVANOSIS)

Granuloma inguinale is a genital ulcerative disease caused by the intracellular Gram-negative bacterium *Calymmatobacterium granulomatis*. The disease is endemic in certain tropical and developing areas, including India, Papua, New Guinea; central Australia; and southern Africa.

## Clinical Features

Clinically, the disease commonly presents as painless, progressive ulcerative lesions without regional lymphadenopathy.

Four varieties of skin lesions occur.

- Ulcerovegetative type (most common): These lesions develop from the nodular type and consist of large, usually painless, spreading, exuberant ulcers. The ulcers have clean, friable bases with distinct, raised, rolled margins. The ulcers are typically beefy red in appearance and bleed easily. Autoinoculation is a common feature, resulting in lesions on adjacent skin.

- Nodular type: Soft, often pruritic, red nodules arise at the site of inoculation and eventually ulcerate and present a bright red granulating surface. (A nodule may be mistaken for a lymph node [a pseudobubo].)
- Cicatricial type: Dry ulcers evolve into cicatricial plaques and may be associated with lymphoedema.
- Hypertrophic or verrucous type (relatively rare): This proliferative reaction with formation of large vegetating masses may resemble genital warts.
  Elephantiasis like swelling of the external genitalia is frequent in later-stage lesions.

## Extragenital Involvement

- Lymphadenopathy does not occur due to GI, but lymph node enlargement due to secondary bacterial infection or pseudobuboes may occur. Extragenital involvement occurs in 6 per cent of cases.
- Autoinoculation may lead to involvement of the oral cavity and the gastrointestinal tract.
- Haematogenous dissemination to the spleen, the lungs, the liver, the bones, and the orbits may occur and occasionally results in death.

## Diagnosis

- Diagnosis requires visualisation of darkstaining Donovan bodies on tissue crush preparation or biopsy.
- The causative organism is difficult to culture.
- Skin tests and complement fixation tests have been used for diagnosis of diagnosis.

## Treatment

Treatment halts progression of lesions, although prolonged therapy may be required to permit granulation and re-epithelialisation of the ulcers. Relapse can occur 6–18 months after apparently effective therapy. Several antimicrobial regimens have been effective, but few controlled trials have been published.

### *CDC Recommended Regimen for Adults*

- Doxycycline 100 mg orally twice a day for at least 3 weeks OR
- Trimethoprim-sulfamethoxazole one double-strength (800mg/160mg) tablet orally twice a day for at least 3 weeks.
- Ciprofloxacin 750 mg orally twice a day for at least 3 weeks, OR
- Erythromycin base 500 mg orally four times a day for at least 3 weeks, OR
- Azithromycin 1 g orally once per week for at least 3 weeks.

Therapy should be continued at least 3 weeks or until all lesions have completely healed. Some specialists recommend addition of an aminoglycoside (e.g. gentamicin 1 mg/kg IV every 8 hours) to the above regimens if improvement is not evident within the first few days of therapy.

### WHO Recommended Regimen for Adults

- Azithromycin, 1 g orally on fi rst day, then 500 mg orally, once a day for a minimum of 14 days or until lesions heal OR
- Doxycycline, 100 mg orally, twice daily for a minimum of 14 days or until lesions heal.
- Alternative regimen
- Erythromycin , 500 mg orally, 4 times daily minimum of 14 days or until lesions heal **OR**
- Tetracycline , 500 mg orally, 4 times daily minimum of 14 days or until lesions heal **OR**
- Trimethoprim 80 mg/sulfamethoxazole 400 mg, 2 tablets orally, twice daily for a minimum of 14 days or until lesions heal.

### Follow-up

Patients should be followed clinically until signs and symptoms have resolved.

### Management of Sex Partners

Persons who have had sexual contact with a patient who has granuloma inguinale within the 60 days before onset of the patient's symptoms should be examined and offered therapy. However, the value of empiric therapy in the absence of clinical signs and symptoms has not been established.

### Special Considerations

#### *Pregnancy*

Pregnancy is a relative contraindication to the use of sulfonamides. Pregnant and lactating women should be treated with the erythromycin regimen, and consideration should be given to the addition of a parenteral aminoglycoside (e.g., gentamicin). Azithromycin may prove useful for treating granuloma inguinale in pregnancy, but published data are lacking. Doxycycline and ciprofloxacin are contraindicated in pregnant women.

#### *HIV Infection*

Persons with both granuloma inguinale and HIV infection should receive the same regimens as those who are HIV negative. Consideration should be given to the addition of a parenteral aminoglycoside (e.g. gentamicin).

## LYMPHOGRANULOMA VENEREUM

Lymphogranuloma venereum (LGV) is a sexually transmitted chlamydial disease that primarily involves the lymphatics. Many synonyms have been used in the past for this condition, such as tropical bubo, climatic bubo, poradenitis inguinale, Durand-Nicolas-Favre disease, lymphopathia venereum and the fourth,fifth or sixth diseases. It is caused by *Chlamydia trachomatis* serovars L1, L2, or L3. LGV occurs in 3 stages.

## Clinical Features

The majority of LGV infections in the primary and secondary stages may go undetected.

*The primary stage* is marked by the formation of a painless herpetiform ulceration at the site of inoculation. The primary lesion is noticed in one-third of affected men but rarely in affected women.

*The secondary stage* classically is described as the inguinal syndrome, and it is characterised by painful inguinal lymphadenitis and associated constitutional symptoms. It occurs after a usual incubation period of 10-30 days, but it may be up to 6 months. This stage is characterised by the formation of enlarged, tender regional lymph nodes, termed buboes. Patients may experience constitutional symptoms, which can include fever, headache, malaise, chills, nausea, vomiting, and arthralgias. Tender inguinal lymphadenopathy, usually unilateral, is the most common clinical manifestation. In women perirectal and pelvic lymph node may be involved as a result of lymphatic spread from the cervix and posterior vaginal wall. Early in the course of the disease, the nodes appear fleshy and show diffuse reticulosis. Later, suppurative granulomatous lymphadenitis and perilymphadenitis occur with matting of the nodes. Frequently, these nodes coalesce to form stellate abscesses. Women and homosexually active men may have proctocolitis or inflammatory involvement of perirectal or perianal lymphatic tissues resulting in fistulas and strictures.

*The tertiary stage* of LGV occurs years after the initial infection. In this stage, an anogenitorectal syndrome may occur with resultant rectal stricture or elephantiasis of the genitalia. This syndrome is found predominantly in women and homosexual men, because of the location of the involved lymphatics. This late stage is characterized by proctocolitis, which is caused by hyperplasia of intestinal and perirectal lymphatic tissue. This inflammation forms perirectal abscesses, ischiorectal abscesses, rectovaginal fistulas, anal fistulas, and rectal stricture. In very late stages, fibrosis and granulomas are characteristic. Chlamydial organisms are scarce at this stage.

*Transmission* is predominantly sexual. However, transmission by fomites, nonsexual personal contact, and laboratory accidents has been documented. The creation of aerosols of this organism has been associated with infection and pulmonary symptoms.

## Diagnosis

- Previously, the Frei test was the only method available to identify a chlamydial infection. Currently, the Frei intradermal test is only of historical interest.
- Complement fixation (CF) is more sensitive than the Frei skin test, but it has some cross-reactivity with other chlamydial species. CF sensitivity is 80 per cent for LGV. A test titer of 1:16 is strongly suggestive of LGV and a titer of > 1:64 indicates active LGV. A 4-fold rise or fall in titer further supports the diagnosis. The microimmunofluorescence test for the L-type serovar of C trachomatis is the most sensitive and specific test. Availability of this test is the limiting factor.
- Definitive diagnosis may be made by aspiration of the bubo and growth of the aspirated material in cell culture. C trachomatis can be cultured in as many as 30 per cent of cases.

## Treatment

Treatment cures infection and prevents ongoing tissue damage, although tissue reaction can result in scarring. Buboes may require aspiration through intact skin or incision and drainage to prevent the formation of inguinal/femoral ulcerations. Doxycycline is the preferred treatment.

### CDC Recommended Regimen for Adults

*Doxycycline* 100 mg orally twice a day for 21 days.

### Alternative Regimen

Erythromycin base 500 mg orally four times a day for 21 days. Some STD specialists believe Azithromycin 1.0 g orally once weekly for 3 weeks is likely effective, although clinical data are lacking.

### WHO Recommended Regimen for Adults

- Doxycycline, 100 mg orally, twice daily for 14 days **OR**
- Erythromycin, 500 mg orally, 4 times daily for 14 days

### Alternative Regimen

- Tetracycline, 500 mg orally, 4 times daily for 14 days.

Fluctuant lymph nodes should be aspirated through healthy skin. Incision and drainage or excision of nodes may delay healing. Some patients with advanced disease may require treatment for longer than 14 days, and sequelae such as strictures and/or fistulae may require surgery.

### Follow-up

Patients should be followed clinically until signs and symptoms have resolved.

### Management of Sex Partners

Persons who have had sexual contact with a patient who has LGV within the 30 days before onset of the patient's symptoms should be examined, tested for urethral or cervical chlamydial infection, and treated.

### Pregnancy and LGV

Pregnant and lactating women should be treated with erythromycin. Azithromycin may prove useful for treatment of LGV in pregnancy, but no published data are available regarding its safety and efficacy. Doxycycline is contraindicated in pregnant women.

#### *HIV Infection*

Persons with both LGV and HIV infection should receive the same regimens as those who are HIV-negative. Prolonged therapy may be required, and delay in resolution of symptoms may occur.

## SYNDROMIC MANAGEMENT

Aetiological diagnosis of STIs is problematic for health care providers in resource poor settings. It places constraints on their time and resources, increases costs and reduces access to treatment. In addition, the sensitivity and specificity of commercially available tests can vary significantly, affecting negatively the reliability of laboratory testing for STI diagnosis. Many health care facilities in developing countries lack the equipment and trained personnel required for etiological diagnosis of STIs. To overcome this problem, a syndrome-based approach to the management of STI patients has been developed and promoted. The syndromic management approach is based on the identification of consistent groups of symptoms and easily recognized signs (syndromes), and the provision of treatment that will deal with the majority of, or the most serious, organisms responsible for producing a syndrome. WHO has developed following flowchart for syndromic management of STIs with genital ulcers:

**Flow Chart 11.1:** Syndromic management of genital ulcer disease (WHO/HIV/20003.09)

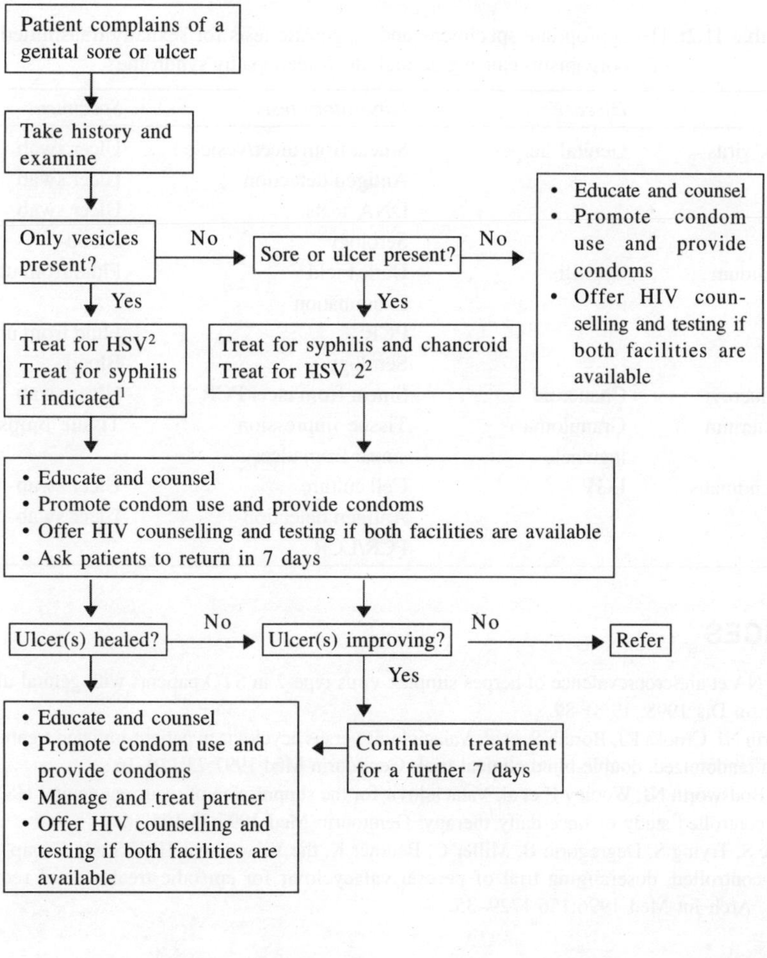
Patient complains of a genital sore or ulcer
Take history and examine
Only vesicles present?
No
Sore or ulcer present?
No
• Educate and counsel
• Promote condom use and provide condoms
• Offer HIV counselling and testing if both facilities are available
Yes
Yes
Treat for HSV[2]
Treat for syphilis if indicated[1]
Treat for syphilis and chancroid
Treat for HSV 2[2]
• Educate and counsel
• Promote condom use and provide condoms
• Offer HIV counselling and testing if both facilities are available
• Ask patients to return in 7 days
Ulcer(s) healed?
No
Ulcer(s) improving?
No
Refer
Yes
• Educate and counsel
• Promote condom use and provide condoms
• Manage and treat partner
• Offer HIV counselling and testing if both facilities are available
Continue treatment for a further 7 days

**Table 11.1:** Diagnostic clinical features of genital ulcers caused by sexually transmitted infections

| | *Genital herpes* | *Syphilis* | *Chancroid* | *LGV* | *Granuloma inguinale* |
|---|---|---|---|---|---|
| Incubation period | 7-10 days | 9-90 days (median 21d) | 1-7 days | 3-30 days | 4-40 days |
| Duration of ulcer | Short | Short | Short | Short | Long |
| Recurrence | Yes | No | No | No | No |
| Pain | Yes | No | Yes | Yes (nodes) | No |
| Pruritus | Possible | No | No | No | No |
| Induration | No | Yes | No | No | Mild |
| Number of lesions | Multiple may colaesce to form single large erosion | Usually one | Multiple | Usually one | Variable |
| Size | Small | Small | Small | Small | Large |
| Destruction | No | Rarely | No | No | Yes |
| Adenopathy | Yes | Yes | Yes | Massive | No |

**Table 11.2:** The appropriate specimens and diagnostic tests for sexually transmitted microorganisms causing genital ulcer-adenopathy syndrome

| *Microorganism* | *Disease* | *Laboratory tests* | *Specimens* |
|---|---|---|---|
| Herpes simplex virus | Genital herpes | Smear from ulcer/vesicle | Ulcer swab |
| | | Antigen detection | Ulcer swab |
| | | DNA tests | Ulcer swab |
| | | Serology | Blood |
| Treponema pallidum | Syphilis | Dark-Field Examination | Fluid from ulcer |
| | | PCR | Fluid from ulcer |
| | | Serology | Blood |
| Haemophilus ducreyi | Chancroid | Smear from ulcer PCR | Ulcer swab |
| Calymmatobacterium granulomatis | Granuloma inguinale | Tissue impression smear from ulcer | Tissue biopsy |
| Chlamydia trachomatis | LGV | Cell culture | Ulcer swab |
| | | Antigen detection-PCR/LCR | Ulcer swab |

## REFERENCES

1. Amhore NA,et al.Seroprevalence of herpes simplex virus type-2 in STD patients with genital ulcers. Indian J Sex Transm Dis 1998; 19:81-89.
2. Bodsworth NJ, Crooks RJ, Borelli S, et al. Valaciclovir versus acyclovir in patient-initiated treatment of genital herpes: a randomized, double-blind clinical trial. Genitourin Med 1997;73:110–16.
3. Patel R, Bodsworth NJ, Wooley P, et al. Valaciclovir for the suppression of recurrent genital HSV infection: A placebo controlled study of once-daily therapy. Genitourin Med 1997;73:105–09.
4. Spruance S, Trying S, Degregorio B, Miller C, Beutner K, the Valaciclovir HSV Study Group. A large-scale, placebo-controlled, doseranging trial of peroral valacyclovir for episodic treatment of recurrent herpes genitalis. Arch Int Med 1996;156:1729–35.

5. Fife KH, Barbarash RA, Rudolph T, Degregorio B, Roth RE.Valaciclovir versus acyclovir in the treatment of first-episode genital herpes infection: Results of an international, multicenter, double-blind randomized clinical trial. Sex Transm Dis 1997;24:481–86.
6. Chosidow O, Drouault Y, Lecontae-Veyriac F, et al. Famciclovir vs. aciclovir in immunocompetent patients with recurrent genital herpes infections: A parallel-groups, randomized, double-blind clinical trial. Br J Dermatol 001:144:818–24.
7. Diaz-Mitoma F, Sibbald RG, Shafran SD, Boon R, Saltzman RL. Oral famciclovir for the suppression of recurrent genital herpes: A randomized controlled trial. JAMA 1998;280:887–92.
8. Loveless M, Harris W, Sacks S. Treatment of first episode genital herpes with famciclovir. In: Programs and abstracts of the 35th Interscience Conference on Antimicrobial Agents and Chemotherapy, San Francisco, California, 1995.
9. Mertz GJ, Loveless MO, Levin MJ, et al. Oral famciclovir for suppression of recurrent genital herpes simplex virus infection in women: A multicenter, double-blind, placebo-controlled trial. Arch Intern Med 1997;157:343–49.
10. Sacks SL, Aoki FY, Diaz-Mitoma F, Sellors J, Shafran SD. Patient initiated, twice-daily oral famciclovir for early recurrent genital herpes: A randomized, double-blind multicenter trial. JAMA 1996;276:44–49.
11. Reiff-Eldridge RA, Heffner CR, Ephross SA, Tennis PS, White AD, Andrews EB. Monitoring pregnancy outcomes after prenatal drug exposure through prospective pregnancy registries: A pharmaceutical company commitment. Am J Obstet Gynecol 2000;182:159–63.
12. Scott LL, Sanchez PJ, Jackson GL, Zeray F, Wendel GD, Jr. Acyclovir suppression to prevent cesarean delivery after first-episode genital herpes. Obstet Gynecol 1996;87:69–73.
13. Brocklehurst P, Kinghorn G, Carney O, et al. A randomised placebo controlled trial of suppressive acyclovir in late pregnancy in women with recurrent genital herpes infection. Br J Obstet Gynaecol 1998;105:275–80.
14. Hawkes S, et al. Diverse realities; sexually transmitted infections and HIV in India. Sex Transm Infect2002; 78(suppl.1): i131-i39.
15. Gjestland T. The Oslo study of untreated syphilis: An epidemiologic investigation of the natural course of syphilitic infection based on a restudy of the Boeck-Bruusgaard material. *Arch Derm Venereol* 35 ([Suppl] (Stockh) 34):1,1955.
16. Hooshmand H, Escobar MR, Kopf SW. Neurosyphilis: A study of 241 patients. *JAMA* 1972; 219:726-29.
17. World Health organization. Guidelines for the management of sexualy transmitted infections. WHO/HIV/ 2003.
18. Centers for Disease Control and Prevention. Sexually transmitted diseases treatment guidelines 2002. MMWR 2002;51(No. RR-6): 11-28.

**CHAPTER 12**

# Sexually Transmitted Infection of Lower Genital Tract

**Raksha Arora, Ruchira Singh**

## INTRODUCTION

Genital tract infections may be classified as endogenous or exogenous. Endogenous infections result from organisms of normal genital flora, whereas exogenous are usually acquired during sexual activity with an infected partner. There has been an ever increasing prevalence of these infections worldwide, especially amongst individuals with increased promiscuity. These infections can be caused by a wide variety of micro-organisms including viruses, bacteria, fungi and parasites.

Following is the list depicting major causes of sexually transmitted infections of the lower genital tract of which HPV, Gonorrhoea, Trichomoniasis, Candidiasis, and Bacterial vaginosis will be discussed in detail.

| *Frequency* | *Disease* | *Agent* | *Organism group* |
|---|---|---|---|
| More common | Genital and warts (condyloma), cervical dysplasia, and cancer | Human papilloma virus | Viruses |
| | Vaginitis | *Gardnerella, Mobiluncus, Trichomonas vaginalis, Candida albicans* | Bacteria |
| | Herpes genitalis | HSV type 2 | Viruses |
| | AIDS | HIV | Viruses |
| | Hepatitis | Hepatitis B virus | Viruses |
| Less common | Lymphogranuloma venerum | *Chlamydia trachomatis* | Bacteria |
| | Granuloma inguinale | *Calymmatobacterium granulomatis* (*Donovani*) | Bacteria |

## HUMAN PAPILLOMA VIRUS

Infections of human papilloma virus have been strongly implicated as the principal sexually transmitted causal agent in development of cervical cancer.

Both epidemiological and molecular evidence implicates HPV as the aetiological agent in 99.8 per cent of cervical cancer. Additionally, HPV is detected in approximately 80 per cent vaginal, 5 per cent vulvar and nearly all penile and anal cancers.[1]

## Aetiological Agent

Papilloma virus are members of Papovaviridae family. They are small non-enveloped, have icosahedral capsid and are composed of double stranded DNA. The viral genome exists in an episomal (circular) configuration. The genome is organised into three major regions:

| | |
|---|---|
| 1. E (early) region | } Protein coding |
| 2. L (late) region | |
| 3. Upstream regulatory region (URR) | Non-coding |

### *HPV Types*

At present more than 100 types of HPV have been identified. Of these, at least 35 primarily infect epithelium of genital tract. The common HPV types can be divided into three major categories based on their oncogenic potential:

- Low risk HPV-6, 11,42,43,44
- Intermediate risk HPV-33,35,39,52,58
- High risk HPV-16,18,31,45

Low risk types most commonly present as genital warts. HPV-6 is the most common type associated with genital warts.

Seventy-five per cent cases of cervical caner are infected with high risk types. HPV-16 is the predominant type in squamous cell cancer. HPV-18 is the predominant type in adenocarcinoma.

Multiple infections are common with prevalence ranging from 2 to 20 per cent.[3]

All types can cause subclinical infection (Fig. 12.1, Plate 2).

## Modes of Transmission

1. *Sexual transmission*—Genital HPV infection are primarily through sexual contact. Infectivity rate is approximately 65 per cent.
   The risk factors for transmission are:
   - Number of lifetime sexual partners
   - Younger age group
   - Cigarette smoking
   - Use of oral contraceptive pills
2. *Extragenital skin transmission:* Skin to skin or genital to skin transmission has been observed in periungual and congenital warts.
3. *Fomites:* Transmission through fomites is a rare documentation, e.g. gloves, surgical instruments.
4. *Vertical transmission:* Genital HPV types appear to be uncommonly transmitted in neonatal period. The only clinically expressed HPV disease that is acquired at birth is laryngeal papillomatosis. This is mainly caused by HPV-6 and 11.

Although neonates delivered vaginally are at a higher risk for exposure to HPV, delivery by caesarean section is also associated with substantial risk.

The risk increases with:

1. High risk type of HPV transmitted.
2. Increased viral load of HPV.

## Pathogenesis

Incubation period is usually 3 to 4 months but it ranges from 1 month to 2 years. All papilloma virus infect epithelial tissues. Approximately, half of all currently identified HPV types infect cutaneous epithelial surface, whereas the remainder preferentially target the mucosal epithelium of anogenital tract.

Access to actively dividing basal epitheial cells is necessary for successful infection. This is facilitated by mucosal abrasions. Replication of virus occurs entirely within the host cell nucleus.

## Histology

Infected cells exhibit nuclear atypia. Koilocytosis, described as a combination of perinuclear halo with pyknotic or shrunken nucleus is a characteristic feature of papilloma virus infection. Other features include dyskeratosis, atypical basal cells, acanthosis and multinucleation. Koilocytosis is the most specific marker except in HPV-16 and 18 where it is often absent.

## Clinical Features

Infection with HPV disease presents with a wide variety of clinical findings. The spectrum of HPV disease includes:

a. *Subclinical (Latent) HPV infection of cervix, vagina vulva, perineum and anus:* HPV transmission also occurs in absence of lesions during latent phase. Subclinical HPV infection may be 10 to 30 times more common than cytologically apparent infections. Latent infection may persist; progress to clinical disease or resolve.

b. *Genital warts:* Gential warts can be divided into four morphological types:
   1. Condyloma acuminata—They are cauliflower-shaped warts usually present initially at fourchette and adjacent labia, then spreads to other parts of vulva.
   2. Papular warts—Dome-shaped (usually skin coloured)
   3. Keratotic genital warts—They are thick horny warts.
   4. Flat-topped papules—May be present on cervix

   Morphological appearance of all warts involving different sites is similar. External genital warts are frequently multifocal (present as one or more lesions at a single anatomic site) or multicentric (present as one or more lesions on different anatomic sites).

   *Lowenstien-Buschke* tumor or "giant condylomata" are extremely large genital warts seen in patient with impaired cell mediated immunity due to HIV, immuosuppressive therapy, lymphoma or pregnancy. These lesions can become locally invasive and destructive but do not metastasize and are usually infected by HPV-6.

c. *Intraepithelial neoplasia of cervix, vulva, perineum, vagina, penis and anus:* High risk HPV are found to be a more common cause of intraepithelial lesions. Leisons with persistant HPV tend to progress more to invasive cancer.

d. *Juvenile respiratory (laryngeal) papillomatosis:* In infants it is caused by HPV-6 and HPV-11. The mode of transmission is not completely understood. Potential routes include transplacental, intrapartum in birth canal or postnatal. The estimated risk of infection from infected mothers to neonates ranges from 1 per 100 to 1 per 1000 cases.

During first several years of life, the juvenile forms tend to be more severe and is characterised by rapid regrowth. This needs frequent surgical excision.

## Diagnosis

I. Genital warts—They can be visualised by gross inspection (Figs 12.2 and 12.3, Plate 2).

II. Subclinical HPV infection is diagnosed by colposcopy.
After application of 3-5 per cent acetic acid, subclinical HPV has shiny-white colour with irregular borders and satellite lesions.
Vaginal subclinical infection may exhibit reverse punctation.

III. Squamous intraepithelial lesions (SIL) of cervix: The are detected mainly by routine cytological screening test Paps smear.

## HPV Detection Techniques

### *Paps Smear*

This cytology test has excellent specificity by only fair sensitivity. This should be done annually in women who become sexually active.

### *Colposcopy*

Colposcopic directed biopsies are often considered 100 per cent accurate.[3] This leads to the opinion that "gold standard" for disease detection is colposocpy (Figs 12.4 and 12.5, Plate 2).

### *Nucleic Acid Detection Tests*

As only certain types of HPV is primarily associated with cervical cancer, HPV typing becomes necessary. The following nucleic acid-based tests have been used for detecting and typing HPV in specimens:

1. Polymerase chain reaction (PCR)
2. Hybrid capture 2 procedure (HC2)
3. *In situ* hybridisation technique (ISH)

The median sensitivity of HPV testing for routine screening of women with CIN2, CIN3 and cervical cancer is 93 per cent compared to 75 per cent for Paps smear. Paps smear is slightly more specific than HPV DNA testing when the presence of high grade cervical disease is considered.[2]

ISH is less-sensitive than PCR or HC2 but is a better confirmatory test.

### *Indications of DNA Testing*

1. To aid the diagnosis of sexually transmitted HPV infections.
2. To screen patients with ASCUS Pap smear and determine the need for colposcopy.
3. To aid risk assessment of women with LSIL or HSIL before colposcopy.

HPV screening for all women is not recommended as it is not cost effective.

## Treatment

1. *Genital warts:* Treatment of external genital warts: (CDC 2001 recommendations).[5]
*Patient applied:*

A. Podofilox 0.5 per cent solution or gel: Apply to visible wart twice daily × 3 days followed by 4 days of no therapy. Such 4 cycles if necessary.

*OR*

B. Imiquimod 5 per cent cream—Apply HS three times a week upto 16 weeks.

*Provider applied:*

A. Cryotherapy: using liquid nitrogen.
B. Podophyllin resin (10-25%) in compound tincture or benzoin-repeat weekly if necessary.
C. Trichloroacetic acid or bichloroacetic (80-90%). Repeat weekly if necessary.
D. Surgical removal—done by tangential scissor excision, curettage or electrocautery.

*Alternative Treatment*

A. Intralesional interferon
B. Laser surgery

2. *Subclinical HPV infection:* It requires follow-up and may not be treated.

## CANDIDIASIS

*Candida* are dimorphic fungi existing in two forms:

1. Blastospores—They are responsible for transmission and asymptomatic colonisation
2. Mycelia—They are formed from blastospore germination and enhance colonisation and facilitate tissue invasion.

At least 75 per cent of women will have one episode of vulvovaginal candidal infection.

### Causative Organisms

- 90% *Candida albicans*
- 10% *Candida tropicalis, Candida glabrator* and other species (Fig. 12.6, Plate 3)

### Predisposing Factors

1. Pregnancy
2. Diabetes mellitus
3. Obesity
4. Recurrent use of following drugs:
   - Corticosteroids
   - Antibiotics, e.g. Ampicillin, Tetracycline, Cephalosporins
   - Immunosupressants

*Other risk factors associated are:*

- Condom use
- Second half of menstrual cycle
- Sexual intercourse more than four per month
- Recent antibiotic use
- Younger age

- Past gonococcal infection
- Absence of current gonorrhoea or bacterial vaginosis.

Role of oral contraceptive use is controversial.

## Clinical Features

| | | |
|---|---|---|
| Symptoms | : | Vulval itching<br>Soreness<br>Vaginal discharge<br>Superficial dyspareunia<br>Dysuria |
| Signs | : | Vulvar or vaginal erythema<br>Vulvar scaling or oedema<br>Vaginal discharge<br>Raised white or yellow adherent vaginal plaques. |

None of the above symptoms are specific for diagnosis of candidiasis.

## Diagnosis

pH of vaginal discharge is 4 to 4.5.

I. *Microscopy*
   1. Gram's stain—for spores and pseudohyphae. May identify 65 to 83 per cent of symptomatic cases.
   2. Saline microscopy—pseudohyphae may be seen.
   3. 10 per cent KOH preparation—to look for pseudohyphae (identifies 70% cases). It is usually sufficient for routine diagnosis.

II. *Culture*—Culture on Sabraoud's dextrose agar (SDA) is considered in:
   1. All symptomatic cases if microscopy is inconclusive.
   2. For identification of species in recent cases which would help in treatment.

III. *Latex agglutination slide tests*—It confers no benefit over microscopy.

## Classification of Candidal Vaginal Infection:

| | *Uncomplicated* | *Complicated* |
|---|---|---|
| 1. Occurrence | 90% | 10% |
| 2. Frequency | Sporadic | Recurrent |
| 3. Severity | Mild to moderate | Severe |
| 4. Host | Normal | Abnormal (e.g. uncontrolled diabetes mellitus) |
| 5. Organisms | *Candida albicans* | Non-albicans species, e.g. *C. glabrator* *C. tropicalis* |
| 6. Treatment | Single dose regimen | Antimycotic agent ≥ 7 days |

## Treatment

According to NACO guidelines[10]

1. Eliminate predisposing factors.
2. Do not treat asymptomatic infections.
3. Intravaginal topical agents:
   Miconazole or Clotrimazole, 100 mg (intravaginally for 6 days )
   Or
   Clotrimazole, 500 mg intravaginally single dose
4. Oral agent:
   Fluconazole 150 mg orally single dose

## Candial Infection in Pregnancy

Symptomatic colonisation is more prevalent during pregnancy although asymptomatic colonisation is found in 30 to 40 per cent of cases. It is more difficult to treat.

Treatment involves topical azole for 7 days. Oral therapy is contraindicated.

## Recurrent Candidal Infection

*Definition*: It is defined as four or more episodes annually.

*Prevalence*: Recurrent candidal infection occurs in < 5 per cent of healthy women of reproductive age group.

*Pathogenesis*—It may be due to:

a. Persistence of *Candida* as an intracellular phase or very low colony counts.
b. An acquired antigen specific immunodeficiency state of vaginal epithelium.

### *Treatment*

1. Reduction or elimination of predisposing factors.
2. Examination of sexual partner.
3. Eradication regimen.
   Fluconazole 150 mg on 1,4,8 days
   Or
   Intravaginal azoles for 10-14 days
   Or
   Ketoconazole 400 mg daily for 14 days
4. Prevention regimen given for 3-6 months
   Fluconazole 150 mg weekly
   Or
   Ketoconazole 100 mg daily
   Or
   Itraconzole 100 mg every alternate day
   Or

Clotrimazole 500 mg intravaginally weekly
Or
Any topical azole applied daily

## TRICHOMONAS VAGINALIS

*Trichomonas vaginalis* is a motile aerobic protozoon that is found in vagina. It is the most prevalent parasite in humans transmitted primarily via sexual intercourse. It is found in 10 per cent healthy women and 50 per cent of patients attending STD clinics. It is responsible for 20 to 30 per cent of vulvovaginitis (Fig.12.7, Plate 3).

### Signs and Symptoms

Approximately 50 per cent are asymptomatic but 30 per cent develop symptoms when observed for 6 months which include.

- Profuse yellow frothy homogenous vaginal discharge
- Pruritis vulvae
- Dyspareunia
- Dysuria and increased frequency of urine
- Abdominal pain and low backache.

#### *Signs*

- Petechial lesions of cervix "strawberry cervix" or "Flea bitten cervix" seen more frequently by colposcopy than naked eye.
- Punctate mucosal haemorrhage of cervix and marked oedema and erythema of cervix.

### Diagnosis

1. Vaginal fluid pH $\geq 4.5$
2. Wet mount examination showing motile trichomonalas is the diagnostic method of choice and has sensitivity of 42 to 92 per cent.
3. Culture of organism on special medium, Fienberg wittington medium might be required if wet mount is negative. Diamond or Kupferberg media is available commercially in a kit.
4. Urine sediment is the preferred method for males.

### New Diagnostic Methods

- Monoclonal antibodies
- ELISA
- Latex agglutination
- PCR

### Treatment

According to CDC 1998 guidelines:

Ideally, treatment should be given for both partners and abstinence should be advocated for 4 weeks.

### *Non-pregnant Females and Males*

- Metronidazole 2000 mg stat.
  Or
- Metronidazole 500 mg BD × 7 days.

### *Pregnant Females*

- Metronidazole 2000 mg single dose.

### *Treatment Failure*

- Metronidazole 2 gm single dose × 3-5 days

### *Prevention*

- Limiting the number of partners
- Using condoms
- Treatment of both partners.

## GONORRHOEA

Gonorrhoea is a sexually transmitted disease affecting epithelium. *Neisseria gonorrhoeae* are gram-negative, non-motile, non-spore bearing diplococci (kidney-shaped) that grow intracellularly in pairs.

It has predeliction for columnar or pseudostratifed epithelium.

*Epidemiology:* Gonorrhoea remains a major public health problem worldwide. It predominately affects young adolescents.

*Transmission:* Transmission is almost entirely by sexual contact.

Risk of transmission is more from male to female (50-90%) as compared to:

Female to male — (20-25%).

Incubation period — 3-5 days.

### Clinical Presentation

The primary site of involvement is genitourinary tract.

1. *Gonococcal cervicitis:* Mucopurulent cervicitis is one of the most common sexually transmitted diseases.

   *The common symptoms*

   - Increased vaginal discharge
   - Increased frequency or urgency in micturition

### *Signs*

- Yellow to green mucopurulent discharge from os
- Oedematous or friable cervix
- Cystitis
- Pyuria

### Complications of Gonococcal Cervicitis

1. Dyspareunia
2. Lower abdominal pain or back pain
3. Ascending infection—seen in approximately 20 per cent cases.
   1. Acute endometritis—This is characterised by:
      Fever, malaise
      Lower abdominal pain and tenderness
      Dyspareunia
      Abnormal menstrual bleeding
   2. Acute salpingitis—There is acute motion tenderness and adnexal mass.

   Tubal scarring is the most devastating sequale leading to infertility and also increases the risk of ectopic pregnancy.
2. *Gonococcal vaginitis:* Vaginal epithelium is usually not affected unlike stratified squamous epithelium but is seen in prepubertal and postmenopausal women.
   *Signs and symptoms include—*
   - Red and oedematous vaginal mucosa
   - Abundant purulent discharge
3. *Disseminated gonococcal infection:*
   Prevalence ranges from 0.1 to 0.3 per cent
   *Female:* male – 4:1
   Predisposing factors
   1. Third trimester of pregnancy
   2. Within 7 days from onset of menstruation.

   *It manifests as two stages:*
   - o Early bacteremic stage
   - o Late stage

### Clinical manifestations of DGI

Early stage—
- Migratory arthritis
- Tenosynovitis
- Dermatitis

Late stage—
- Arthritis
- Perihepatitis
- Osteomyelitis
- Pericarditis
- Endocarditis
- Meningitis

4. Anorectal gonorrhoea
5. Pharyngeal gonorrhoea
6. Ocular gonorrhoea

## Gonococcal Infection and Pregnancy

Incidence of gonorrhoea in pregnancy—Ranges from rare to 10 per cent.

1st trimester—Salpingitis and PID are associated with high rate of foetal loss.

2nd and 3rd trimester—Gonococcal infection is less common

Acquisition of gonococcal infection late in pregnancy can adversely affect labour by causing:

- Prolonged rupture of membranes
- Premature delivery
- Chorioamnionitis
- Fumsitis (infection of unbillical cord stump)
- Sepsis of infant

In neonates, most common form of gonorrhoea is ophthalmia neonatorium which results from cervical secretions during parturition. Ocular neonatal instillation of prophylactic agent (e.g. 1% silver nitrate) is a cost-effective measure for prevention.

## Diagnosis

Sample should be collected by Dacron or rayon swabs.

1. *Gram's stain of cervical discharge:*
   a. $\geq 30$ PMN per high power field in 5 fields indicates mucopurulent cevicitis.
   b. The presence of gonococcal intracellular diplococci in cervical smear does not accurately predict gonorrhoea.
2. *Culture:* Sensitivity of single endocervical culture is ~ 80-90 per cent.
   - Clinical isolation is best performed using Thayer-Martin medium containing antibiotics Vancomycin, Colistin and Nystatin which inhibit growth of contaminating organisms.
   - *Neisseria gonorrhoeae* do not tolerate drying and thus require immediate innoculation on appropriate media and placement in an incubator. Ideal growth occurs in 35 to 37°C, in 5% $CO_2$ atmosphere.
     Transport media as Stuart, Aimes, etc can be used if culture media are not available.
   - All gonococcal cultures should be tested for antimicrobial susceptibility.
   - For optimal yield either two endocervical or an endocervical and an anal specimen should be obtained. A single swab can miss 10 per cent of endocervical infection.
3. *Serology*—Serodiagnosis is not helpful because of persistence of antibody due to previous gonococcal disease.
   *Gonozyme test*—It is a solid phase immunoassay which has high sensitivity and specificity for infections in men but not for cervical infections. So, it cannot be used as a screening test for low prevalence women.
4. *Other methods:*
   a. Non-amplified DNA probe test (PACE 2 system)
   b. Nuclei acid amplification tests as—
      - Ligase chain reaction—90 to 95 per cent sensitivity
      - Polymerase chain reaction
      - Transcription mediated amplification

## Treatment

I. CDC guidelines (2002) for uncomplicated gonorrhoeal infection:[5]
Cefixime 400 mg single dose per orally

*Or*

Ceftriaxone 125 mg single dose per orally

*Or*

Ciprofloxacin 500 mg single dose per orally

*Or*

Ofloxacin 400 mg single dose

*Or*

Levofloxacin 250 mg single dose

plus

Azithromycin 1 gm orally single dose

Or

Doxycycline 100 mg perorally BD × 7 day
Quinolone resistant *N. gonorrhoeae* (QNRG) continue to spread making treatment with quinolones inadvisable.

II. Recommendations for disseminated gonococcal infection (2001).
Recommended initial regimen
Ceftriaxone 1 gm I.M. or I.V. every 24 hrs
Alternate initial regimens-
Cefotaxime 1 gm I.V. every 8 hrs hours

Or

Ceftizoxime 1 gm I.V. every 8 hours
For patient allergic to b-lactam drugs-
Ciprofloxacin 500 mg I.V. every 12 hours

Or

Ofloxacin 400 mg I.V. every 12 hours

Or

Levofloxacin 250 mg I.V. daily.

Or

Spectinomycin 2 gm IM every 12 hours
All regimens should be continued for 24-48 hours
After improvement begins, the therapy may be shifted to
Cefixime 400 mg BD

Or

Ciprofloxacin 500 mg BD

Or

Ofloxacin 400 mg BD

O r

Levofloxacin 500 mg OD

## BACTERIAL VAGINOSIS

Bacterial vaginosis is clinical syndrome in which there is alternation of normal bacterial vaginal flora. It is the commonest cause of vaginitis. It is characterised by shift in vaginal flora from dominant flora of Lactobacillus sps to mixed vaginal flora that included *Gardnerella vaginalis*, *Bacteriodes* sps, *Mobilincus* sps and *Mycoplasma hominis*. In women with bacterial vaginosis the concentration of anaerobes and *Gardnerella* is 100 to 1000 times higher in normal women. Lactobacilli are usually absent.

### Clinical Features

Vaginal discharge is the chief complaint as compared to pruritis.

Clinical criteria for diagnosis of bacterial vaginosis (Amsel's criteria):

Presence of three out of four criteria is necessary for diagnosis.

- Homogenous, milky or creamy discharge.
- Presence of clue cells on microscopic examination
- pH of secretion above 4.5
- Fishy or amine odour with or without addition of 10 per cent KOH.

### Diagnosis

1. pH > 4.5
2. Gram's stain of vaginal discharge with three types of bacterial morphotypes are most reliable in establishing diagnosis of Bacterial vaginosis.
   a. Large gram-positive rods—*Lactobacilli*
   b. Small gram-negative or gram-variable rods—*Gardnerella* and *Bacteriodes* sps.
   c. Curved gram-negative or gram-variable rods—*Mobilincus* sps.

   These morphotypes have been used to establish 10 point Bacterial vaginosis score—
   - 0-3 Normal
   - 4-6 Intermediate
   - 7-10 Bacterial vaginosis

   Gram stain has 62 to 100 per cent sensitivity and 70 to 100 per cent positive predictive value
3. *Saline microscopy:* This shows clue cells which are diagnostic.
4. *Whiff test:* Release of fishy odour on adding alkali.
5. *Other diagnostic tests:*
   - Pap smear
   - Oligonucleotide probe
   - Enzymes detection

### Treatment

According to CDC 1998 guidelines:

I *Non-pregnant women*

Recommended regimen

Metronidazole 500 mg BD × 7 days

Or

Clindamycin 2 percent cream (5 gm) intravaginally

Or

Metronidazole 0.75 percent (5 gm) intravaginally

*Alternative regimens:*

- Metronidazole 2 gm single dose

  Or

- Clindamycin 300 mg orally BD × 7 days
- Efficacy of single dose regimen is lower as compared to 7 days regimen.

II. *Pregnant women*:

1. Patients at low risk for preterm birth are only treated if they are symptomatic. All patients who are high risk for preterm birth are screened in early second trimester. They are treated only if symptomatic bacterial vaginosis develops.

*Recommended Treatment*

- Metronidazole 250 mg TDS × 7 days
- Alternative treatment
- Metronidazole 2 gm single dose

  Or

- Clindamycin 300 mg BD × 7 days

  Or

- Metronidazole 0.75 (5 gm) intravaginally

➢ Use of clindamycin vaginal cream is not recommended.
Vaginal treatment appears to be not as effective in preventing preterm labour.

## Syndromic Management of Vaginal Discharge

Vaginal discharge is caused by either vaginitis which is due to *Trichomonas vaginalis*, *Candidiasis*, *Bacterial vaginosis* or due to cervicitis which is caused by *Neisseria gonorrhoeae* and *Chlamydia trachomatis*.

Routine STI care should be delivered through general health services. In developing countries; due to absence of cheap, simple and accurate diagnostic tests or comprehensive laboratory services for microbiological diagnosis, WHO has developed syndromic guidelines for treatment of sexually transmitted infections. NACO has advocated similar guidelines for Indian set up.

The essential components of syndromic management includes-

❖ Diagnosis and treatment based on syndromes
❖ Education on risk reduction
❖ Condom provision
❖ Counselling
❖ Partner notification
❖ Follow up

*Trichomonas vaginalis*, *Candida albicans*, *Bacterial vaginosis* are common causes of vaginal discharge. *Neiserria gonorrhoeae* along with *Chlamydia trachomatis* cause cervicitis which is a more serious cause of vaginal discharge. The clinical management of patients with vaginal discharge based on syndromic approach is as follows:

***Syndromic Management of Vaginal Discharge (with speculum examination) NACO- 2004***[9]

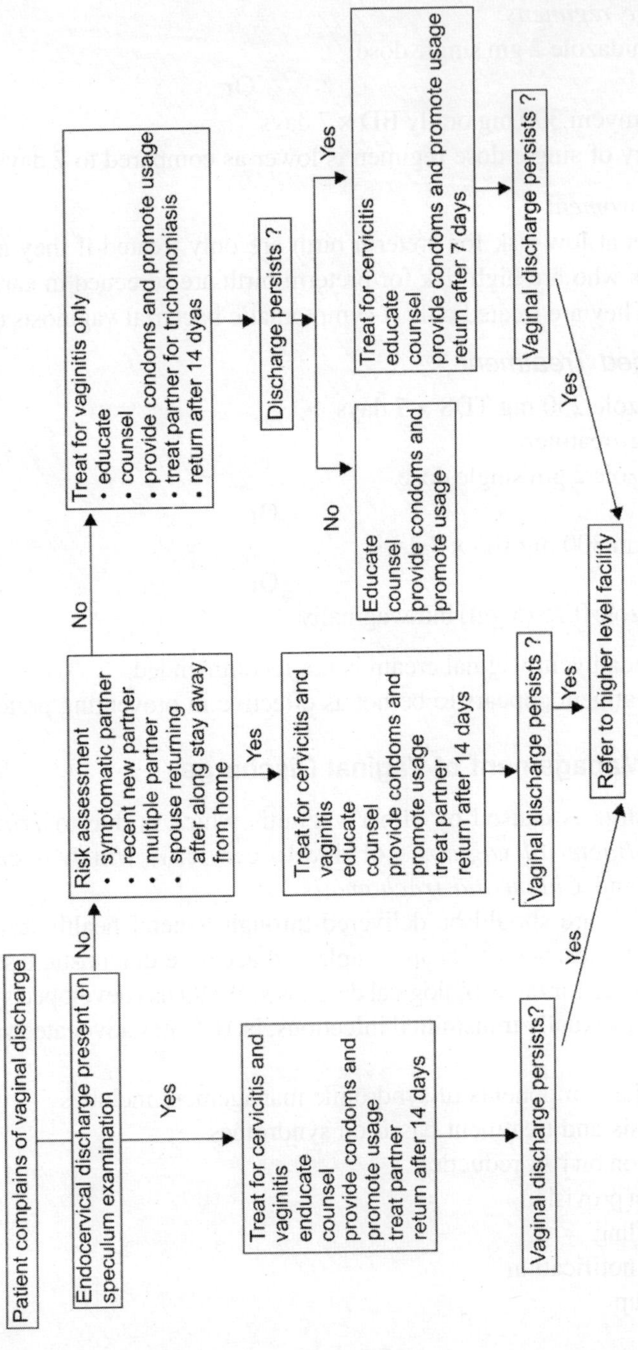

### *Recommended Treatment*

- Cervicitis (Gonococcal and Chlamydial infection)
- Azithromycin 2 gm orally single dose under supervision
- Vagnitis
- Metronidazole 2 gm orally single dose (Trichomoniasis and Bacterial vaginosis)
  Plus
- Fluconazole 150 mg orally single dose (Candidiasis)
  Plus
- Clotrimazole pessary 100 mg intravaginally once for 6 days (Candidiasis)

## Key Points

1. Human papilloma virus, *Garnedella vaginalis, Trichomonas vaginalis* and *Candida albicans* are some of the common sexually transmitted infections.
2. Low risk HPV types (HPV-6, 11, 42, 43 and 44) are commonly cause genital warts where as high risk types (HPV-16, 18, 37, 45) are detected in cervical cancer.
3. Sexual transmission is the primary mode of transmission of HPV. Infectivity rate is 65 percent.
4. Koilocytosis is the most specific histological marker of HPV infection except HPV-16 HPV-18 where it is often absent.
5. Lowenstien—Buschke tumor or "giant condylomata" are large genital warts seen in patients with impaired cell mediated immunity and are usually caused due to infection by HPV-6.
6. Gold standard for detection of HPV infection of cervix is colposcopy.
7. Nucleic acid detection techniques for detection of HPV are polymerase chain reaction, hybrid capture 2 procedure and In situ hybridization technique.
8. At least 75 percent of women will have one episode of vulvovaginal candidal infection.
9. 10% KOH preparation is usually sufficient for routine diagnosis of *Candida*. Culture on Sabroaud's Dextrose Agar (SDA) is indicated in recurrent cases and in all asymptomatic cases if microscopy is inconclusive.
10. Recurrent candidal infection is defined as four or more episodes annually. It is treated by eradication regimen which includes Tab. Fluconazole 150 mg on 1,4, 8 days or Ketaconazole 400 mg OD × 14 days. This is followed by prevention regimen for 3 to 6 months.
11. Trichomoniasis is responsible for 20 to 30 percent of vulvovaginitis.
12. For optimal yield of *Gonococcus* either 2 endocervical or an endocervical and anal specimen should be obtained.
13. For uncomplicated gonococcal infection recommended treatment is cefixime 400 mg single dose.
14. Recommended treatment for disseminated gonococcal infection is Ceftriaxone 1 gm IM or IV every 24 hours.
15. Bacterial vaginosis is the commonest cause of vaginitis. Amsel's criteria is a set of clinical criteria for diagnosis of Bacterial vaginosis, which are - homogenous milky discharge, presence of clue cells, pH > 4.5 and fishy or amine odour after addition of 10 percent KOH.
16. Gram's stain has 62 to 100 percent sensitivity and 70 to 100 percent positive predictive value in diagnosis of Bacterial vaginosis.

## REFERENCES

1. Human papillomavirus and cervical cancer. Clinical proceedings www.arhp.org/health care providers/ on line publications/clinical proceedings/ephpv/contents.
2. HPV testing. Barbara S. Apgar, Gregory L. Brotzman, Mark Spitzer(eds). Colposcopy, Principles and Practice: An Integrated Textbook and Atlas. W.B. Saunders com.2002.

3. Epidemiology of genital tract human papilloma virus infections. Barbara S. Apgar, Gregory L. Brotzman, Mark Spitzer(eds). Colposcopy, Principles and Practice: An Integrated Textbook and Atlas. W.B. Saunders com.2002;1-22.
4. Human papillomaviruses: Molecular aspects of viral life cycle and pathogenesis. Barbara S. Apgar, Gregory L. Brotzman, Mark Spitzer(eds). Colposcopy, Principles and Practice: An Integrated Textbook and Atlas. W.B. Saunders com.2002; 23-37.
5. Sexually transmitted diseases. Richard L. Sweet, Ronald S. Gibbs(eds) Infectious diseases of female genital tract. Fourth edition. Lippincott Williams and Wilkins. 2002;119-68.
6. Genital tract Infections. Betty A Forbes, Daniel F. Salim, Alice S. Weissfeld (eds). Bailey and Scott's Diagnostic Microbiology. Eleventh edition. Mosby Inc. 2002;939-53.
7. Human papillomavirus. Braunwald, Fauci, Kasper, Hauser, Longe, Jameson(eds). Harrison's Priciples of Internal Medicine. Fifteenth edition 1118-20.
8. Sexually transmitted diseases in the female. V.G. Padubidri, Shirish. N. Daftary (Eds). Shaws Textbook of Gynaecology. Thirteenth edition 135-45.
9. Flowchart on Syndromic Management of Sexually Transmitted Infection. NACO, Ministry of Health and Family Welfare, New Delhi 2004. http://www. nacoonline.org/publication/flowchart.pdf.
10. Sexually transmitted infections—Treatment Guidelines. NACO. http://www.nacoonline.org/publication/stiguideline.pdf.
11. Genitourinary infections and sexually transmitted diseases. Jonathan S. Berek (eds). Novak's Gynaecology.Thirteenth Edition 453-71.
12. Vaginal discharge-cause, diagnosis and treatment. Clinical review. BMJ Vol May 2004;29:328.
13. Infectious vulvovaginitis. Richard L. Sweet, Ronald S. Gibbs (eds) Infectious diseases of female genital tract. Fourth edition. Lippincott Williams and Wilkins. 2002;337-58.

# CHAPTER 13

# Pelvic Inflammatory Disease

Deepti Goswami

Pelvic Inflammatory Disease (PID) refers to inflammatory disorders of upper female genital tract comprising of endometrium, uterus, fallopian tubes and the adenexa. It occurs most frequently secondary to sexually transmitted infections (STIs) in the lower genital tract and is a major cause of morbidity in women in reproductive age group. The clinical spectrum varies from being asymptomatic to endometritis, salpingitis, tubo-ovarian abscess, pelvic peritonitis, generalised peritonitis, septicaemia and death. It can lead to late sequelae in the form of tubal block causing infertility and ectopic pregnancy, and chronic pelvic pain causing much physical and psychological suffering to the woman.[1] Early diagnosis and treatment reduces the incidence of complications associated with PID.

## EPIDEMIOLOGY

### Sexually Transmitted Infections

The risk factors for PID are similar to those for sexually transmitted infections. Ascent of organisms from the lower to the upper genital tract is believed to be the cause of PID. However there may be role of genetic factors as well since not all women with lower genital tract infection develop PID. Other risk factors include past history of STIs, cigarette smoking, vaginal douching and recent insertion of an intrauterine contraceptive device (IUCD).

### Iatrogenic

Procedures involving instrumentation of the cervix may introduce cervical infection to the upper genital tract and can cause PID; for example, termination of pregnancy, hysterosalpingography, or embryo transfer.

### HIV

In the early days of the HIV epidemic it was thought that concomitant PID might be more severe. However subsequent studies have disputed this. Women with PID who are HIV-positive are treated in the same manner as women without HIV and response rates to treatment are comparable.

### Intrauterine Contraceptive Devices (IUCDs)

The risk of PID associated with IUCDs has been shown to be limited to the first few weeks after insertion, reflecting the introduction of bacteria into the upper genital tract during insertion.

The risk of PID in such cases therefore depends on the prevalence of STIs specially *Chlamydia trachomatis* and *Neisseria gonorrhoeae*, which varies among different populations.[2] Even if the relative risk of PID is higher in IUCD users the absolute risk remains very low (one in 1000) and there does not appear to be an increased risk of tubal infertility.[3]

### Oral Contraceptive Pills

The association between the oral contraceptive pill and PID is poorly understood. It was thought that it may reduce the incidence of PID by preventing the ascent of infection by progesterone-induced thickening of cervical mucus and endometrial suppression or a direct steroid effect reducing immune-related damage to the tubal mucosa. However, it may just reduce the prevalence of symptomatic infection and its protective effect has not been conclusively proven.[4]

## AETIOLOGY

A large number of micro-organisms that comprise the vaginal flora (e.g., anaerobes, *Gardnerella vaginalis*, *Haemophilus influenzae*, enteric Gram-negative rods, and *Streptococcus agalactiae*) have been isolated from the upper genital tract of women with PID. However sexually transmitted organisms, especially *Neisseria gonorrhoeae* and *Chlamydia trachomatis* are the primary causes of PID.[5] *Chlamydia* is the more common cause and the risk of PID in young women with chlamydia in the lower genital tract is about 10 per cent.[6]

*Anaerobes* are almost universally found in PID. The enzymes produced by them may weaken the cervical mucous plug favouring ascent of micro-organisms. A higher rate of bacterial vaginosis has been found in women with PID, but its role in pathogenesis is not established. In addition, cytomegalovirus, *Mycoplasma hominis*, and *Ureaplasma urealyticum* may be the etiologic agents in some cases of PID.

*Mycobacterium tuberculosis* can infect the pelvic organs but is not usually found in the lower genital tract. In over 20 percent of cases no organism are isolated from the upper genital tract due to clearance or overgrowth of original chlamydial or gonococcal infection by anaerobic organisms.

*Actinomyces*-like organisms (ALOs) live in the gastrointestinal system as harmless commensals. When found in the female genital tract they are almost exclusively in association with foreign bodies like IUCDs. They can be a rare cause of pelvic infection. The longer the IUCD is in place, the greater the likelihood of finding ALOs on a cervical smear. Limited evidence suggests that an IUCD should be removed in symptomatic women and appropriate antibiotics prescribed. However, there is no evidence to support routine removal in asymptomatic women or to screen those without symptoms.[7]

## PATHOGENESIS

Pathogenesis essentially involves ascending infection along the mucosal surfaces of vagina and cervix to the endometrial cavity and fallopian tubes followed by spill into the abdominal cavity. Adherence of organisms to spermatozoa may facilitate spread of organisms to the upper genital tract. Loss of the cervical mucus plug at the time of menstruation may also facilitate access of bacteria to the endometrium.

The gonococcal infection affects the ciliated cells of fallopian tube which lose their motility and slough with a neutrophilic inflammatory response. *Chlamydia trachomatis* attaches to the tubal epithelium and is engulfed into the tubal cells where it escapes immune recognition. A Th 1-type response occurs initially with production of a range of cytokines, but much of the inflammatory response is secondary to a delayed type hypersensitivity response.

There may be some degree of strain-specific immune protection with gonococcal reinfection and this may reduce the risk of repeated upper genital tract infection. However, with recurrent chlamydial infection there is a greater degree of tubal damage. The inflammation causes fibrosis and occlusion of the tubal lumen. Tubo-ovarian abscess formation is a late manifestation and occurs due to anaerobic bacteria and not due to *N. gonorrhoeae* or *Chlamydia trachomatis*.

## CLINICAL FEATURES

Diagnosis of PID is largely based on clinical findings; however the symptoms and signs associated with PID may be nonspecific while some cases may be asymptomatic. The common symptoms include lower abdominal pain, dyspareunia, vaginal discharge, and abnormal bleeding. Clinical signs include lower abdominal tenderness, mucopurulent cervical or vaginal discharge, adnexal tenderness, and cervical motion tenderness. The signs and symptoms are more severe in cases with tubo-ovarian abscess and pelvic peritonitis. About 60 percent of cases are subclinical, 36 percent have mild to moderate disease, and 4 percent have severe disease. Gonococcal PID often has a more acute presentation in terms of duration and severity of symptoms while long-term sequelae are more common with *Chlamydia*.

## INVESTIGATIONS

### Blood Tests

Inflammatory markers such as white blood cell count, erythrocyte sedimentation rate or C-reactive protein, while correlating with the severity of PID, are not specific and neutrophil counts may not be raised in mild disease. Therefore no individual or combination of blood tests can reliably diagnose PID.[8]

*Endocervical swabs* taken for *N. gonorrhoeae* (culture) and *C. trachomatis* (nucleic acid amplification test—NAAT) can be helpful. Negative tests for these do not exclude diagnosis of PID but, if positive, will support it. In suspected cases the woman is also screened for other sexually transmitted infections.

### Imaging

*Transvaginal ultrasound* scanning is the preferred method but its diagnostic sensitivity will depend upon operator's experience. Transvaginal ultrasound can detect tubo-ovarian abscess or pyosalpinx, but cannot visualise the fallopian tube wall which limits its use in diagnosing less severe disease. Therefore routine use is not justified but it will help detect tubal abscesses.

The newer technique, *power Doppler* imaging may be sensitive enough to detect tubal

The newer technique, *power Doppler* imaging may be sensitive enough to detect tubal hyperaemia suggestive of salpingitis in mild to moderate PID but high level of expertise is required to interpret the scans.[9] Potential limitations include difficulties in differentiating between endometriosis associated masses.

*Magnetic resonance imaging* has also been employed to diagnose PID but is not used in clinical practice due to cost, lack of access and limited experience with this modality.

*Laparoscopy* is considered to be the "gold standard" for diagnosing PID as it can be used to obtain a more accurate diagnosis of salpingitis and a more complete bacteriologic diagnosis; however it is invasive, expensive and impractical in an outpatient setting. The findings are subjective and one may miss subtle inflammation of the fallopian tubes where there is little visible hyperaemia on the serosa of the tube. Moreover it will not detect endometritis. Thus, it is not 100 percent sensitive and is subject to interoperator and intraoperator variability.[10] Often it is not readily available, and its use is not easy to justify when symptoms are mild or vague. Consequently, a diagnosis of PID usually is based on clinical findings. Indications for laparoscopy are rather limited and include cases where the diagnosis remains in doubt, the woman is unwell and there is no response to antibiotics within 72 hours.

*Others* If urinary tract infection is suspected, urine microscopy should be performed and a midstream urine sample should be sent for culture. Endometrial sampling is not helpful.

## DIAGNOSIS

Diagnosis of PID is largely based on clinical findings even though the sensitivity and specificity of a clinical diagnosis is around 50 per cent. The traditional triad of lower abdominal pain, cervical motion tenderness, and adnexal pain are still taught as the classic findings for diagnosing PID. However there is insufficient evidence to support existing diagnostic criteria, which have been based on a combination of empirical data and expert opinion.[11] Many episodes of PID may well be asymptomatic and go unrecognised. There is no cheap, simple and accurate diagnostic test and laboratory criteria are neither highly specific nor sensitive.[12] The clinical and investigational parameters which, often in combination, aid in diagnosing PID are summarised in Box 13.1.

**Box 13.1**

Uterine/adnexal or cervical motion tenderness

- Oral temperature >101 degrees F (> 38.3 degrees C)
- Abnormal cervical or vaginal mucopurulent discharge
- Presence of white blood cells on saline microscopy of vaginal secretions
- Elevated erythrocyte sedimentation rate
- Elevated C-reactive protein
- Laboratory documentation of cervical infection with *N. gonorrhoeae* or *C. trachomatis*
- Histopathological evidence of endometriosis on endometrial biopsy
- Transvaginal sonography or magnetic resonance imaging techniques showing pyosalpinx or tubo-ovarian mass with or without free pelvic fluid
- Laparoscopic abnormalities consistent with pelvic inflammatory disease

## DIFFERENTIAL DIAGNOSIS

It is vital to exclude the possibility of an *ectopic pregnancy*. There may be a history of amenorrhoea with lower abdominal pain, initially unilateral. Therefore it is advisable to perform a pregnancy test on all sexually active women of childbearing age presenting with these symptoms. *Endometriosis* and *ovarian cyst accidents* (like torsion and haemorrhage) are other differential diagnosis. *Gastrointestinal* or *urinary tract pathology* should be excluded by enquiring about bowel and urinary symptoms.

## MANAGEMENT

Empiric treatment of PID should be initiated in sexually-active young women and other women at risk for STDs if the following minimum criteria are present and no other cause for the illness can be identified:

- Uterine/adnexal tenderness
- Cervical motion tenderness

Additional criteria that support a diagnosis of PID are given in Box 13.1.Aims of treatment include achievement of microbiologic cure, alleviation of signs and symptoms, and prevention of sequelae and transmission.

PID treatment regimens must provide empiric, broad-spectrum coverage of likely pathogens that is *N. gonorrhoeae*, *C. trachomatis* and anaerobes.[13,14] Common antimicrobials used include quinolones, cephalosporins, metronidazole, doxycycline, and azithromycin. *C.trachomatis* is rarely resistant but gonococcal resistance is common, where third generation cephalosporins may be preferred. Choice of regimen is influenced by local strain sensitivities, patient tolerance, history of allergy, severity of disease, availability of drug and its cost. Most patients prefer oral therapy.

Antibiotic treatment should be commenced as soon as possible, ideally within two days of the onset of symptoms. Delay or inadequate treatment is associated with long term sequelae including tubal infertility and chronic pelvic pain.[15] Supportive measures would include pain management for which ibuprofen or diclofenac can be used.

Most cases can be managed on an *outpatient* basis. The combination of doxycycline and metronidazole is widely used. Some recent studies have reported that 1 gram of azithromycin as a single dose is highly effective in eradicating *C. trachomatis*.[16] Azithromycin alone (1 gram as a single dose) or in combination with metronidazole is effective in treating PID. Caution should be exercised while prescribing ofloxacin as there have been some reports of significant psychiatric adverse effects with this drug. All patients who are treated on an outpatient basis must be followed within 72 hours. They should demonstrate substantial clinical improvement (e.g. defervescence; reduction in abdominal tender-ness; and reduction in uterine, adnexal, and cervical motion tenderness) within 3 days after initiation of therapy. Any patient who does not show significant clinical improvement with oral regimen should be re-evaluated and given parenteral therapy on inpatient basis.

## Syndromic Management

The syndromic approach to STD and resulting PID case management is based on the identification of a relatively constant combination of symptoms and signs (Syndrome) and on knowledge of the most common causative organisms of these syndromes and their antimicrobial susceptibility. This approach offers no definitive diagnosis; the patient is treated for all the possible infections that could cause the syndrome.

Symptomatic management has been advocated in the developing countries. Clinical algorithms based on symptoms and signs are used to select patients who should receive antimicrobial therapy. Even in resource-rich environments, syndromic management is sometimes practiced as in cases where the offending pathogens become undetectable in the lower genital tract necessitating treatment based on the presumed cause (including *C. trachomatis*).

Advantages in resource poor settings include immediate treatment and avoidance of the costs associated with laboratory tests. The main disadvantage is the cost of over diagnosis and over treatment when multiple antimicrobials are given to the patient with no infection and also there is a potential for developing antibiotic resistance. This approach is unable to identify persons with asymptomatic infection.

Syndromic approach for PID as advocated by the National AIDS Control Organisation (NACO) is given below in Box 13.2 and 13.3.[17]

*Hospitalisation* Indications for *inpatient* management with parenteral therapy are summarised in Box 13.4. Duration of treatment should be 14 days. Review at 48 to 72 hours is advised. Most patients on parenteral treatment show clinical improvement by this time and can be switched to oral regimen. Failure to respond would indicate a change to parenteral therapy, the possible need for surgical intervention or an incorrect diagnosis.

Some specialists also recommend rescreening for *C. tra-chomatis* and *N. gonorrhoeae* 4 to 6 weeks after therapy is completed in women with documented infection with these pathogens to assess compliance and outcome. Patients should desist from sexual intercourse until they, and their partners, have completed treatment and follow-up. An explanation of the condition and the possibility of long-term sequelae should be emphasised. Rest in bed is advised in moderate or severe cases.

The drug regimens for parenteral therapy as suggested by Center for Disease Control and Prevention (CDC), USA are given below.[18]

### *Parenteral Regimen A*

- Cefotetan or cefoxitin plus doxycycline
- Other second-or third-generation cepha-losporins such as ceftizoxime, cefotaxime, ceftriaxone in place of cefotetan or cefoxitin
- Clindamycin or metronidazole in addition to doxycycline.

- *Cefotetan* 2 g intravenously every 12 hours

or

- *Cefoxitin* 2 g intravenously every 6 hours

## Box 13.2

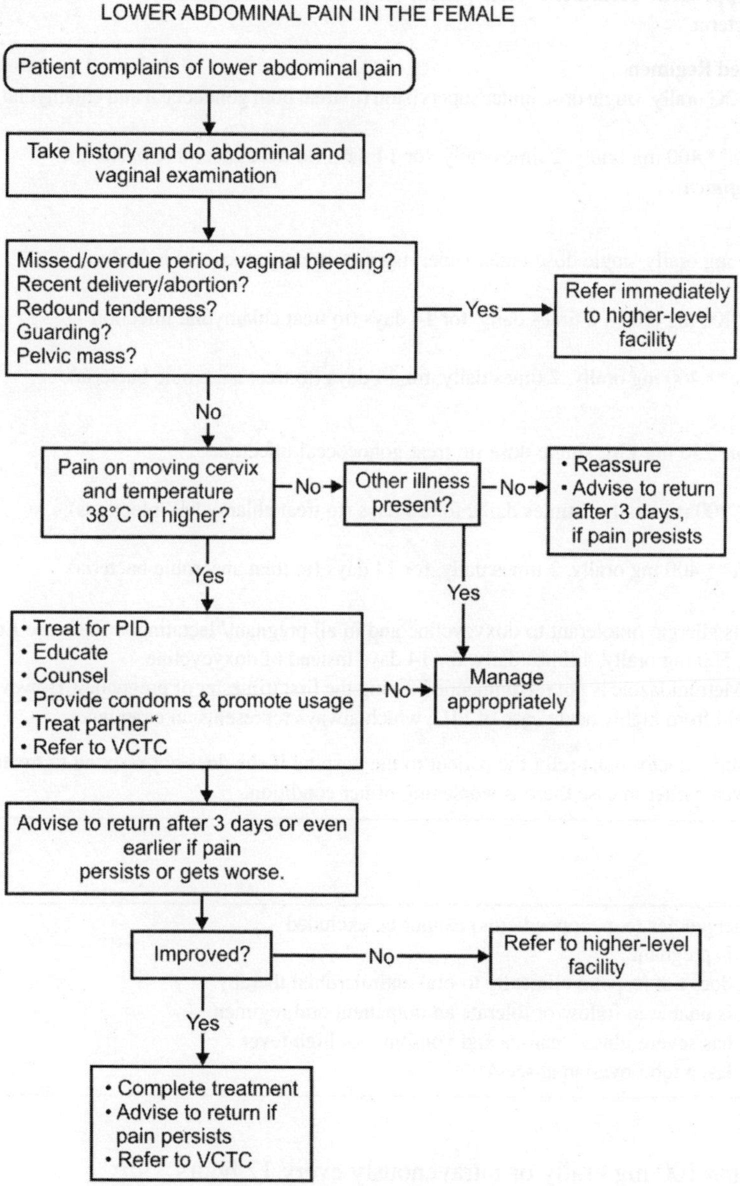
LOWER ABDOMINAL PAIN IN THE FEMALE
Patient complains of lower abdominal pain
Take history and do abdominal and vaginal examination
Missed/overdue period, vaginal bleeding? Recent delivery/abortion? Redound tendemess? Guarding? Pelvic mass?
Yes
Refer immediately to higher-level facility
No
Pain on moving cervix and temperature 38°C or higher?
No
Other illness present?
No
• Reassure • Advise to return after 3 days, if pain presists
Yes
Yes
• Treat for PID • Educate • Counsel • Provide condoms & promote usage • Treat partner* • Refer to VCTC
No
Manage appropriately
Advise to return after 3 days or even earlier if pain persists or gets worse.
Improved?
No
Refer to higher-level facility
Yes
• Complete treatment • Advise to return if pain persists • Refer to VCTC

* Treat partner for gonococcal and chlamydial infections.

**VCTC**—Voluntary Counselling and Testing Centre

## Box 13.3

**Syndromic approach: Treatment** Treat patient for gonococcal and chlamydial infection as well as for anaerobic bacteria.

**Recommended Regimen**
*Azithromycin* 2G orally, single dose under supervision (to treat both gonococcal and chlamydial infections).
*Plus*
*Metronidazole*** 400 mg orally, 2 times daily, for 14 days (to treat anaerobic bacteria).
***Alternate Regimen***

**Option 1**
*Cefixime* 400 mg orally single dose under supervision (to treat gonococcal infection)
*Plus*
*Doxycycline** 100 mg orally, 2 times daily, for 14 days (to treat chlamydial infection )
*Plus*
*Metronidazole*** 400 mg orally, 2 times daily, for 14 days (to treat anaerobic bacteria).

**Option 2**
*Inj. ceftriaxone* 250 mg I.M, single dose (to treat gonococcal infection)
*Plus*
*Doxycycline** 100 mg orally, 2 times daily, for 14 days (to treat chlamydial infections),
*Plus*
*Metronidazole*** 400 mg orally, 2 times daily, for 14 days (to treat anaerobic bacteria)

*In individuals allergic /intolerant to doxycycline and in all pregnant/ lactating women use Erythromycin base/stearate, 500 mg orally, 4 times daily, for 14 days instead of doxycycline.
**Generally, Metronidazole is not recommended during the first trimester of pregnancy. However, it should not be withheld from highly acute case of PID, which always represents an emergency.

*Caution*: Treating doctor must refer the patient to the hospital if she does not respond to treatment within 3 days and even earlier in case there is worsening of her condition.

## Box 13.4

- Surgical emergencies (e.g., appendicitis) cannot be excluded
- The patient is pregnant
- The patient does not respond clinically to oral antimicrobial therapy
- The patient is unable to follow or tolerate an outpatient oral regimen
- The patient has severe illness, nausea and vomiting, or high fever
- The patient has a tubo-ovarian abscess

PLUS

- *Doxycycline* 100 mg orally or intravenously every 12 hours

Because of pain associated with infusion, doxycycline should be administered orally when possible, even when the patient is hospitalised. Both oral and intravenous administration of doxycycline provides similar bioavailability. Parenteral therapy may be discontinued 24 hours after a patient improves clinically, and oral therapy with doxycycline (100 mg twice a day) should continue to complete 14 days of therapy.

When tubo-ovarian abscess is present, clindamycin or metronidazole with doxycycline can be used for continued therapy rather than doxycycline alone, because it provides more effective anaerobic coverage.

Clinical data are limited regarding the use of *other second- or third-generation cephalosporins (e.g., ceftizoxime, cefotaxime, and ceftriaxone)*, which also may be effective therapy for PID and may replace cefotetan or cefoxitin. However, these cephalosporins are less active than cefotetan or cefoxitin against anaerobic bacteria.

### *Parenteral Regimen B*

- Clindamycin plus gentamicin intravenously
- Doxycycline or clindamycin orally following intravenous therapy

- *Clindamycin* 900 mg intravenously every 8 hours

PLUS

- *Gentamicin* loading dose intravenously or intramuscularly (2 mg/kg of body weight) followed by a maintenance dose (1.5 mg/kg) every 8 hours. Single daily dosing may be substituted.

### *Alternative Parenteral Regimens*

- Ofloxacin or levofloxacin with or without metronidazole
- Ampicillin/sulbactam plus doxycycline

- *Ampicillin/Sulbactam* 3 g intravenously every 6 hours

PLUS

- *Doxycycline* 100 mg orally or intravenously every 12 hours

Preliminary data suggest that levofloxacin is as effective as ofloxacin and its single daily dosing improves compliance.

Intravenous ofloxacin has been investigated as a single agent; however because of concerns regarding its spectrum, metronidazole may be included in the regimen.

## Oral Treatment

The following regimens provide coverage against the frequent etiologic agents of PID.

### *Regimen A*

- Ofloxacin or levofloxacin with or without metronidazole

- *Ofloxacin* 400 mg orally twice a day for 14 days

OR

- *Levofloxacin* 500 mg orally once daily for 14 days with or without
- *Metronidazole* 500 mg orally twice a day for 14 days

Oral ofloxacin has been found to be effective against both *N. gonorrhoeae* and *C. trachomatis*, though lack of anaerobic coverage with ofloxacin is a concern. Addition of metronidazole to the treatment regimen provides this coverage. Preliminary data suggest that levofloxacin is as effective as ofloxacin and its single daily dosing improves compliance.

In the earlier CDC recommendations, oral *ciprofloxacin* 500 mg twice a day was included but not in the latest guidelines due to increasing resistance of gonococci to this drug. In India ciprofloxacin is still commonly used in management of PID. Ultimately the drug resistance pattern in a population should guide choice of antibiotics for PID.

*Regimen B*

- Ceftriaxone intramuscularly once
- Cefoxitin intramuscularly plus probenecid orally
- Other parenteral third-generation cephalosporins (e.g., ceftizoxime or cefotaxime) plus doxycycline orally
- Addition of metronidazole to above regimens

- *Ceftriaxone* 250 mg intramuscularly in a single dose

OR

- *Cefoxitin* 2 g intramuscularly in a single dose and *Probenecid*, 1 g orally administered concurrently in a single dose

OR

- Other parenteral third-generation *cephalosporin* (e.g., *ceftizoxime* or *cefotaxime*)

PLUS

- *Doxycycline* 100 mg orally twice a day for 14 days

WITH or WITHOUT

- *Metronidazole* 500 mg orally twice a day for 14 days

The optimal choice of a cephalosporin for Regimen B is unclear; although cefoxitin has better anaerobic coverage, ceftriaxone has better coverage against *N. gonorrhoeae*. Clinical trials have demonstrated that a single dose of cefoxitin is effective in obtaining short-term clinical response in women who have PID; however, the theoretical limitations in its coverage of anaerobes may require the addition of metronidazole to the treatment regimen. The metronidazole also will effectively treat bacterial vaginosis, which is frequently associated with PID. No data have been published regarding the use of oral cephalosporins for the treatment of PID. Limited data suggest that the combination of oral metronidazole plus doxycycline after primary parenteral therapy is safe and effective.

*Alternative Oral Regimens*

- Amoxycillin/clavulanic acid plus doxycycline
- Azithromycin
- Amoxicillin/clavulanic acid plus doxycycline was effective in obtaining short-term clinical response in a single clinical trial; however, gastrointestinal symptoms might limit compliance with this regimen. Azithromycin with or without metronidazole is also used as oral treatment regimen for PID.

### Management of Sex Partners

Evaluation and treatment of male partner are imperative because of the risk for reinfection of the patient and the strong likelihood of urethral gonococcal or chlamydial infection in the sex partner. Repeated chlamydial infection has been shown to increase the risk of PID and long-term sequelae. The relative risk of an ectopic pregnancy following one episode of *C. trachomatis* is 1, increasing to a relative risk of 11 with three episodes of infection. Male partners of women who have PID caused by *C. trachomatis* and/or *N. gonorrhoeae* often are asymptomatic. They should ideally be screened for chlamydia and gonorrhoea. They are treated empirically with regimens effective against both of these infections, regardless of the etiology of PID or pathogens isolated from the infected woman. Azithromycin 1 g stat is commonly used for this purpose.

## PREVENTION

Prevention of *Chlamydia* infection by screening and treating high-risk women reduces the incidence of PID.[19] Theoretically, most cases of PID can be prevented by screening all women or those determined to be at high-risk (based on age or other factors) using deoxyribonucleic acid (DNA) amplification on cervical specimens (in women receiving pelvic examination) and on urine (in women not undergoing this check up). In some of the western countries viz, Sweden, in some US states and in UK screening programmes for *C. trachomatis* are in place since majority of women with chlamydial infection present with atypical symptoms or are asymptomatic. However there is no such screening program in our country.

Although *bacterial vaginosis* is associated with PID, whether the incidence of PID can be reduced by identifying and treating women with bacterial vaginosis is unclear.

The effectiveness of antibiotic prophylaxis in women having an *IUCD insertion* remains unproved. A Cochrane review suggests that administration of doxycycline 200 mg immediately did not reduce an already low rate of PID following IUCD insertion.[20] The World Health Organisation expert working group on recommendations for contraceptive use concluded that there was no additional benefit to be gained by removing an IUCD in a woman diagnosed with mild to moderate PID who had been commenced on antibiotics.[21] If the woman wants it to be removed, this should take place only after antibiotics have been started. It should however be removed if, at review, there is no clinical improvement.

Education, use of barrier methods, and provision of preventive health care to sex workers are some of the *public health measures* that will help reduce the incidence of sexually transmitted infections and PID.

## SPECIAL CONSIDERATIONS

### Pregnancy

Because of the high risk for maternal morbidity, fetal wastage, and preterm delivery, pregnant women who have suspected PID should be hospitalised and treated with parenteral antibiotics.

There is no consensus on the optimal antibiotic regimen, though treatment with ceftriaxone, cefixime, or procaine penicillin plus probenecid is effective. This is combined with erythromycin, 500 mg, 4 times daily for seven days, to eliminate chlamydia. Azithromycin is a Class B pregnancy drug and would be effective monotherapy. Quinolones (e.g., ciprofloxacin and ofloxacin) are to be avoided as these are contraindicated during pregnancy.

## HIV Infection

HIV-infected women with PID have similar symptoms as uninfected controls. The microbiologic findings for HIV-positive and HIV-negative women are reported to be similar, except for higher rates of concomitant *M. hominis*, *Candida*, streptococcal, and human papilloma virus (HPV) infections among those with HIV infection. They are more likely to have a tubo-ovarian abscess, but respond equally well to standard parenteral and oral antibiotic regimens. Whether the management of immunodeficient HIV-infected women with PID requires more aggressive interventions (e.g., hospitalisation or parenteral antimicrobial regimens) has not been determined. At present it is advocated that women with PID who are HIV positive may be treated in the same manner as women without HIV.[22]

## Key Points

- PID occurs due to ascending infection from lower genital tract. Sexually transmitted organisms, especially *Neisseria gonorrhoeae* and *Chlamydia trachomatis* are the primary causes of PID. Subsequently anaerobes take over.
- Clinical diagnosis of PID is often imprecise as there is no single historical, physical, or laboratory finding that is both sensitive and specific for the diagnosis of acute PID.
- It is vital to exclude the possibility of an ectopic pregnancy.
- Because of the difficulty in diagnosis and the potential for long term sequelae even following mild or atypical PID, clinicians should maintain a low threshold for the diagnosis of PID.
- Antibiotics for treatment should provide broad-spectrum coverage of likely pathogens that is *N. gonorrhoeae*, *C. trachomatis* and anaerobes.
- Symptomatic management has been advocated in the developing countries for the management of STDs and PID using clinical algorithms based on symptoms and signs without laboratory investigations. Antibiotics likely to cover the major causal agents are prescribed.
- Patient should be reviewed at 72 hours and any worsening requires hospitalisation and treatment with parenteral antibiotics.
- Evaluation and treatment of male partner are imperative.
- Prevention of *Chlamydia* infection by screening and treating high-risk women reduces the incidence of PID.

## REFERENCES

1. Westrom L, Joesoef R, Reynolds G, Hagdu A, Thompson SE. Pelvic inflammatory disease and fertility. A cohort study of 1,844 women with laparoscopically verified disease and 657 control women with normal laparoscopic results. Sex Transm Dis 1992;19(4):185-92.
2. Steen R, Shapiro K. Intrauterine contraceptive devices and risk of pelvic inflammatory disease: standard of care in high STI prevalence settings. Reprod Health Matters 2004;12(23):136-43.
3. Ross JDC. An update on pelvic inflammatory disease. Sex Transm Inf 2002;78:18-19.
4. Ness RB, Soper DE, Holley RL, et al. Hormonal and barrier contraception and risk of upper genital tract disease in the PID Evaluation and Clinical Health (PEACH) study. Am J Obstet Gynecol 2001;185:121–27.

5. Bevan CD, Johal BJ, Mumtaz G, Ridgway GL, Siddle NC. Clinical, laparoscopic and microbiological findings in acute salpingitis: report on a United Kingdom cohort.Br J Obstet Gynaecol 1995;102(5):407-14.
6. Westrom L, Svensson L, Wolner-Hansen P, Mardh PA. Chlamydial and gonococcal infections in a defined population of women.Scand J Infect Dis Suppl 1982;32:157-62.
7. Penney G, Brechin S, de Souza A, et al. Faculty of Family Planning and Reproductive Health Care Clinical Effectiveness Unit. FFPRHC Guidance (January 2004). The copper intrauterine device as long-term contraception. J Fam Plann Reprod Health Care. 2004;30(1):29-41.
8. Hall MN, Leach L, Beck E. Clinical inquiries. Which blood tests are most helpful in evaluating pelvic inflammatory disease? J Fam Pract 2004;53(4):326,330-1.
9. Molander P, Sjoberg J, Paavonen J, et al. Transvaginal power Doppler findings in laparoscopically proven acute pelvic inflammatory disease. Ultrasound Obstet Gynecol 2001;17:233–38.
10. Molander P, Finne P, Sjoberg J, Sellors J, Paavonen J. Observer agreement with laparoscopic diagnosis of pelvic inflammatory disease using photographs.Obstet Gynecol 2003;101(5 Pt 1):875-80.
11. Simms I, Warburton F, Westrom L. Diagnosis of pelvic inflammatory disease: time for a rethink. Sex Transm Infect 2003;79(6):491-4.7.
12. Gaitan H, Angel E, Diaz R, Parada A, Sanchez L, Vargas C. Accuracy of five different diagnostic techniques in mild-to-moderate pelvic inflammatory disease. Infect Dis Obstet Gynecol 2002;10(4):171-80.
13. Beigi RH, Wiesenfeld HC. Pelvic inflammatory disease: new diagnostic criteria and treatment. Obstet Gynecol Clin North Am 2003;30(4):777-793.
14. Ross JD. Pelvic inflammatory disease: how should it be managed? Curr Opin Infect Dis 2003;16(1):37-41.
15. Hillis SD, Joesoef R, Marchbanks PA, et al. Delayed care of pelvic inflammatory disease as a risk factor for impaired fertility. Am J Obstet Gynecol 1993;168:1503–9.
16. Rustomjee R, Kharsany AB, Connolly CA, Karim SS. A randomized controlled trial of azithromycin versus doxycycline/ciprofloxacin for the syndromic management of sexually transmitted infections in a resource-poor setting. J Antimicrob Chemother 2002;49(5):875-78.
17. Flow Charts on the Syndromic Management of Sexually Transmitted Infections. National AIDS Control Organisation, Ministry of Health and Family Welfare, Government of India. New Delhi 2004.
18. Centers for Disease Control and Prevention. Pelvic inflammatory disease. Sexually transmitted diseases treatment guidelines. MMWR Recomm Rep 2002;51(RR-6):48-52.
19. Honey E, Templeton A. Prevention of pelvic inflammatory disease by the control of C. trachomatis infection. Int J Gynaecol Obstet 2002;78(3):257-61.
20. Grimes DA, Schulz KF. Antibiotic prophylaxis for intrauterine contraceptive device insertion. Cochrane Database Syst Rev 2000;(2):CD001327.
21. Grimes DA. Intrauterine device and upper-genital-tract infection. Lancet 2000;356(9234):1013-9.
22. Bukusi EA, Cohen CR, Stevens CE, et al. Effects of human imunodeficiency virus 1 infection on microbial origins of pelvic inflammatory disease and on efficacy of ambulatory oral therapy. Am J Obstet Gynecol 1999;181(6):1374-81.

CHAPTER 14

# Antimicrobials in Pregnancy

Swaraj Batra, Poonam Sachdeva, Neha Gami

Pregnancy is a normal physiological state. However, infections may occur in pregnancy and in such cases antibiotic administration becomes unavoidable. All antibiotics have the potential to affect the foetus and our knowledge about the long term effect of drugs on the foetus is still meagre and evolving. Also due to altered pharmacokinetics of all drugs during pregnancy, the unwanted effects of the drugs may be more severe during pregnancy as compared to the non-gravid state. Hence, there should be a rational use of antibiotics in pregnancy in indicated situations.

## Physiological Changes Affecting Metabolism during Pregnancy

A pregnant woman undergoes a number of physiological changes. There is an increase in total body water of approximately 8 litres.[1] Total body fat and body weight are also increased significantly. Plasma volume expands and albumin concentration decreases while $\alpha$ 1 acid glycoprotein increases. Due to the effect of progestogens gastrointestinal motility is decreased resulting in decreased gastric emptying and thus delayed absorption of drugs. Pregnancy related nausea and vomiting aggravates the situation.There is increase in renal blood flow resulting in faster elimination of polar drugs. The hepatic microsomal enzymes undergo induction resulting in faster metabolism of drugs. All these physiological changes contribute to altered absorption, distribution and elimination during pregnancy.

Knowledge of the altered pharmacokinetics in pregnancy is useful for calculating maternal dosages. The altered metabolism in pregnancy may result in a change in the amount or frequency of the dose.

Another important aspect is the route of administration. Antibiotics are distributed more rapidly after an intravenous injection than an intramuscular route. As mentioned, delayed gastric emptying and concomitant nausea and vomiting during pregnancy may significantly affect absorption of oral antibiotics. Serum levels of the antibiotics have been found to be lower in gravidas than in nonpregnant women. This difference is attributed to altered gastrointestinal motility and change in volume of distribution, coupled with an increase in glomerular filteration and renal clearance that occurs during pregnancy. Because of this change higher levels of antibiotics have been found in the urine of gravidas as compared to non-pregnant women.

An additional compartment, i.e. placenta and foetus removes the antibiotics from maternal serum, significantly affecting the distribution of antibiotics administered to the mother. Also, cellular response to infection is decreased during pregnancy and humoral response is increased. Thus, diseases which evoke a cellular response can become more virulent in pregnancy, e.g. Tuberculosis, malaria, coccidiomycosis, listeriosis and in HIV-positive patients, the CD4 count can fall.

## Placental Transfer

Placental transfer of various drugs occurs by several methods including simple diffusion and active transport system. Most drugs transfer across the placenta by simple diffusion. Drugs which have low molecular weight,high lipid solubility and low protein binding are most readily transferred.

Protein binding of antibiotics is an important aspect. Protein binding is reversible and albumin is the primary protein involved in the process. The bound portion of the antibiotic depends on the protein concentration, antibiotic concentration, competition with other drugs for binding sites and displacement from binding sites. Clinical significance of protein binding lies in the fact that only unbound portion of the drug is available to act against the organism. In addition, displacement of other molecules such as bilirubin with the administration of sulpha drugs is also extremely important.

Foetal pharmacokinetics are difficult to ascertain as most of the blood in the umbilical vein bypasses the liver, allowing higher concentrations of antimicrobials to arrive at the fetal heart and central nervous system. Therefore a drug safe for the mother may result in toxic doses to the foetus.

## Possible Role of Antimicrobials on Fertilised Ovum

From fertilisation to implantation ( i.e. conception to implantation) the deleterious effect on the foetus will/may result in abortion.

The teratogenic risk period in human beings lasts from 31 days through 10 weeks from the last menstrual period, during which the drugs may affect organogenesis.

## Types of Antibiotics and Their Effects

The Food and Drug Adminstration (FDA) has divided the drugs into categories according to foetal risk involved (Table 14.1). Currently no antibiotic comes under category A (safe). Most fall into categories B and C. Category B drugs are relatively safe in pregnancy and if possible an antibiotic should be chosen from category B. When maternal infection requires treatment with category C, the risks and benefits should be considered. Category D drugs should be avoided. However, sometimes even drugs in category D are required, e.g.

- For immunosuppression in gravidas undergoing renal allograft.
- Antiepileptic agents for pregnant patients

**Table 14.1:** Food and Drug Administration foetal risk drug categories

| *Category* | *Description* |
|---|---|
| A | No foetal risk; proven safe for use during pregnancy |
| B | Foetal risk not demonstrated in animal or human studies |
| C | Foetal risk unknown; not adequate human studies |
| D | Some evidence of foetal risk; may be necessary to use this drug |
| X | Proven foetal risk; contraindicated for use in pregnancy |

**Table 14.2:** Antimicrobials and antiparasitic drugs' safety profile during pregnancy

| *Type of drug* | *Category* | | | | |
|---|---|---|---|---|---|
| | *A* | *B* | *C* | *D* | *X* |
| ***Antibacterial*** | | Penicillins | Gentamicin | Tetracyclins | |
| | | Cephalosporins | Amikacin | Streptomycin | |
| | | Erythromycin[i] | Vancomycin | Tobramycin | |
| | | Clindamycin | Chloramphenicol | | |
| | | Sulphonamides | Fluoroquinolones | | |
| | | Nitrofurantoin | Nitrofurantoin [ii] | | |
| | | Rifampicin | | | |
| | | Ethambutol | Isoniazid | | |
| | | | p-aminosalicylic acid | | |
| | | | Pyrazinamide | | |
| | | | Cycloserine | | |
| | | | Trimethoprim-sulpha Methoxazole | | |
| ***Antivirals*** | | Ritonavir | Lamivudine | | |
| | | Saquinavir | Stamuvidine | | |
| | | Valacyclovir | Acyclovir | | |
| | | | Amantadine | | |
| | | | Vidarabine | | |
| | | | Idoxuridine | | |
| | | | Ganciclovir | | |
| | | | Nevirapine | | |
| ***Antifungals-vaginal*** | | Nystatin | Butoconazole | | |
| | | | Clotrimazole | | |
| | | | Miconazole | | |
| ***-Oral or IV Preparations*** | | Amphotericin B | Ketoconazole | | |
| | | | Fluconazole | | |
| | | | Griseofulvin | | |
| ***Antiparasitic*** | | Metronidazole | Mebendazole | Metronidazole[iii] | Quinine |
| | | | Albendazole | | |
| | | | Ivermectin | | |
| | | | Chloroquine | | |
| | | Praziquantel | Mefloquine | | |
| | | Piperazine | Primaquine | | |
| | | | Pyrimethamine | | |
| ***Vaccines*** | | | All vaccines | | |

i. Except Erythromycin estolate[2]

ii. In the third trimester Nitrofurantoin may cause hemolytic anaemia in the newborn which is related to immature liver and G6PD deficiency.[2]

iii. In the first trimester.[2]

## Choice of Drugs

Antimicrobial drugs can be started based on clinical diagnosis, e.g. tuberculosis, malaria, venereal diseases. In severely ill patients like patients in septicemia broad spectrum antibiotics can be started. In cases with bacteriological diagnosis like in urinary tract infection specific antibiotics can be stared depending upon the sensitivity reports.

Failure to respond to antimicrobials may take place in wrongly- selected patients or in patients where there is a barrier to access of the drug like in multiple pus pockets with loculi or in patients with low host resistance, as integrity of the host defence plays a critical role in overcoming an infection, inadequate dosages, and resistant organisms. Sometimes spurious drugs may add to the problem.

## Prophylactic Antibiotics

There is a definite role of antibiotics for preventing the setting in of an infection or suppressing contacted infection before it becomes clinically evident. In pregnancy prophylactic antibiotics are used to prevent intrapartum and postpartum infections in patients with Rheumatic heart disease, diabetes, anaemia, patients in need of surgical intervention and patients who have undergone lower segment caesarian section(LSCS). In a study conducted in Lok Nayak Hospital, Sulbacin ( Ampicillin 1 gm + Sulbactam 0.5 gm) given half hour before LSCS was more effective than postoperative Ampicillin + gentamicin given for 7 days.[3] Another indication for antibiotics is before termination of pregnancy where even drugs usually contraindicated during pregnancy can be given. In a study in Lok Nayak Hospital, a single shot of Ciprofloxacin before MTP was as effective in preventing postoperative morbidity as postoperative oral ciprofloxacin for 7 days.[4]

When indicated vaccines may be administered to pregnant patients. Although all vaccines belong to FDA category C, vaccines based on inactivated bacterial toxins, inactivated bacteria or bacterial components or inactivated virus may be administered. However live attenuated bacterial and live viral vaccines are contraindicated in pregnancy.

**Table 14.3:** Indications for use of antimicrobials during pregnancy with few examples

| *Bacterial infections* | *Sexually transmited diseases* | *Protozoal and helminthic infestations* |
|---|---|---|
| Rheumatic fever | Syphilis | Ascariasis |
| Urinary tract infection | Gonorrhoea | Hookworm |
| Chorioamnionitis | *Chlamydia* | Tapeworm |
| Bacteremia | Bacterial vaginosis | Malaria |
| Septic shock | Granuloma inguinale | Toxoplasmosis |
| Septic abortion | Chancroid | |
| Postpartum endometritis | Trichomoniasis | |
| Infective endocarditis | | |
| Listeriosis | | |
| Group B β hemolytic *Streptococcus* | | |
| Tuberculosis | | |
| *Fungal infections* | *Viral* | *Cancer chemotherapy* |
| Superficial candidiasis | Herpes simplex | Germ cell tumours |
| Systemic candidiasis | HIV | |

**Table 14.4:** Prescriptions in common usage

| *Condition* | *Prescription* |
|---|---|
| Syphilis [5] | Primary, Secondary and Early Latent (upto 1 year)—Benzathine penicillin G 2.4 MU i/m single dose<br>Late Latent ( > 1 year)—Benzathine penicillin G 2.4 MU i/m weekly × 3 weeks<br>Neurosyphilis—Aqueous crystalline Penicillin G 3-4 MU i/v every 4 hours for 10-14 days<br>Or<br>Aqueous procaine penicillin 2.4 MU i/m daily + Probenecid 500 mg orally 4 times a day × 10-14 days<br>Penicillin sensitive patients should undergo desensitization.<br>Tetracyclines are effective but are not recommended because of risk of yellow brown discolouration of the foetal decidual teeth. |
| Gonorrhoea | Ceftriaxone 125 mg i/m single dose<br>Or Cefixime 400 mg orally single dose<br>Or Spectinomycin 2 gm i/m single dose |
| Toxoplasmosis | Spiramycin 3g/day or 3 MIU twice or three times a day for three weeks. Repeat the course at two weeks interval till delivery.<br>OR<br>Pyrimethamine (25 mg/day )+ Sulfadiazine (50-100 mg/ day) +<br>Folinic acid 5 mg/day<br>OR<br>Pyrimethamine 25 mg/day + sulphadoxine (500 mg )<br>2 tablets weekly till delivery. |
| *Chlamydia trachomatis* [5] | Erythromycin base 500 mg orally 4 times daily for 7 days<br>Or Amoxicillin 500 mg orally three times daily for 7 days |
| Bacterial vaginosis [5] | Clindamycin 300 mg twice a day for 7 days<br>Metronidazole 250 mg three times a day for 7 days or 2 gms orally single dose. |
| Malaria [5] | Tab Chloroquine 800 mg stat followed by<br>400 mg 6-8 hours later and<br>400 mg OD for 2 days. |
| Chorioamnionitis and Postpartum endometritis [5] | Amoxicillin 500 mg IV 8 hourly or Ampicillin 500 mg IV 6 hourly<br>+ Gentamicin 1-1.5 mg/kg IM or IV 8 hourly<br>+ Metronidazole 500 mg IV 8 hourly<br>OR<br>Amoxicillin 500 mg IV 8 hourly or Ampicillin 500 mg IV 6 hourly<br>+ Cefuroxime 0.75 gm- 1.5 gm IM or IV 8 hourly<br>+ Metronidazole 500 mg IV 8 hourly<br>OR<br>Clindamycin 200-600 mg IV 8 hourly<br>+ Gentamicin 1-1.5 mg/kg IM or IV 8 hourly |

## Penicillins

Penicillins are considered the safest antibiotics in pregnancy. They are bactericidal acting through inhibition of bacterial cell wall synthesis. Penicillin group covers gram-positive cocci and bacilli. However, gram-negative bacilli (except for *E.coli* and *Proteus*) *M.tuberculosis*, *Chlamydia*, *Rickettsia*, protozoa, fungi and viruses are totally insensitive to penicillins.

Penicillin G remains the drug of choice for syphillis and group B streptococcal infections in pregnancy.[6] Pregnant women with syphillis who are allergic to penicillin should undergo desensitization and then receive treatment with penicillin G.

Many aerobic and anaerobic bacteria contain beta lactamase enzymes which may render a specific antibiotic ineffective. Because of increasing resistance to bacteria to some of the penicillins, newer agents have been developed that contain a beta lactamase inhibitor such as clavulanic acid, sulbactam and tazobactam.They provide excellent coverage against the mixed aerobic and anerobic "polymicrobial" infections encountered in post caesarian metritis.[6]

Penicillins may cause adverse maternal effects such as hypersensitivity reactions, nausea, diarrhoea, central nervous system irritability and phlebitis. Anaphylaxis occurs in 0.004 to 0.4 percent. And upto 10 percent of these patients have a similar reaction to cephalosporins and carbapenems.[6]

Penicillin is among the least expensive of all antibiotics.

## Ampicillin and Amoxycillin

Like Penicillin, Ampicillin and Amoxicillin are beta lactam antibiotics under category B of FDA classification. Mechanism of action is similar to Penicillin. Their spectrum of activity is also almost similar to that of Penicillin. In addition, they are active against many strains of *Haemophilus influenzae*, most strains of Enterococci and many aerobic gram-negative bacilli. Because of indiscriminate use of these drugs over many years, a number of strains of coliform organisms have become resistant to these antibiotics, as has also been noted in a study conducted by Dunlow and Duff.[7] where 20 percent of strains of *E.coli* and 30 percent of strains of *Klebsiella* were resistant to Ampicillin.

Four major uses of Ampicillin and Amoxicillin in obstetrics are:

1. Drug of choice for confirmed enterococcal UTIs.
2. Intrapartum prophylaxis against group B streptococcal infections.
3. In combination with Gentamicin, Ampicillin is suitable for treatment of Chorioamnionitis.
4. Same combination may be used as prophylaxis against endocarditis to selected patients with heart disease who are undergoing obstetric procedures.

## Amoxycillin Clavulanate

Amoxycillin Clavulanate ( Augmentin ) is an oral beta lactam antibiotic that inhibits cell wall synthesis. Clavulanate is a beta lactamase inhibitor that, when combined with Amoxicillin, expands the spectrum of activity of the latter significantly. Compared to ampicillin and amoxicillin, this combination has enhanced activity against staphylococcal species, *H.influenzae* and anaerobic organisms.

In obstetrics, this drug has three major indications –

1. In treatment of sinusitis, when other less expensive antibiotics have failed.
2. Treatment of lower UTIs, and mild pyelonephritis caused by resistant organisms.
3. Treatment of mild postoperative infections (wound infections or endometritis)

Amoxycillin clavulanate combination is quite expensive therefore it should be used only when less expensive antibiotics are not likely to be effective.

## Cephalosporins

Like penicillins, cephalosporins contain the four member beta lactam ring. They are also bactericidal, acting through inhibition of bacterial cell wall synthesis. Cephalosporins have been classified as first, second and third generation, based on their spectrum of activity. They are listed as FDA category B.

First generation cephalosporins are commonly used for post- caesarian delivery prophylaxis and for treatment of urinary tract infection, typically caused by aerobic gram-negative bacilli ii none of the cephalosporins are effective against *Enterococcus*. Third generation cephalosporins are ten fold less active against *Staphylococcus aureus* than the first generations. However, they adequately cover all aerobic streptococci except *Enterococcus*.[6] They provide excellent coverage against the aerobic gram-negative rods and many of them are active against the gram-positive and gram-negative anaerobes. Almost all cover *Pseudomonas* except for Cefotetan.

Limited spectrum cephalosporins have four major applications in obstetrics.

1. One gram cefazolin 8 hourly for acute pyelonephritis in pregnant women.
2. Cefazolin in same dose is excellent treatment of a surgical wound infection.
3. It is particularly good for surgical prophylaxis in patients having caesarean delivery (one gram immediately after cord is clamped).
4. Oral cephelexin 500 mg. q.i.d. is the drug of choice for puerperal mastitis.

The intermediate spectrum cephalosporins are used mainly for the treatment of Gonorrhoea ( Ceftriaxone 125 mg as a single i.m. dose or oral cefixime 400 mg in a single dose)

Extended spectrum cephalosporins are best used as single agents for the treatment of polymicrobial postoperative pelvic infections such as Chorioamnionitis or puerperal endometritis.

Side effects include hypersensitivity and diarrhoea. Others are thrombophlebitis at the site of intravenous injection, pain at site of I.M. injection, bleeding diathesis due to platelet dysfunction or hypoprothrombinemia.

## Macrolides

Macrolide antibiotics, for example Erythromycin, Clindamycin, Azithromycin and Clarithromycin are bacteriostatic antibiotics. They act by attaching to the 50 S ribosome and inhibiting bacterial protein synthesis.

Erythromycin is FDA category B drug. It is the drug of choice for *Legionella*, *Mycoplasma* and *Chlamydia* infection in pregnancy. As it crosses the placenta minimally, it is not the first line treatment for syphilis in pregnancy. Side effects include GI upset, pain at injection site, hypersensitivity reaction and infrequent liver function test abnormality.[6]

Azithromycin is a relatively new macrolide with an extended spectrum against gram-positive cocci, some gram-negative rods, and many anaerobes as well as *Mycoplasma* and *Chlamydia*. Azithromycin has two major applications in obstetrics

1. It is an excellent antibiotic for community acquired pneumonia or severe bronchitis in pregnancy (500 mg initially, then 250 mg dialy for four days).

**Table 14.5:** Cephalosporins

| *Generation* | *Route of administration* | *Dosage* |
|---|---|---|
| *First generation* | | |
| Cephalothin | The only Parenteral drug | 0.5–2 gm 8 hourly |
| Cefazolin | Oral | 0.5–2 gm QID |
| Cephalexin | Oral | 0.25–0.5 gm QID |
| Cephradine | Oral | 0.25–0.5 gm QID |
| Cefadroxil | Oral | 0.5–1 gm BD |
| *Second generation* | | |
| Cefaclor | Oral | 10–15 mg/kg/ day in two or four divided doses |
| Cefuroxime axetil (Ceftum) | Oral | 250–500 mg BD |
| Cefoxitin | Parenteral | 50–200 mg/ kg /day, 6–8 hourly |
| Cefotetan | Parenteral | 50–200 mg /kg /day, 12 hourly |
| Cefprozil | Parenteral | 50–200 mg/ kg/day, once a day |
| *Third generation* | | |
| Cefixime | Oral | 200 mg BD |
| Cefibuten | Oral | 400 mg OD |
| Cefoperazone | Parenteral | 25–100 mg/kg/day, 8–12 hourly |
| Cefotaxime (Omnatax) | Parenteral | 1–2 gm, 6-8 hourly |
| Ceftazidime (Fortum) | Parenteral | 0.5–2 gm, 8 hourly |
| Ceftizoxime | Parenteral | 15–50 mg /kg/day, once daily |
| Moxalactam | Parenteral | – |
| Ceftriaxone (Monocef) | | 15–50 mg/kg/day, once daily |
| *Fourth generation* | | |
| Cefepime | Parenteral | 0.5–2 gm, 12 hourly |

2. Azithromycin also finds application in the treatment of lower genitourinary tract infections caused by *Chlamydia* (Azithro-mycin powder in a dose of 1gram).[8]

Azithromycin is listed as FDA category B drug. G.I. Side effects are less common as compared to erythromycin. Other side effects include headache, dizziness and mild liver function abnormalities.

Clindamycin is a FDA category B drug. It has excellent coverage against many anaerobes including *Clostridium* and *Bacteroides* along with many aerobic gram-positive cocci but it does not cover gram-negative rods.

Its primary obstetric indication is postpartum metritis and is also the drug of choice for group B streptococcal prophylaxis. Pseudomembranous colitis (1 in 10,000) is a side effect of clindamycin as are minor GI. Upsets and infrequent liver function test abnormalities. Oral metronidazole constitute the treatment if this condition develops.

Clarithromycin, a FDA category C drug, is most often used during pregnancy for the treatment and prophylaxis of *Mycobacterium avium* complex in women who are HIV-positive.

## Aminoglycosides

Aminoglycosides are bactericidal antibiotics that bind the 30s ribosomes and inhibit bacterial protein synthesis. Members of this group are streptomycin, gentamycin, tobramycin, kanamycin, amikacin and netilmicin. Gentamycin, the most widely used aminoglycoside in pregnancy is a FDA category C drug. It covers a wide range of aerobic gram-negative rods, and has activity against *S. aureus* and has synergistic activity with Ampicillin against *Enterococcus*. Aminoglycosides are not active against streptococcal organisms and anaerobes. Gentamycin rapidly crosses the placenta, however there are no reports of congenital anomalies in fetus or neonatal ototoxicity or nephrotoxicity following in utero exposure.

The principal obstetric indications are:

1. To treat pyelonephritis in patients allergic to β lactam antibiotics.
2. In combination with Clindamycin for treatment of mixed aerobic and anaerobic pelvic infections such as post operative and puerperal metritis.
3. In combination with ampicillin for SABE prophylaxis.
4. Treatment of chorioamnionitis

Three major side effects are nephrotoxicity, ototoxicity and neuromuscular blockage and the dosage may need to be reduced in the setting of renal insufficiency.

## Sulphonamides

Trimethoprim Sulphamethoxazole.

Sulphonamides are bacteriostatic drugs and when combined with trimethoprim they sequentially block biosynthesis of folic acid.

This combination has excellent activity against most aerobic gram negative bacilli with the exception of *Pseudomonas aeruginosa*. Also, it is effective against *H. influenzae* and *S. pneumoniae* and is drug of choice for *Pneumocystis carinii* infections.

If given shortly before delivery, sulphonamides can bind to albumin and displace bilirubin causing neonatal hyperbilirubinemia with kernicterus.

The main uses in obstetrics are for the treatment of:

1. UTIs
2. Otitis media and sinusitis especially in patients allergic to beta lactam antibiotics.
3. Traveller's diarrhoea caused by *Shigella* organisms.
4. Acute *Pneumocystis carinii* infection and for prevention of recurrent infections.

Sulphonamides are FDA category B drugs and trimethoprim is FDA category C.

## Metronidazole

It is a FDA category B drug except in first trimester when it is a category D drug. It has excellent activity against several genital tract pathogens namely anaerobic organisms,

*Trichomonas vaginalis*, *Giardia lamblia*, *Entamoeba histolytica* and *Clostri-dium difficile*. Metronidazole is not effective against aerobic gram- negative bacilli. Although it has not been associated with adverse fetal effects, it is currently recommended for use in the second and third trimester only.

Metronidazole is the treatment of choice for trichomoniasis. Along with Vancomycin it is highly effective for treatment of pseudo-membranous colitis. It can also be combined with penicillin or ampicillin plus gentamycin for treatment of puerperal endometritis.

The principal adverse effects of metronidazole are nausea, vomiting, diarrhoea and skin rash. The drug also exerts a disulfiram like reaction when taken with alcohol.

## Nitrofurantoin

It is a bactericidal antibiotic which is highly active against most of the common uropathogens, i.e. *E.coli*, *Klebsiella*, *Staphylococcus saprophyticus*, *S. aureus* and *E. faecalis*. It is not active against most strains of *Proteus*, *Serratia* or *Pseudomonas*. In obstetric patients it is mainly used for treatment of UTI and prophylaxis against recurrent UTI. Rare but potentially serious side effects include pulmonary hypersensitivity, hepatitis, peripheral neuropathy and anaemia due to G-6 PD deficiency in the mother with no effect on foetus. It is listed as FDA Category B drug except in third trimester when it is considered category C drug.

## Vancomycin

It is a bactericidal drug used for treatment of *C. difficile* induced pseudomembranous colitis and for treatment of methicillin resistant *S. aureus*. In penicillin allergic patients, vancomycin is the drug of choice for treatment of *Enterococcus* and for prophylaxis of SABE. Although it appears that standard doses pose no threat to the foetus, it is listed as FDA category C.

## Tetracyclines

They are bacteriostatic antibiotics that have a broad spectrum of activity against many gram positive and gram-negative aerobes and anaerobes including *Chlamydia*, *Mycoplasma* and the *Spirochetes*. Being FDA category D drugs, they should be avoided in pregnancy and lactation. One potential indication is the treatment of syphillis in a penicillin allergic patient who cannot be desensitized.

## Fluoroquinolones

They are bactericidal antibiotics that act by inhibiting DNA gyrase (bacterial toposomerase II) thus dissipating bacterial protein synthesis. They have excellent activity against aerobic gram-negative bacilli including *H. influenzae*, *N. gonorrhoeae*, *N. meningitidis*, *M. catarrhalis* and staphylococci. However, since the fluoroquinolones may cause injury to the developing cartilage of the foetus, these drugs should not be used in pregnant or lactating women.[6]

## Antitubercular Agents

According to the Revised National Tuberculosis Control Program, all pregnant patients diagnosed with tuberculosis should start or continue their antitubercular therapy. Short course chemotherapy is the treatment of choice. Isoniazid (H), Rifampicin (R), Pyrizinamide (Z), Ethambutol (E) for two months followed by HR for four months is the usual treatment. No harmful effect is observed even if the drugs are given in the first trimester.

**Table 14.6:** Antitubercular drugs safety in pregnancy

| *Drug* | *Category* |
|---|---|
| Ethambutol | B |
| Rifampicin | C |
| INH | C |
| Para-amino salicylic acid | C |
| Pyrizinamide | C |
| Cycloserine | C |

Streptomycin is not recommended for use during pregnancy as eighth cranial nerve abnormalities have been identified in up to 15 per cent of exposed infants.

Breastfeeding is recommended. If the mother is sputum-positive, the neonate should receive chemoprophylaxis with Isoniazid for three months. Tuberculin test should be done at three months. If positive the infant does not require vaccination with BCG and chemoprophylaxis should be continued for 3 more months. If however, the tuberculin test is negative the child should be given BCG vaccination. If the mother is sputum negative, BCG should be administered to the neonate and there is no need for chemo-prophylaxis.

## Newer Antibiotics

### *Linezolid*

It is an oxazolidine antibiotic which is effective against strains of enterococci, staphylococci, and *S. pneumoniae* which are resistant to other antibiotics such as methicillin and penicillin.

### *Quinupristin/Dalfopristin*

Quinupristin and Dalfopristin are streptogramin antibiotics.This combination is effective against *E.faecium*, methicillin resistant *S. aureus* and *S. epidermidis* and strains of *S. pneumoniae* that are resistant to penicillin.

## Antiviral

Acyclovir, a category C drug is antiherpes in activity. It is also active against varicella zoster. Although no adverse effects on the fetus have yet been observed its use should be limited to varicella zoster pneumonia and severe herpetic infections.

Ganciclovir, it is a category C drug that is used to treat cytomegalovirus retinitis. Its benefit to the mother outweighs possible foetal effects.

Didanosine, it is a category B drug, indicated for use in HIV patients who are unable to tolerate AZT.

## Antiretroviral Therapy during Pregnancy

Antiretroviral therapy is given for two reasons during pregnancy; firstly for prevention of mother to child transmission (therapy usually discontinued at or soon after delivery) and secondly for treatment of the mother to prevent maternal disease progression (therapy continued indefinitely after delivery).

In 1994 the ACTG 076 protocol demonstrated that zidovudine monotherapy, administered 5 times daily and initiated between 14 and 34 weeks of pregnancy, intravenously during labour and to infants for 6 weeks reduced the risk of HIV infection in non-breastfeeding populations from 25 percent to 7.6 percent.[9]

Potent combinations of three or more antiretroviral drugs, known as Highly-active antiretroviral therapy (HAART), have now become the standard of care for all HIV-positive individuals requiring therapy for their own health.

According to British HIV Association guidelines pregnant women with CD4 counts of 200–350 × $10^6$ should be treated with HAART in the same way as nonpregnant adults.[10] However, the start of treatment should be deferred until after first trimester, if possible, and should be continued after delivery.

In India, NACO has recommended use of Nevirapine 200 mg tablet as a single dose for mother in labour four hours before delivery for preventing vertical transmission to the foetus and Nevirapine syrup 2 mg/kg for the neonate as a single dose.

**Table 14.7:** Commonly used antiretroviral drugs[11]

| *Drug* | *FDA category* | *Oral dosage* | *Major toxicity in adult* |
|---|---|---|---|
| Zidovudine (ZDV) | B | Usual – 200 mg TDS<br>Low dose – 100 mg 5 times daily | General: transient headache, GI upset, fatigue, nail pigmentation Hematological: anemia, neutropenia<br>Other: myopathy, cardiomyopathy, hepatic dysfunction |
| Didanosine (ddI) | B | 200 mg twice daily, now 300 mg per day is used for increased compliance | General: GI upset, diarrhea, headache, peripheral neuropathy. Pancreatitis, Hepatitis, elevated uric acid, triglycerides. |
| Zalcitabine (ddC) | C | 0.75 mg 3 times daily | General: rash, stomatitis, esophageal ulcer, peripheral neuropathy Hematological: anemia, leukopenia<br>Pancreatitis, cardiomyopathy |
| Stavudine (d4T) | C | 40 mg twice daily<br>if < 60 kg: 30 mg twice daily | Peripheral neuropathy, hepatic toxicity, Pancreatitis, Hematological |
| Lamivudine (3TC) | C | 150 mg twice daily | Headache, diarrhea, nausea, fatigue. Pancreatitis, Hematologic |
| Indinavir | C | 800 mg 3 times a day | Renal stones, increased bilirubin, nausea, vomiting, diarrhea. Hematologic: anemia, neutropenia |

*Contd...*

*Contd...*

| | | | |
|---|---|---|---|
| Ritonavir | B | 600 mg twice daily | Bitter aftertaste, vomiting, diarrhea, circumoral parasthesia |
| Saquinavir | B | 600 mg twice daily | GI side effects |
| Nelfinavir | B | 750 mg 3 times daily | Diarrhea, flatulence, rash, altered liver function |
| Nevirapine | C | 200 mg daily for 14 days, if no rash then 200 mg twice daily | Rash, rarely toxic epidermal necrosis, nausea, headache, drowsiness, fatigue, fever, hepatitis |

**Table 14.8:** Antiretroviral therapy regimens[12]

*Paediatric AIDS Clinical Trials Group (PACTG) 076 Zidovudine (ZDV ) Regimens*[12]

| *Time of ZDV administration* | *Regimen* |
|---|---|
| Antepartum | Oral administration of 100 mg ZDV five times daily,* initiated at 14-34 weeks* gestation and continued throughout the pregnancy |
| Intrapartum | During labour, intravenous administration of ZDV in a 1 hour initial dose of 2 mg/kg body weight, followed by a continuous infusion of 1 mg/kg body weight per hour until delivery |
| Postpartum | Oral administration of ZDV to the newborn (ZDV syrup at 2 mg/kg body weight dose every 6 hours) for the first 6 weeks of life, beginning at 8-12 hours after birth.** |

* Oral ZDV, administered as 200 mg three times daily or 300 mg twice daily, is used in general clinical practice and is an acceptable alternative regimen to 100 mg orally five times daily.

** Intravenous dosage for infants who cannot tolerate oral intake is 1.5 mg/kg body weight intravenously every 6 hours.

The use of Efavirenz (EFV) is contraindicated in pregnant women and women of child-bearing age who are not using contraception because of its teratogenic potential.[11] In patients with HIV – TB co-infection Nevirapine should not be used in combination with Rifampicin. This is because Rifampicin causes enzyme induction which makes it a physiologic antagonist of Nevirapine.

## Antifungals

Nystatin is a polyene category B antibiotic and is available as vaginal cream or suppository. The category C drugs Clotrimazole and Miconazole are available as suppositories, creams and lotions. Amphotericin B has been demonstrated to cross the placenta, however it has not been associated with foetal anomalies. It is a category B drug. Ketoconazole and Fluconazole are category C drugs and should be used only when indicated and when other safer drugs have been tried. Griseofulvin is a category C drug of which placental transfer has been observed. Its use should be limited to severe infections not responsive to safer antifungals.

## Antibiotic Use in Lactating Mothers

Lactating mothers can pass on the antibiotics to foetus as most of these are secreted in milk. Thus, antibiotics adversely affecting the foetus should be avoided during lactation and to minimise the adverse effects on the neonate such drugs should be stopped 3 weeks before delivery.

**Table 14.9:** Comparison of intrapartum/postpartum regimens for HIV–1 infected women in labour who have had no prior antiretroviral therapy[12]

| *Drug regimen* | *Source of evidence* | *Maternal intrapartum* | *Infant postpartum* | *Transmission* | *Advantages* | *Disadvantages* |
|---|---|---|---|---|---|---|
| Nevirapine | Clinical trial, Africa; compared with oral ZDV* given intrapartum and for 1 week to the infant | Single 200 mg oral dose at onset of labour | Single 2 mg/kg oral dose at age 48-72 hours** | Transmission at 6 weeks 12% with nevirapine vs 21% with ZDV a 47% reduction (95% CI*, 20-64%) | Inexpensive<br>Oral regimen<br>Simple, easy to administer<br>Can give directly observed treatment | Unknown efficacy if mother has nevirapine-resistant virus |
| ZDV-3TC* | Clinical trial, Africa; compared with placebo | ZDV 600 mg orally at onset of labour, followed by 300 mg orally every 3 hours until delivery and 3TC 150 mg orally at onset of labour, followed by 150 mg orally every 12 hours until delivery | ZDV 4 mg/kg orally every 12 hours and 3TC 2 mg/kg oraly every 12 hours for 7 days | Transmission at 6 weeks 9% with ZDV-3TC vs. 15% with placebo, a 40% reduction | Oral regimen<br>Adherence easier than 6 weeks of ZDV | Potential toxicity of multiple drug exposure |
| ZDV | Epidemiologic data, US: compared with no ZDV treatment | 2 mg/kg intravenous bolus, followed by continuous infusion of 1 mg/kg/hr until delivery | 2 mg/kg orally every 6 hours for 6 weeks | Transmission 10% with ZDV vs. 27% with no ZDV treatment, a 62% reduction (95% CI, 19-82%) | Has been standard recommendation before clinical trial results | Requires intravenous administration and availability of ZDV intravenous formulation; Adherence to 6 week infant regimen |

*Contd...*

*Contd...*

| *Drug regimen* | *Source of evidence* | *Maternal intrapartum* | *Infant postpartum* | *Transmission* | *Advantages* | *Disadvantages* |
|---|---|---|---|---|---|---|
| ZDV-nevirapine | Theoretical | ZDV 2 mg/kg intravenous bolus, followed by continuous infusion of 1 mg/kg/hr until delivery and Nevirapine single 200 mg oral dose at onset of labour | ZDV 2 mg/kg orally every 6 hours for 6 weeks and Nevirapine single 2 mg/kg oral dose at age 48-72 hours | No data | Potential benefit if maternal virus is resistant to either nevirapine or ZDV; synergistic inhibition of HIV replication with combination in vitro | Reguires intravenous administration and availability of ZDV intravenous formulation; Adherence to 6 week infant ZDV regimen; Unknown efficacy and limited toxicity data |

* ZDV, zidovudine; Cl, confidence interval; 3TC lamivudine

** If the mother received nevirapine less than 1 hour before delivery, the infant should be given 2 mg/kg oral nevirapine as soon as possible after birth and again at 48-72 hours

**Table 14.10:** Treatment of HIV–TB coinfection

*ART Recommendations for Individuals with Tuberculosis Disease and HIV Coinfection (WHO- Dec, 2003)*[13]

| *CD4 Cell count* | *Recommended regimen* | *Comments* |
|---|---|---|
| CD4<200 cu mm | Start TB treatment. Start ART as soon as TB treatment is tolerated (between 2 weeks and 2 months).[1] EFV containing regimens[2,3,4] EFV is | Recommend ART. contraindicated in pregnant women or women of child bearing potential without effective contraception |
| CD4 between 200-350/cu mm | Start TB treatment. Start one of the below regimens after initiation phase (if severely compromised start earlier): EFV containing regimens[2] or NVP containing regimen in case of rifampicin free continuation phase TB treatment regimen | Consider ART |
| CD4>350 cu mm | Start TB treatment | Defer ART[5] |
| CD4 not available | Start TB treatment | Consider ART[6] |

1. Timing of ART initiation should be up to clinical judgement based on other signs of immunodeficiency. For extra-pulmonary TB, ART should be started as soon as TB treatment is tolerated irrespective of CD4 cell count.
2. Alternatives to the EFV portion of the regimen include SQV/r(400/400 mg bid or 1600/200 qd in sgc), LPV/RTV(400/400 mg bid) and ABC (300 mg bid).
3. NVP (200 mg qd for 2 weeks followed by 200 mg bid) may be used in place of EFV in absence of other options. NVP containing regimens include: d4T/3TC/NVP or ZDV/3TC/NVP.
4. EFV containing regimens include d4T/3TC/EFV or ZDV/3TC/EFV.
5. Unless non-TB stage IV conditions are present. Otherwise start ART upon completion of TB treatment.
6. If no other signs of immunodeficiency are present is improving on TB treatment, ART should be started upon completion of TB treatment.

**Table 14.11:** Drugs used as Prophylaxis of Opportunistic Infections in HIV-infected Pregnant Women[11]

| *$CD_4$ Lymphocyte count* | *Pathogen* | *Drug* |
|---|---|---|
| < 350/ mm$^3$ | *Mycobacterium tuberculosis* | INH 300 mg+ Pyridoxine 50 mg daily for 12 months |
| < 200/ mm$^3$ | *Pneumocystis carinii* | Trimethoprim-sulfamethoxazole (TMP/SMX) double strength tablets daily or three times a week OR Aerosolized Pentamidine 300 mg monthly up to 600 mg weekly OR Dapsone 100 mg once daily |
| < 100/ mm $^3$ | Toxoplasmosis | TMP/ SMX (as above) |
| < 50/ mm $^3$ | *M. avium* complex | Clarithromycin 500 mg twice daily OR Azithromycin 1200 mg weekly OR Rifabutin 300 mg once daily |

Also, certain antibiotics interact with contraception and doses may need alteration, e.g. patients receiving ATT using oral contraception need an increase in the dose of rifampicin.

## CONCLUSION

Most antibiotics can be used with relative safety during pregnancy and many antibiotics are now available to the physician for management of infections in pregnancy. However, while choosing among these agents obstetricians must consider not only their therapeutic effectiveness but also their toxicity profile, both for the mother and the foetus (immediate as well as long term), ease of administration and cost. Preferably, only those drugs should be used which have been used for a long time and which have a proven safety profile.

## REFERENCES


1. Hedstrom S, Martens MG. Antibiotics in pregnancy COG 1993;36(4):886-92.
2. www.fpnotebook.com/ID120.htm
3. Gandhi G, Batra S. Antibiotic prophylaxis in gynaecologic surgery. Paper presented at the XV FIGO Congress of Gynaecology and Obstetrics, Copenhagen. August 1997;3-8.
4. Khera N, Sachdeva J, Batra S.Antibiotic prophylaxis in lap ligation (single dose parentral versus multidose oral Ciprofloxacin ) Poster presented at the VIth World Conference of NARCHI, Taj Hotel, Delhi, 20-22 September, 2002.
5. Pedler SJ, Orr KE. Bacterial, Fungal, and Parasitic Infections. In: Barron WM, Lindheimer MD editors. Medical Disorders in Pregnancy, Third edition. Mosby USA.2000;411-65.
6. Dashe JS, Gilstrap LC. Antibiotic use in pregnancy. N Am Clinics Obs Gyn 1997;24:617-29.
7. Dunlow SG, Duff P. Prevelance of antibiotic resistant uropathogens in obstetric patients with acute pyelonephritis. Obstet Gynaecol 1990;76:241-5.
8. Duff P. Antibiotic selection in obstetrics : making cost-effective choices. COG 2002;45(1):59-72.
9. Conner EM, Sperling RS, Gelber R, Kiselev P, Scott G, et al. Reduction of maternal infant transmission of human deficiency virustype 1 with Zidovudine treatment. Pediatrics AIDS clinical Trials group Protocol 076 Study Group. N Eng J Med 1994;33:1173-80.
10. Lyall EG, Blott M, de Ruiter A, Hawkins D, Mercy D, et al. Guidelines for the management of HIV infection in pregnant women and the prevention of mother to child transmission. HIV Med 2001;2:3114-34.
11. Peiris JSM, Madeley CR. Viral Infections. In: Barron WM, Lindheimer MD editors. Medical Disorders in Pregnancy, Third edition. Mosby USA.2000: 466-515.
12. Perinatal HIV Guidelines working group members: US Public Health Service Task Force Recommendations for the use of antiretroviral drugs in pregnant women infected with HIV 1 for maternal health and reduced perinatal HIV 1 transmission in the United States. USPHS, February 25, 2000.
13. HIV-TB co-infection. Program co-ordination, Guidelines for clinicians and standard operating Procedures. National AIDS control Organisation, Ministry of Health and Family Welfare, India.

CHAPTER 15

# Maternal Immunisation

Sumita Mehta, Renu Tanwar, Gauri Gandhi

## DEFINITION

Immunisation is the process by which extra immunity is artificially- induced or protection from disease is provided.

## TYPES

Immunisation can be active or passive.

### Active Immunisation

Active immunisation induces the body to develop defences against infection. It is accomplished with vaccines or toxoids that stimulate the immune system to produce antibodies, cell-mediated immunity, or both, which in turn protects against an infectious disease.

### Passive Immunisation

Passive immunisation is a process that provides temporary protection against an infectious agent by administration of exogenously produced antibody. The most common methods of passive immunisation are transplacental passage of maternal antibodies to the foetus and the use of immunoglobulin (Ig) to prevent specific infectious disease.

*Immunising agents*: Include the following:

a. Vaccine which is a suspension of attenuated live or killed organisms or factors there of administered to induce immunity.
b. Toxoid—A modified bacterial toxin that has been rendered nontoxic but is still capable of producing antitoxin.
c. Immunoglobulin—A solution containing antibody from human blood that can provide passive immunisation against certain infections (e.g. Measles and hepatitis A) or protection of immunodeficient patients.
d. Specific immunoglobulin—Special preparations obtained from donor pools with high antibody content against a specific disease (e.g. Hepatitis B immunoglobulin (HBIG) and Varicella zoster immunoglobulin (VZIG).

The introduction of vaccines has controlled the following ten major infectious disease in at least some areas of the world—Smallpox, diphtheria, tetanus, pertussis, yellow fever, poliomyelitis, measles, mumps, rubella and *Haemophilus influenzae* type B disease.

*Currently Five Major Types of Vaccines are Available*

a. Live attenuated viruses or bacteria (e.g. Cowpox, oral polio vaccine, typhoid, cholera, measles mumps rubella)
b. Killed whole viruses (e.g. Salk poliovirus vaccine and influenza virus vaccine)
c. Killed bacteria (e.g. Pertussis, typhoid and cholera)
d. Purified component vaccines such as polysaccharide vaccine (e.g. Pneumococcal and *Haemophilus influenzae* type B vaccine or toxins (e.g. Tetanus toxoid)
e. Genetically engineered proteins produced by recombinant technology (e.g. Hepatitis B vaccine)

The decision to use a vaccine must take into account the risk of disease, the benefits of vaccination and the risks associated with vaccination.

In pregnancy the benefit is greater than the risk when:

a. The risk for disease exposure is high (e.g. Travel to endemic area)
b. Infection would pose a special risk to pregnant women (e.g. Influenza)
c. Vaccine is unlikely to cause harm.

## Tetanus Toxoid

There is no increased risk to mother or foetus following vaccination with tetanus toxoid or combined tetanus—diphtheria toxoid vaccine during pregnancy including in the first trimester. ACOG recommends the use of tetanus toxoid in pregnancy for those women who lack the primary series of immunisation or in whom no booster has been given in the past ten years.[2] According to National Immunisation Scheme two doses of tetanus toxoid are recommended in pregnancy:

First dose (0.5 ml IM) – 16 to 20 weeks

Second dose (0.5 ml IM) – 20 to 24 weeks

Minimum interval between the doses should be one month. Second dose should preferably be given one month before the expected date of delivery.

For a woman who has been immunised earlier, one booster dose is sufficient which will provide immunity for the next five years.

## MMR (Measles-Mumps-Rubella)

MMR is a trivalent vaccine which contains live attenuated viruses. If immunity to one or more components can be demonstrated, monovalent or bivalent vaccines can be used.

MMR vaccines can produce a viraemia with the potential for transplacental passage to the foetal compartment, hence women of child bearing age group should avoid pregnancy for 3 months after vaccination but with the currently available RA27/3 strain vaccine the risk of congenital rubella syndrome (CRS) is between 0 to 1.6 per cent.[3] This risk is considerably lower than the 20 per cent or greater risk associated with wild rubella virus infection during the first trimester.[4] CDC recommends that women should avoid being pregnant for three months after receiving this vaccine. However, if vaccination does occur within three months of conception or pregnancy, considering the low risk of CRS, it should not be an indication for termination of pregnancy.[5]

### *Dose*

Single dose subcutaneously.

*Adverse reactions* are usually mild, upto 40 per cent patients experience joint pains which are often worst than that associated with natural infection. Symptoms are self-limiting, lasting 3 to 10 days.

### *Contraindications*

Immunosuppressed women.

Patients with history of anaphylaxis to neomycin (since the vaccine contains trace amounts of neomycin).

### *Breastfeeding*

Vaccination of susceptible women with MMR vaccine in the immediate postpartum period is recommended by ACOG and CDC.[2,4]

## Hepatitis B Vaccine

Hepatitis B virus vaccine inactivated (recombinant) is a non- infectious surface antigen vaccine. It is safe to use in pregnancy and there is no risk to the foetus or breast-fed infants.[7]

One source recommends that administration after the first trimester is preferred because of a theoretical risk of teratogenicity.[8] CDC states that there is no apparent risk of foetal adverse effects and the pregnancy is not a contraindication to vaccination. Pre- and postexposure prophylaxis is indicated in women at high risk of infection.[8] All pregnant women should be screened for HBsAg early in prenatal care. HBsAg (–)ve women at high risk of HBV infection should be retested during the early third trimester.

### Dose

3 doses (20 μg) IM at 0, 1, 6 months.

After 3 doses 95 to 99 per cent, persons have productive antibody titre, which provides protection against serious HBV infection for at least 12 years.[9]

Infants born to HBsAg (+) ve women should receive the first dose of vaccine + Hepatitis B immunoglobulin within 12 hours of birth.

## Hepatitis A Vaccine

Hepatitis A vaccine is inactivated virus vaccine. Any risk to the foetus from maternal vaccination is minimal. Based on the experience of other inactivated viral vaccines, hepatitis A vaccine can be given to pregnant women at risk of infection (travellers or persons living in high risk areas).[6]

### Dose

1 ml IM followed by a booster at 6 months after primary dose.
Provides protection for at least 10 years.

### Adverse Effects

Local inflammatory reaction, headache, fatigue, anorexia.

### Contraindication

History of allergy to any vaccine component.

### Breastfeeding

Hepatitis A vaccine can be given to nursing mothers.

## Varicella Vaccine

Varicella vaccine is a live attenuated viral vaccine. Because of a theoretical risk of viraemia and transplacental passage of vaccine virus the risk to the foetus pregnant women should not be inoculated with the vaccine virus.

The risk of congenital varicella syndrome with natural (wild) varicella virus is approximately 1 to 2 percent during the first 20 weeks of gestation. Moreover, there is a significant risk for infectious morbidity and mortality in the neonate, if maternal varicella occurs after the first trimester. The risk from vaccine is much less because of the low virulence of the attenuated viruses used in the vaccine. Because of this the ACIP recommends that the decision to terminate a pregnancy should not be based on whether the vaccine was given during pregnancy.[10] No case of varicella vaccine induced foetal harm has been identified till date.

### Dose

Two doses with second dose 4 to 8 weeks after the first dose.

### Breastfeeding

Varicella vaccine can be administered to nursing mothers.

## Pneumococcal Vaccine

Pneumococcal vaccine polyvalent is a killed bacteria vaccine that contains a mixture of purified capsular polysaccharides from 23 types of *Streptococcus pneumoniae*. The safety of pneumococcal vaccine for use in pregnant women has not been determined. Pneumococcal vaccine use in not contraindicated in pregnancy but ACOG limits the use of this vaccine to pregnant women at high risk:

A. Persons with functional or anatomic asplenia, e.g. Sickle cell disease, splenectomy
B. Persons with chronic cardiovascular or pulmonary disease
C. Those with diabetes mellitus
D. Alcoholic and those with chronic liver failure
E. Person inhabiting special environments.

### Dose

Single dose 0.5 ml IM or subcutaneous.

## Breastfeeding

Pneumococcal vaccine is safe to use in breastfeeding women.

## Influenza Vaccine

Human influence vaccines are classified into 3 types A,B and C. Influenza A infection in the most frequent associated with most morbidity and mortality and is responsible for worldwide pandemics.[11]

Influenza B causes regional epidemics.

Influenza C rarely causes epidemics.

Influenza vaccine is inactivated viral vaccine. It is considered safe for use during all stages of pregnancy but vaccination during the second trimester can avoid a coincidental association with spontaneous abortions that is common in the first trimester.[12]

In 1999 the Advisory Committee on Immunisation Practices (ACIP) recommended that the vaccine should be administered to:

A. Women who will be beyond the first trimester of pregnancy (no less than 14 weeks of gestation) during the influenza season (beginning of October to mid November)

B. Women who have medical conditions (diabetes, chronic pulmonary disease, asthma, renal disease) that increase their risk for complications from influenza.

## Dose

0.5 ml subcutaneous single dose.

## Adverse Reaction

Local inflammation at site of injection, fever, very rarely Guillain- Barré syndrome.

## Breastfeeding

Influenza vaccine is safe to use in breastfeeding women.

## Typhoid Vaccine

Three types of typhoid vaccine are available.

A. Vi polysaccharide vaccine—given IM

B. Live attenuated Ty 21a (Typhoral) given orally

C. Inactivated (killed bacteria) given subcutaneous.

The risk of the foetus from vaccine is unknown. ACOG recommends vaccination only in those pregnant patients who have been in close / continued exposure or travelled to endemic areas.

## Dose

0.5 ml subcutaneous, two doses 4 to 6 weeks apart.

### Adverse Reactions

Local pain and swelling at injection site, headache, pyrexia which subsides in 36 hours.

### Breastfeeding

No data is available.

## Rabies Vaccine

Rabies vaccine (human) is an inactivated virus vaccine.

As rabies is nearly 100 per cent fatal if contracted, the vaccine should be given for post-exposure prophylaxis.[2] Foetal risk from the vaccine is unknown but indications for prophylaxis are not altered by pregnancy.

In a prospective study done by Chutivongse S et al in 1995, no increase in maternal (spontaneous abortion, hypertension, placental previa or gestational diabetes) or foetal (stillbirth, minor birth defects or low-birth weight) complications were observed in exposed vaccinated women in comparison with a control group of non- vaccinated, non-exposed women.[13]

### Dose

Days 0, 3, 7, 14, 28, 90 intramuscular.

### Adverse Reaction

Local reaction at injection site (25%), arthropathy (6%).

## Cholera Vaccine

Cholera vaccine is a killed bacterial vaccine.

The risk to the foetus from maternal vaccination is unknown because there is no specific information on the safety of vaccine during pregnancy. ACOG and CDC recommend that vaccine should only be given in unusual outbreak situations.[2]

### Dose

Two doses IM 2 to 6 weeks apart.

### Breastfeeding

Maternal vaccination with cholera increases specific immunoglobulin-A antibody titres in breast milk.

## Polio Virus Vaccine

Polio virus vaccine inactivated (Salk vaccine, IPV) is an inactivated virus vaccine administered by injection.

Polio virus vaccine live ( Sabin, OPV) is a live, trivalent (types I, II and III ) attenuated virus administered orally.

No adverse effects attributable to the use of inactivated virus vaccine has been reported. Both the ACOG and ACIP recommend the use of vaccine during pregnancy only if an increased risk of exposure exists.[2] Inactivated form is preferred over the oral form because of a lower risk of vaccine associated paralysis.

### Dose

Three doses of 0.5 ml subcutaneous. First two doses 4 to 8 weeks apart and third dose 6 to 12 months after the second dose.

### Breastfeeding

No data available.

## IMMUNE THERAPY

### Hepatitis A

In case of exposure to hepatitis A immunoglobulin is effective in preventing disease when administered within 14 days of exposure.[9]

### Dose

0.02 ml/kg of body weight to family contacts.

3.2 ml/kg of body weight in institutional outbreaks.

It is an alternative to hepatitis A vaccine on prophylaxis for short- term exposure (single international trip of less than 2 to 3 months duration).

The efficacy of hepatitis A Ig for prevention of hepatitis A infection is 80 to 90 per cent if given in early incubation period.

### Breastfeeding

Immunoglobulin is safe for use in lactating mothers.

### Hepatitis B Immune Globulin

Recommended for post-exposure prophylaxis in susceptible persons who have been exposed to blood or body fluids containing HBsAg by percutaneous or mucous membrane routes or by Hepatitis B infected sexual partners.

### Dose

0.05 to 0.07 ml/kg body weight or 8 to 11 mg/kg of body weight IM.
To be repeated in one month.

For newborn—0.5 ml given within 12 hours of delivery.

## Breastfeeding

The use of HBIG is safe in breastfeeding women.

## Varicella Zoster Immune Globule (VZIG)

Recommended for post-exposure prophylaxis in:

Susceptible pregnant women exposed to varicella zoster.

Infants delivered to mothers who developed clinical varicella within 5 days before to 48 hours after delivery.[10]

## Dose

1.25 to 5 ml given IM.

VZIG should be administered within 72 hours of exposure.

## Tetanus Immunoglobulin

In pregnant patient not immunised during pregnancy or for post- exposure prophylaxis tetanus immunoglobulin is used.

## Dose

Prophylaxis—250 IU IM, single dose used in conjunction with tetanus toxoid .

Therapeutic—3000 to 6000 units.

## Measles

Measles immunoglobulin should be given within 3 to 4 hours of exposure.

## Dose

0.25 ml/kg of body weight.

The person passively immunised should be given live measles vaccine 8 to 12 weeks later.

## Rabies

In women exposed to rabid animals rabies immunoglobulin is used in conjunction with rabies killed.

## Dose

20 IU/KG of body weight. Half dose at injury site, half dose at deltoid.

## Rh Isoimmunisation

Rh immunoglobulin (anti-D) given to Rh-negative women following:

- Delivery of Rh-positive infant.
- First or second trimester abortion.

- Prenatal diagnostic procedures (e.g. cordocentesis, amniocentesis, chorionic villus sampling).
- Transfusion of Rh-positive blood.

## Key Points

- MMR vaccine is contraindicated in pregnancy and pregnancy should be avoided for three months following vaccination.
- Risk of CRS following vaccination with the RA 27/3 MMR vaccine is between 0-1.6 per cent.
- Hepatitis B vaccine is inactivated (recombinant) surface antigen vaccine. It can be given during pregnancy and pre- and post- exposure prophylaxis is indicated in pregnant women at high risk of infection.
- Hepatitis A vaccine is inactivated viral vaccine. Given in pregnancy only if clearly indicated.
- Varicella vaccine is live attenuated viral vaccine. It is contraindicated in pregnancy but ACIP recommends that pregnancy not to be terminated if it has been given inadvertently during pregnancy.
- Pneumococcal vaccine is a killed bacterial vaccine. It is given only to women in special high risk situations.
- Influenza vaccine contains inactivated viral vaccines. It is safe for use in pregnancy.
- Typhoid vaccine used contains killed bacteria. Not recommended routinely during pregnancy.
- Rabies vaccine (human) is an inactivated viral vaccine. It is given for post- exposure prophylaxis in pregnancy.
- Cholera vaccine is a killed vaccine and is only given in unusual outbreak situations during pregnancy.
- Inactivated Salk polio vaccine is preferred over oral polio vaccine in pregnancy. This is because of lower risk of vaccine associated paralysis with the inactivated vaccine.
- Hepatitis A Ig if administered within 14 days of exposure prevents hepatitis A in 80-90 per cent cases.
- Hepatitis B Ig (HBIG) is recommended for post-exposure prophylaxis in susceptible pregnant women.
- Tetanus Ig (TIG) given to pregnant women not immunised during pregnancy for post-exposure prophylaxis.

## REFERENCES

1. American College of Obstetricians and Gynaecologists. Immunisation during pregnancy. Technical bulletin No. 160 October 1991.
2. CDC Measles , Mumps and Rubella. Vaccine use and strategies for elimination of measles , rubella and congenital rubella syndrome. Recommendations of the ACIP. MMWR:1998;47:1-57.
3. CDC . Rubella vaccination during pregnancy-United states , 1971-82.MMWR 1983;32:429-32.
4. Linder N, Obel G. In utero vaccination. Cl Perinatology 1994;21:663-74.
5. Duff B, Duff P. Hep A vaccine : ready for prime time. Obstet Gynecol 1998;91:468-79.
6. CDC Hepatitis B virus: a comprehensive strategy for eliminating transmission in US through universal childhood vaccination. ACIP MMWR 1991;40:1-25.
7. Faix RG Maternal immunisation to prevent fetal and neonatal infection. Clin Obstet Gynecol 1991;34:277-87.
8. Ender G , Miller G Craddock –Watson J, et al. Consequences of varicella and herpes zoster in pregnancy: a prospective study of 1739 cases. Lancet 1994;343:154-58.
9. CDC. Prevention of varicella. MMWR 1996;45:1-36.
10. Schnab LZ, Glizer WP. Influenza virus. In Gonik B. Viral disease in pregnancy.1994;215-23.
11. CDC. Prevention and control of influenza: Recommendations of ACIP.MMWR 1999;48:1-28.
12. Product information: Typhim vi. Aventis Pasteur, 2001.
13. Chutivongse S,Wilde H, et al. Post-exposure rabies vaccination during pregnancy: effect on 202 women and their infants. Clin Infect Dis 1995;20:818-20.

**Table 15.1:** Immunisation during pregnancy

| *Immunobiologic agent* | *Risk from disease to pregnant woman* | *Risk from disease to foetus or neonate* | *Type of immunising agent* | *Risk from immunising agent to foetus* | *Indications for immunising during pregnancy* | *Dose schedule** | *Comments* |
|---|---|---|---|---|---|---|---|
| | | | ***LIVE VIRUS VACCINES*** | | | | |
| Measles | Significant morbidity, low mortality; not altered by pregnancy | Significant increase in abortion rate; may cause malformations | Live attenuated virus vaccine | None confirmed | Contraindicated (see immune globulins) | Single dose SC preferably as measles-mumps-rubella[1] | Vaccination of susceptible women should be part of postpartum care. Breastfeeding is not a contraindication |
| Mumps | Low morbidity and mortality; not altered by pregnancy | Possible increased rate of abortion in first trimester | Live attenuated virus vaccine. | None confirmed | Contraindicated | Single dose SC, preferably as measles-mumps-rubella | Vaccination of susceptible women should be part of postpartum care |
| Poliomyelitis | No increased incidence in pregnancy but may be more severe if it does occur | Anoxic foetal damage reported; 50% mortality in neonatal disease | Live attenuated virus (oral polio vaccine) and enhanced-potency inactivated virus vaccine | None confirmed | Not routinely recommended for women in the United States except women at increased risk of exposure | *Primary*: Two doses of enhanced potency inactivated virus SC at 4-8 week intervals and a third dose 6-12 months after the second dose *Immediate protection* one dose oral polio vaccine (in out-break setting) | Vaccine indicated for susceptible pregnant women travling in endemic areas or in other high-risk situations |
| Rubella | Low morbidity and mortality; not altered by pregnancy | High rate of abortion and congenital rubella syndrome | Live attenuated virus vaccine | None confirmed | Contraindicated but congenital rubella syndrome has never been described after vaccine | Single dose SC, preferably as measles-mumps-rubella | Teratogenicity of vaccine is theoretic, not confirmed to date; vaccination of susceptible women should be part of postpartum care |

*Contd...*

*Contd...*

| *Immunobiologic agent* | *Risk from disease to pregnant woman* | *Risk from disease to foetus or neonate* | *Type of immunising agent* | *Risk from immunising agent to foetus* | *Indications for immunising during pregnancy* | *Dose schedule** | *Comments* |
|---|---|---|---|---|---|---|---|
| Yellow fever | Significant morbidity and mortality, not altered by pregnancy | Unknown | Live attenuated virus vaccine | unknown | Contraindicated except if exposure is unavoidable | Single dose SC | Postponement of travel preferable to vaccination, if possible. |
| Varicella | Possible increase in severe pneumonia | Can cause congenital varicella in 2% of foetuses infected during the second trimester | Live attenuated virus vaccine | None confirmed | Contraindicated, but no adverse outcomes reported if given in pregnancy | Two doses needed with second dose given 4-8 weeks after first dose. Should be strongly encouraged | Teratogenicity of vaccine is theoretic, outcomes reported weeks 4-8 not confirmed to date. Vaccination of susceptible women should be considered postpartum |
| Influenza | Increase in morbidity and mortality during epidemic of new antigenic strain | Possible increased abortion rate; no malformations confirmed | Inactivated virus vaccine | None confirmed | All women who are pregnant in the second and third trimester during the flu season (October-March); women at high risk for pulmonary complications regardless of trimester | One dose IM every year | — |
| Rabies | Near 100% fatality; not altered by pregnancy | Determined by maternal disease | Killed virus vaccine | Unknown | Indications for prophylaxis not altered by pregnancy; each case considered individually | Public Health Authorities to be consulted for indications, dosage and route of administration | — |
| Hepatitis B | Possible increased severity during third trimester | Possible increase in abortion rate and preterm birth; neonatal hepatitis can | Purified surface antigen produced by recombinant technology | None reported | Pre-exposure and postexposure for women at risk of infection | Three-dose series IM at 0,1 and 6 months | Used with hepatitis B immune globulin for some exposures; exposed newborn needs |

*Contd...*

*Contd...*

| *Immunobiologic agent* | *Risk from disease to pregnant woman* | *Risk from disease to foetus or neonate* | *Type of immunising agent* | *Risk from immunising agent to foetus* | *Indications for immunising during pregnancy* | *Dose schedule** | *Comments* |
|---|---|---|---|---|---|---|---|
| | | occur; high risk of newborn carrier state | | | | | birth dose vaccination and immune globulin as soon as possible. All infants should receive birth dose of vaccine |
| Hepatitis A | No increased risk during pregnancy | — | Inactivated virus | None reported | Pre-exposure and postexposure for women at risk of infection; international travelers | Two-dose schedule 6 months apart | — |
| | | | ***INACTIVATED BACTERIAL VACCINES*** | | | | |
| Pneumococcus | No increased risk during pregnancy; no increase in severity of disease | Unknown but depends on maternal illness | Polyvalent polysaccharide vaccine | None reported | Recommended for women with asplenia; metabolic, renal, cardiac, pulmonary diseases; smokers immunosuppressed. Indications not altered by pregnancy | In adults, one SC or IM dose only, consider repeat dose in 6 years for high-risk women | — |
| Meningococcus | Significant morbidity and mortality; not altered by pregnancy | Unknown but depends on maternal illness | Quadrivalent polysaccharide vaccine | None reported | Indications not altered by pregnancy; vaccination recommended in unusual outbreak situations | One SC dose; Public Health Authorities consulted | — |
| Typhoid | Significant morbidity and mortality; not altered by pregnancy | Unknown | Killed or live attenuated oral bacterial vaccine | None confirmed | Not recommended routinely except for close, continued exposure or travel to endemic areas | Killed *Primary*: Two injections SC at least 4 weeks apart *Booster*: Single dose SC or ID (depending on type of product) | Oral vaccine preferred |

*Contd...*

*Contd...*

| *Immunobiologic agent* | *Risk from disease to pregnant woman* | *Risk from disease to foetus or neonate* | *Type of immunising agent* | *Risk from immunising agent to foetus* | *Indications for immunising during pregnancy* | *Dose schedule** | *Comments* |
|---|---|---|---|---|---|---|---|
| | | | | | | *Booster*: Schedule not yet determined | |
| Anthrax | Significant morbidity and mortality not altered by pregnancy | Unknown, but depends on maternal illness | Preparation from cell-free filtrate of *B anthracis,* no dead or live bacteria | None confirmed | Not routinely recommended unless pregnant women work directly with *B anthracis,* imported animal hides, potentially infected animals in high incidence areas (not United States) or military personnel deployed to high-risk exposure areas | Six-dose primary vaccination SC, then annual booster vaccination | Teratogenicity of vaccine theoretical |
| ***TOXOIDS*** | | | | | | | |
| Tetanus-diphtheria | Severe morbidity; tetanus mortality 30% diphtheria mortality 10%; unaltered by pregnancy | Neonatal tetanus mortality 60% | Combined tetanus-diphtheria toxoids preferred; adult tetanus-diphtheria formulation | None confirmed | Lack of primary series or no booster within past 10 years | *Primary*: Two doses IM at 1-2 month interval with a third dose 6-12 months after the second. *Booster*: Single dose IM every 10 years after completion of primary series | Updating of immune status should be part of antepartum care |
| ***SPECIFIC IMMUNE GLOBULINS*** | | | | | | | |
| Hepatitis B | Possible increased severity during third trimester | Possible increase in abortion rate and preterm birth; neo- | Hepatitis B immune globulin | None reported | Postexposure prophylaxis | Depends on exposure: consult Immunization | Usually given with hepatitis B virus vaccine; |

*Contd...*

*Contd...*

| *Immunobiologic agent* | *Risk from disease to pregnant woman* | *Risk from disease to foetus or neonate* | *Type of immunising agent* | *Risk from immunising agent to foetus* | *Indications for immunising during pregnancy* | *Dose schedule** | *Comments* |
|---|---|---|---|---|---|---|---|
| | | natal hepatitis can occur, high risk of carriage in newborn | | | | Practices Advisory committee recommendations (IM) | exposed newborn needs immediate postexposure prophylaxis |
| Rabies | Near 100% fatality; not altered by pregnancy | Determined by maternal disease | Rabies immune globulin | None reported | Postexposure prophylaxis | Half dose at injury site half dose in deltoid | Used in conjunction with rabies killed virus vaccine |
| Tetanus | Severe morbidity; mortality 60% | Neonatal tetanus mortality 60% | Tetanus immune globulin | None reported | Postexposure prophylaxis | One dose IM | Used in conjunction with tetanus toxoid |
| Varicella | Possible increase in severe varicella pneumonia | Can cause congenital varicella with increased mortality in neonatal period; very rarely causes congenital defects | Varicella-zoster immune globulin (obtained from the American Red Cross) | None reported | Should be considered for healthy pregnant women exposed to varicella to protact against maternal, not congenital, infection | One dose IM within 96 hours of exposure | Indicated also for newborns of women who developed varicella within 4 days before delivery or 2 days following delivery; approximately 90-95% of adults are immune to varicella; not indicated for prevention of non-genital varicella |
| | | | ***STANDARD IMMUNE GLOBULINS*** | | | | |
| Hepatitis A | Possible increased severity during third trimester | Probable increase in abortion rate and preterm birth; possible transmission to neonate at delivery if woman is incubating the virus or is acutely ill at that time | Standard immune globulin | None reported | Postexposure prophylaxis, but hepatitis A virus vaccine should be used with hepatitis A immune globulin | 0.02 mL/kg IM in one dose of immune globulin | Immune globulin should be given as soon as possible and within 2 weeks of exposure; intants born to women who are incubating the virus or are acutely ill at delivery should receive one dose of 0.5 mL as soon as possible after birth |

*Abbreviations: ID intradermally, IM, intramuscularly, PO, orally and SC subcutaneously.
Data from General recommendations on immunization. Recommendations of the Advisory Committee on Immunization Practices (ACIP) and the American Academy of Family Physicians (AAFP) 2003.

CHAPTER 16

# Antibiotic Prophylaxis in Obstetrics and Gynaecology

*Vijay Zutshi*

## INTRODUCTION

Antibiotic prophylaxis is defined as the use of antibiotics for the prevention of infection in the absence of current signs or symptoms of infection.

The role of prophylactic antibiotics for the prevention of postoperative morbidity in terms of an abdominal wound infection, wound discharge or abscess, pelvic cellulitis, pelvic abscess, postoperative pelvic inflammatory disease (PID), and postoperative septicaemia has been extensively studied.[1-5]

Infection continues to be the most important cause of the failure of surgical operations despite the development of more and more powerful antimicrobial drugs. It is accepted that infection can occur only when pathogens invade the tissues in sufficient numbers to overcome defenses of the body. The role of antimicrobials is to reduce the number of invaders to a manageable level. It is equally true that the host's ability to resist infection can be reduced by gross malnutrition, by prolonged anesthesia, and by ischaemia, whereas the only proven way of enhancing host resistance is to ensure an adequate supply of oxygenated blood to the tissues that are contaminated by bacteria.[6]

Infections in surgical patients arise as a result of exogenous or endogenous bacterial contamination, either in the operating theatre or in the wards. They may affect the tissues at the site of operation—wound infections and intra-abdominal or intrathoracic infections—or they may occur at distant sites, most often, in the respiratory and urinary systems. The prophylaxis of each of these infections differs in detail, but the principles are the same—to avoid or minimize bacterial contamination, to use antibiotics intelligently, and to do nothing to compromise the host's ability to defeat the invaders.

Infection of the incised skin or soft tissues is a common but potentially avoidable complication of any surgical procedure. Some bacterial contamination of a surgical site is inevitable, either from the patient's own bacterial flora or from the environment. In a survey of antibiotic use in one district general hospital, this indication accounted for approximately one third of all antibiotics prescribed.[7] Administration of antibiotics also increases the prevalence of antibiotic-resistant bacteria and predisposes the patient to infection with organisms such as *Clostridium difficile*, a cause of antibiotic-associated colitis.[8]

A survey of antibiotic control measures published by the British Society for Antimicrobial Chemotherapy in 1994 found that policies for surgical prophylaxis existed in only 51 percent of the hospitals surveyed and compliance was monitored in only half of these.[9]

**There are special conditions regarding the use of antibiotic prophylaxis in an obstetric and most gynaecological population:**

- Nearly all obstetric and most gynaecologic patients are healthy and free of serious underlying disorders.
- Lower genital tract is a contaminated field, operation through or adjacent to this field leads to a moderate-to-high incidence of infection in the absence of prophylaxis, but generally serious infections are unusual.
- Use of certain antimicrobials for prophylaxis in pregnancy is often contraindicated because of the potential for adverse effects on the foetus, newborn, or mother.

*Endogenous pathogens commonly present preoperatively at different sites: Knowledge about these microorganisms is important for use of antibiotic prophylaxis.*

*Skin*:

1. *Staphylococcus epidermidis*.
2. *Staphylococcus aureus* (small number).
3. *Micrococcus* species.
4. Nonpathogenic *Neisseria* species.
5. Alpha haemolytic and nonhaemolytic streptococci.
6. Diphtheroids.
7. *Propionobacterium* species.
8. *Peptostreptococcus* species.
9. Small number of other organisms (*Candida* sp), *Acinetobacter* species.

### *GI Tract and Rectum*

1. Upper intestine: Lactobacilli and Enterococci.
2. Lower ileum, caecum, colon: About 96 to 99 per cent anaerobes, bacteroides sp: *B. fragilis*, Fusobacterium species, anaerobic lactobacilli- bifido bacteria, *Clostridium perfringens*, anaerobic gram + cocci –*Peptostreptococcus*.
3. About 1 to 4 per cent facultative aerobes: Gram-negative coliform, enterococci, small number of protei, pseudomonas, lactobacilli, *Candida*.

### *Vagina*

1. Aerobic—lactobacilli till four to six months of birth ( pH—acidic)
2. Puberty—anaerobic and aerobic lactobacilli.
3. Childbearing age: About 25 per cent group B streptococci, anaerobic strep (peptostreptococci), alpha haemolytic strep- *Strep viridans*, *Prevotella binia*, *P disiens*, Clostridia, *Gardnerella vaginalis*, *Ureaplasma urealyticum*.

### *Urethra*

1. Lightly colonised 100 to 10,000: *Staph epidermidis*, *Strep faecalis*, diphtheroids, *Staph saprophyticus*.

**Factors associated with increased risk of surgical infection.**

### *Host Factors*

1. Older age.
2. Obesity.

3. Malnutrition.
4. Diabetes mellitus.
5. Immunocompromising diseases or therapies.
6. Presence of other infections.
7. Skin diseases.

### *Preoperative Factors*

1. Prolonged preoperative stay.
2. Shaving of skin.
3. Inadequate antibiotic prophylaxis.

### *Surgical Factors*

1. Inadequate skin antiseptics.
2. Emergency procedures.
3. Prosthetic implants.
4. Prolonged procedures.
5. Use of drains.
6. Poor techniques.
7. Unexpected contamination.

### *Environmental Factors*

1. Staphylococcal or streptococcal carrier.
2. Excessive activity in operation room.
3. Contaminated antiseptics.
4. Inadequate ventilation.
5. Inadequately sterilised equipment.

## Clinical Use of Antibiotics

- *Prophylactic therapy*: Given to patients prior to contamination or infection.
- *Anticipatory therapy*: Includes situations where contamination has already occurred and therapy is aimed at minimising postoperative infection.
- *Empiric therapy*: Non-directed therapy in the absence of pathogen identification.
- *Directed therapy*: Pathogen identified.

## Fundamental Principles of Surgical Prophylaxis

- The antibiotic must be in the tissue before the bacteria are introduced, i.e. antibiotic must be given intravenously shortly before surgery to ensure high blood/tissue levels. Prophylaxis failure may be due to antibiotics given too late or more often, given too early. **The knowledge about half-life of the particular antibiotic used is therefore important.**
- There is no data to support more than a single dose. Further doses generally constitute treatment. Note the waste of resources, the increased risk of complications and the fact that multiple doses are not associated with increased efficiency.

- The chosen antibiotics must be active against the most common expected pathogens.
- Deviations from these guidelines may be warranted in certain situations, e.g. MRSA (methicillin-resistant *Staphylococcus aureus*) outbreak in an individual hospital.
- High-risk patients, e.g. patients with jaundice or diabetics, or patients who undergo any procedures to insert prosthetic devices, generally warrant antibiotic prophylaxis.

Over the last three decades, a large body of data have accumu-lated to allow for the establishment of practical recommendations for use in many procedures.

Searches were initially carried out on the Cochrane Library, Embase, Healthstar, and Medline from 1987 to 1998, and were updated during the course of development. In view of the volume of literature in this area, searches were initially restricted to existing guidelines, meta-analyses, and systematic reviews. Subsequently, searches for additional papers on audit of guideline effectiveness, and on the impact of haemodilution following intravenous administration of antibiotics were carried out. All search strategies were subject to independent review.

In addition to the initial search, members of the guideline development group searched the Medline database from 1960 to find the best evidence of the role of prophylactic antibiotics in surgical site infection prophylaxis. If a good meta-analysis was found, this was used as the sole evidence. Failing this, good quality randomised trials were sought. Some of the references are old, but these were used when they were judged to be "practice changing" papers. In the absence of good randomised trials, other published evidence (e.g. other trials, audits, expert opinion, etc.) was used as a guide to prophylaxis.

## Goals of Antibiotic Prophylaxis

- The aim of prophylaxis is to augment host defence mechanism at the time of bacterial invasion, thereby decreasing the size of the bacterial inoculum.
- Use antibiotics in a manner that is supported by evidence of effectiveness.
- Minimize the effect of antibiotics on the patient's normal bacterial flora.
- Minimize adverse effects.
- Cause minimal change to the patient's host defences.

**It is important to emphasise that surgical antibiotic prophylaxis is an adjunct to, not a substitute for, good surgical technique. Antibiotic prophylaxis should be regarded as one component of an effective policy for the control of hospital-acquired infection.**

## Factors Affecting the Incidence of Surgical Site Infection

### *a. Classification of Operation*

Operations can be categorised into four classes (Table 16.1) with an increasing incidence of bacterial contamination and subsequent incidence of postoperative infection.[10]

**Table 16.1:** Classification of operation

| *Class* | *Definition* |
|---|---|
| Clean | Operations in which no inflammation is encountered and the respiratory, alimentary or genitourinary tracts are not entered. There is no break in aseptic operating theatre technique. |
| Clean-contaminated | Operations in which the respiratory, alimentary or genitourinary tracts are entered but without significant spillage. |
| Contaminated | Operations where acute inflammation (without pus) is encountered, or where there is visible contamination of the wound. Examples include gross spillage from a hollow viscus during the operation or compound/open injuries operated on within four hours. |
| Dirty | Operations in the presence of pus, where there is a previously perforated hollow viscus, or compound/open injuries more than four hours old. |

### *b. Duration of Surgery*

Duration of surgery is positively associated with risk of wound infection, and this risk is additional to that of the classification of operation. With prolonged duration, chances of infection increase.

## Benefits of Prophylaxis

- *Decreased incidence of infection (wound/distal)*
  In many ways, the value of surgical antibiotic prophylaxis in terms of the incidence of surgical site infection (SSI) after elective surgery is related to the severity of the consequences of SSI. For example, in the presence of an anastomosis of the colon, prophylaxis reduces postoperative mortality.[11] However, for most operations, prophylaxis only decreases short-term morbidity. *(Evidence level III).*
- *Reduce overall costs and prolonged stay*
  Surgical wound infection increases the length of hospital stay.[12] The additional length of stay is dependent on the type of surgery. For example, about three days for cholecystectomy or hysterectomy but 11 to 16 days for major orthopaedic procedures.[13,14] Prophylaxis, therefore, has the potential to shorten hospital stay. However, there is little direct evidence that it does so as few randomised trials have included hospital length of stay as an outcome measure. Nonetheless, there is limited evidence to show that prevention of wound infection is associated with faster return to normal activity after discharge from hospital.[15] *(Evidence level III).*

## Risks of Prophylaxis

- Toxic reactions
- Allergic reactions
- Emergence of resistant bacteria
- Drug interaction.
- Superinfection.

One of the aims of rationalising surgical antibiotic prophylaxis is to reduce the inappropriate use of antibiotics thus minimising the consequences of misuse.

Rates of antibiotic resistance are increasing in all hospitals. The prevalence of antibiotic resistance in any population is related to the proportion of the population that receives antibiotics, and also the total antibiotic exposure.[16] *(Evidence level IIa)*.

An additional problem is the dramatic increase in the number of cases of colitis caused by *Clostridium difficile* in the UK from 1993 to 96. The prevalence of *C. difficile* infection is related to total antibiotic usage and, in particular, to the use of third generation cephalosporins.[17-19] In epidemiological studies of *C. difficile* colitis, surgical antibiotic prophylaxis is the single most common indication for use of antibiotics.[8] Although even single dose prophylaxis increases the risk of carriage of *C. difficile*,[20] in a case-control study of patients all of whom received surgical prophylaxis carriage of *C. difficile* was more common in patients who received prophylaxis for >24 hours (56% versus 17%). *(Evidence level IIa)*.

The consequences of *C.difficile* infections include increased morbidity and mortality and prolonged hospital stay, leading to an overall increase in health care costs. The estimated cost of treating a single episode of *C.difficile* in hospital is £4000, largely due to prolongation of hospital stay.[19] Moreover, one study has shown a statistically significant increase in the frequency of bacteraemia and line infections in surgical patients who received prophylactic antibiotics for more than four days in comparison with those who received prophylaxis for one day or less.[21]

Validity of recommendations is based on the following two methods:

1. Grades of recommendations.
2. Statements of evidence.

## Grades of Recommendations

a. Requires at least one randomised controlled trial as part of a body of literature of overall good quality and consistency addressing the specific recommendation. (*Evidence levels Ia, Ib*).
b. Requires the availability of well-conducted clinical studies but no randomised clinical trials on the topic of recommendation. (*Evidence levels IIa, IIb, III*).
c. Requires evidence obtained from expert committee reports or opinions and/or clinical experiences of respected authorities. Indicates an absence of directly applicable clinical studies of good quality. (*Evidence level IV*)

## Statements of Evidence

- *Ia*: Evidence obtained from meta-analysis of randomised controlled trials.
- *Ib*: Evidence obtained from at least one randomised controlled trial.
- *IIa*: Evidence obtained from at least one well-designed controlled study without randomization.
- *IIb*: Evidence obtained from at least one other type of well-designed quasi-experimental study.

- *III*: Evidence obtained from well-designed non-experimental descriptive studies, such as comparative studies, correlation studies and case studies.
- *IV*: Evidence obtained from expert committee reports or opinions and/or clinical experiences of respected authorities.

## Four Different Recommendations have been made Regarding Surgical Antibiotic Prophylaxis

*Highly recommended*: Prophylaxis unequivocally reduces major morbidity, reduces hospital costs and is likely to decrease overall consumption of antibiotics.

*Recommended*: Prophylaxis reduces short-term morbidity, but there are no RCTs that prove that prophylaxis reduces the risk of mortality or long-term morbidity. However, prophylaxis is highly likely to reduce major morbidity, reduce hospital costs and may decrease overall consumption of antibiotics.

*Recommended but local policy makers may identify exceptions*: Although prophylaxis is recommended for all patients, local policy makers may wish to identify exceptions, as prophylaxis may not reduce hospital costs and could increase consumption of antibiotics, especially if given to patients at low risk of infection. However, any local policy that recommends restriction of prophylaxis to "high-risk" patients must specify and justify the threshold of risk. Moreover, such a policy requires continuous documentation of wound infection rates in order to provide evidence that the risk of SSI in patients who do not receive prophylaxis is below the specified risk threshold. In addition, for clean-contaminated procedures or procedures involving insertion of prosthetic device, evidence for the clinical effectiveness of surgical antibiotic prophylaxis is lacking. This is either because trials have not been done or have been done with such small numbers of patients that important treatment effects cannot be excluded. A local policy that does not recommend prophylaxis for these operations can be justified on the basis that there is no conclusive evidence of effectiveness. However, policy makers must be aware that their policy represents a minority of professional opinion.

**As per these grades, grade A is only given for use of pro-phylactic antibiotic for the procedures like caesarean section, hysterectomy (abdominal and vaginal) and induced abortion.**

## Route of Administration

Intravenous (IV) administration of antibiotic prophylaxis immediately before or after induction of anaesthesia is the most reliable method for ensuring effective serum antibiotic concentrations at the time of surgery.

Serum concentrations after oral or intramuscular administration are determined in part by the rate of absorption, which varies between individuals. There is relatively little evidence about the effectiveness of orally or intramuscularly administered antibiotic prophylaxis. A further problem is that often the correct time of administration is difficult to guarantee in practice. **Administration of antibiotic prophylaxis by the intravenous route is the only method that is supported by a substantial body of evidence.**

## Timing of Administration

The period of risk for SSI begins with the incision. The time taken for an antibiotic to reach an effective concentration in any particular tissue reflects its pharmacokinetic profile and the route of administration.[22] *(Evidence level Ia).*

Administration of prophylaxis more than three hours after the start of the operation significantly reduces its effectiveness.[23] For maximum effect, it should be given just before or just after the start of the operation. *(Evidence level Ia).*

In most circumstances, prophylaxis should be started preoperatively, ideally within 30 minutes of the induction of anaesthesia.

However, there may be situations where over-riding factors alter the normal timing of administration. For example, during a caesarean section prophylaxis should be delayed until the cord is clamped in order to prevent the drug reaching the neonate. Then a tourniquet is to be applied, the necessary tissue concentration must be achieved prior to its application rather than at the time of incision. This probably occurs within 10 minutes of administration of an IV antibiotic injection.

Antibiotics should also be administered immediately after unexpected contamination of the tissues.

### *Current Recommendations*

- Parenteral antibiotics used in prophylaxis should be given in sufficient dosage within 30 minutes preceding incision.
- This results in near maximum drug levels in the wound and the surrounding tissues during the operation.
- This can be facilitated, by having the anaesthetist administer the antibiotic in the operating room, when the intravenous lines are inserted shortly before operative incision.
- A single preoperative dose of antibiotic has the same efficacy as multiple doses and the current recommendation is to administer a second dose only if the operation lasts for longer than 2 to 3 hours.
- With the oral preoperative antibiotic preparation commonly used before elective colonic resection, the chosen agents should be given during the 24 hours before the operation in order to attain significant intraluminal (local) and serum (systemic) levels.

## Choice of Antibiotic

### *Type of Antibiotic*

Classification of antibiotics can be done as follows:

1. Cephalosporins
   - *First generation* (for example, cefazolin, cephradine, cephazolin, cephalexin, cefadroxil)
   - *Second generation* (for example, cefoxitin, cefuroxime, cephamandole, cefaclor, cefprozil, loracarbef)
   - *Third generation* (for example, cefotaxime, cefotetan, ceftazidime, ceftriaxone, cefixime, cefpodoxime proxetil, ceftibuten, cefdinir, cephoperazone, ceftizoxime)
   - *Fourth generation* (for example, cefepime)

2. Penicillins (for example, penicillin, amoxicillin)
3. Macrolides (for example, erythromycin, calrithromycin, azithromycin)
4. Fluoroquinolones (for example, ciprofloxacillin, levofloxacin, ofloxacin)
5. Sulfonamides (for example, cotrimoxazole, trimethoprim)
6. Tetracyclines (for example, tetracycline, doxycycline)
7. Aminogylocosides (for example, gentamicin, tobramycin)
8. Glycopeptides (for example, vancomycin)
9. Antiprotozoals (for example, metronidazole)
10. Combination drugs
11. Augmentin (amoxycillin and clavulanic acid).

Although a wide range of organisms can cause infection in surgical patients, SSI is usually due to a small number of common pathogens (except in the presence of implanted biomaterial).[24] **The antibiotics selected for prophylaxis must cover the common pathogens.**

The antibiotics chosen for prophylaxis can be those used for active treatment of infection. However, the chosen antibiotics must reflect local, disease-specific information about the common pathogens and their antimicrobial susceptibility. In patients who develop infection after prophylaxis, same antibiotic should not be used to treat. In addition, extended-spectrum antibiotics should not be used for prophylaxis but should be reserved for treatment.[25] Half-life of the particular antibiotic and spectrum of the activity should be known (Table 16.2).

**Table 16.2:** Half-life of the commonly used drugs

| *Drug* | *Half-life* |
|---|---|
| Cefazolin | 1.8 hours |
| Cefoxitin | 60 minutes |
| Cefotetan | 4 hours |
| Ampicillin | 1 hour |
| Ciprofloxacin | 3–4.5 hours |
| Gentamicin | 2–3 hours |
| Metronidazole | 7.5 hours |
| Clindamycin | 3 hours |

A past history of a serious adverse event should preclude administration of a particular antibiotic.

A comprehensive risk assessment should be part of the process of choosing the appropriate antibiotic.[26] This should include economic considerations, such as the acquisition costs of the drug and costs of administration and preparation, set against conse-quences of failure of prophylaxis and the possible adverse events.

Prescribers need to be aware of that bacteria that remain sensitive to the prophylactic regimen usually cause infections, that occur in patients who receive prophylaxis. Implementation of prophylaxis should not be accompanied by radical changes in treatment policy because such changes may wipe out the benefits of prophylaxis. For example, changing to third generation cephalosporins for routine treatment of postoperative infection because of implementation of prophylaxis with first or second generation cephalosporins may lead to major drug-resistance problems.[25] Treatment policies should be based on local information about the epidemiology of drug-resistant bacteria. Implementation of a prophylaxis policy should not trigger an automatic change in treatment policy.

## Penicillin Allergy

Reactions to penicillin may occur because of allergy to the parent compound or its metabolites. In descending order of association, the previous symptoms most allied with a subsequent immediate hypersensitivity reaction to penicillin are,[27-29] anaphylaxis urticaria, rash. *(Evidence level IIb).*

Other symptomatologies show either no or extremely weak associations with subsequent allergic reactions.

In patients allergic to penicillins, challenge tests can be used to demonstrate cross-reactions with cephalosporins[30] and carba-penems.[31] However, the frequency of these relationships and their clinical significance is uncertain. *(Evidence level IIb).*

Patients with a history of rash occurring more than 72 hours after administration of penicillin are probably not allergic to penicillin. Patients with a history of anaphylaxis or urticaria or rash occurring immediately after penicillin therapy are at increased risk of immediate hypersensitivity to penicillins and should not receive prophylaxis with a beta-lactam antibiotic.

For patients who have documented immediate hypersensitivity reactions to penicillin, antibiotic choices for prophylaxis are limited. In such cases, cephalosporins are contraindicated, as are penicillin-type antibiotics. One recommendation is for the use of single dose clindamycin (900 mg), perhaps with a single dose of gentamicin (1.5–2.0 mg/kg).[32]

Vancomycin may be used for prophylaxis of caesarean section endometritis in patients with an immediate hypersensitivity reaction to penicillin.

## Duration of Prophylaxis

### *Additional Doses of Antibiotic*

Many of the drugs used in prophylaxis have relatively short half-lives (1–2 hours in studies of normal volunteers). In such situations, it may, therefore, seem logical to give an additional dose of prophylaxis during operations that last for more than 2 to 4 hours.[33] However, in comparison with normal volunteers, patients undergoing surgery have slower clearance of drugs from their blood.[34,35] This is probably due to a combination of factors. For example, in comparison with normal volunteers, surgical patients are older (and, therefore, have poorer renal function) and have more co-morbidities. The limited data available show that drugs such as cefuroxime, which has a half-life of 1 to 2 hours in normal volunteers has a half-life of 2 to 4 hours in patients at the time of surgery, and that effective concentrations are maintained for at least five hours after the start of surgery.

The search strategy used in the development of this guideline, found only two clinical studies that explicitly compared a single dose preoperatively with a preoperative dose plus an additional intraoperative dose.[36] One randomised trial did not support the effectiveness of a second intraoperative dose.[36] In this study, Timentin, a combination of ticarcillin and clavulanic acid, was administered intravenously (3.1 g) at the commencement of operation to all patients, and this was repeated after two hours in those patients randomised to receive a second dose. The wound infection rate was 11 percent in those patients receiving a single dose, and 13 percent in the patients receiving two doses of Timentin. The second study[32] did support the use of second intraoperative doses of cefazolin when patients were still in the operating theatre three hours after the start of surgery. The odds ratio (OR) of wound infection was 0.21 (95% CI 0.04–0.98) in comparison with patients who only received a single, preoperative dose. However, there are important methodological flaws in this evidence. The data were collected ten years before the study was published, the method of allocation to treatment regimens is not stated, the study was not blinded and the definition of wound infection is not given.

### *Additional Doses After the End of the Operation*

In all operations, the administration of additional doses after the end of surgery does not provide any additional prophylactic benefit.[24,37-39] Individual studies claiming to support additional postoperative doses are methodologically flawed. For example, not blinding observers to treatment allocation and including culture of bacteria from a wound swab as an indication of wound infection.[40] This is specifically excluded from most definitions of wound infection, as the test does not distinguish between colonisation and infection. Moreover, patients who are continuing to receive antibiotics are clearly less likely to have bacteria grown from swabs than patients who are not receiving antibiotics.

Prophylaxis should be confined, therefore, to the perioperative period (i.e. administration immediately before or during the procedure). Postoperative doses of antibiotic for prophylaxis should not be given for any operation. Any decision to prolong prophylaxis beyond a single dose should be explicit and supported by an evidence base. Antibiotic prophylaxis should be confined to the perioperative period.

## Blood Loss, Fluid Replacement and Antibiotic Prophylaxis

Serum antibiotic concentrations are reduced by blood loss and fluid replacement, especially in the first hour of surgery when drug levels are high.[41,42] *(Evidence levels IIa and IIb).*

The precise effects of blood loss and fluid replacement are difficult to predict, depending on the timing and rate of loss and replacement.[24] However, in adults, the impact of intraoperative bleeding and fluid replacement on serum drug concentrations is usually negligible.[43,44] *(Evidence level IIb).* **In adults, blood loss of up to 1500 ml during surgery or haemodilution up to 15 ml/kg does not require an additional dose of prophylactic agent.**

*In the event of major intraoperative blood loss (>1,500 ml), additional doses of prophylactic antibiotic should be given after fluid replacement.* Fluid replacement bags should not be primed with prophylactic antibiotics because of the potential risk of contamination and calculation errors.

Types of outcome measures one looks for after giving antibiotic prophylaxis:

## *Primary Outcomes*

1. *Infection*:
   Measured as the proportion of women who develop one of the following (according to the study definition) within eight weeks of surgery:
   - Any postoperative infection
   - Abdominal wound infection (for example, wound cellulitis, abscess, dehiscence)
   - Pelvic infection [including vaginal cuff (vault) infection, pelvic inflammatory disease, pelvic abscess, infected haematoma]
   - Urinary tract infection (UTI)
   - Other serious infection or infectious complication, such as septicaemia, septic shock, distant infections (for example, pneumonia)
   - Postoperative fever of > 38°C on at least two occasions more than four hours apart, excluding the day of surgery.
2. Morbidity (for example, allergic reaction, diarrhoea, bacterial resistance or as defined by the study) and mortality (infection-related and all-cause)
   Primary outcomes will be classified as either early (before discharge from hospital or within seven days of surgery), late (at follow-up: within eight weeks of surgery), or total (early and late).

## *Secondary Outcomes*

1. Asymptomatic infection, diagnosed solely by lab test with no clinical signs or symptoms (e.g. asymptomatic bacteriuria), either early (before discharge from hospital or within seven days of surgery), late (at follow-up: within eight weeks of surgery) or total (early and late).
2. Any requirement for systemic antibiotics, either early (before discharge from hospital or within seven days of surgery), late (at follow-up: within eight weeks of surgery) or total (early and late).
3. Length of hospital stay.
4. Readmission to hospital.
5. Cost (including both public and private costs).
6. Quality of life.

## Evidence-based Results on the use of Prophylactic Antibiotics, Cochrane Data Base Reviews

### *Uses in Obstetrics*

**Antibiotic prophylaxis for caesarean section**

Review of the literature regarding use of prophylactic antibiotics in caesarean section has been done. Eighty-one trials that enrolled close to 12,000 women were identified that met the inclusion criteria for this review. All these trials were included from 1972 onwards.

The main comparison of any treatment versus no treatment was stratified by whether the caesarean section was elective, non-elective or a combination of both/unspecified, resulting in four main comparisons:

1. Any antibiotic versus placebo/no treatment (elective caesarean deliveries).
2. Any antibiotic versus placebo/no treatment (non-elective caesarean deliveries).
3. Any antibiotic versus placebo/no treatment (a combination of both elective and non-elective/unspecified caesarean deliveries).
4. Any antibiotic versus placebo/no treatment (all caesarean deliveries).

The antimicrobial agents most often used in the trials included ampicillin, a first generation cephalosporin (usually cefazolin), a second generation cephalosporin (cefoxitin, cefotetan or cefuroxime), metronidazole, an extended-spectrum penicillin (e.g. ticarcillin, or a beta-lactamase inhibitor combination) and an aminoglycoside-containing combination. Antibiotics for prophy-laxis were usually administered intravenously after the cord was clamped. Nine studies were included where irrigation of the peritoneal or uterine cavity with an antibiotic-containing solution was compared with either saline irrigation or no irrigation. The duration of the postoperative treatment course varied from a single dose (n = 22) to as long as a week. In 32 studies, antibiotics were continued for up to 24 hours following the procedure. While most studies were published in the 1980s, new studies have continued to be performed in the 1990s and published as recently as 2001.

### *Message*

The results of the trials included in this review are, however, remarkably consistent, both in direction of effect and in effect size. Overall, the use of prophylactic antibiotics with caesarean section results in a major, clinically important, and statistically significant reduction in the incidence of episodes of fever, endometritis, wound infection, urinary tract infection (UTI) and serious infection after caesarean section. Only in nine studies that reported the incidence of UTI in women undergoing an elective caesarean section, there were the differences in the rate of UTIs not statistically significant and there were too few serious infectious outcomes in women undergoing an elective caesarean section to analyse.

Despite the theoretic need to cover gram-negative and anaerobic organisms, studies have not demonstrated a superior result with broad-spectrum antibiotics (BSAs) compared with first and second generation cephalosporins.

Both ampicillin and first generation cephalosporins represent good choices for prophylaxis in women undergoing caesarean section. More costly extended-spectrum penicillins, second or third generation cephalosporins and combination regimens have not been demonstrated to be more effective. There is no evidence to suggest that a multiple dose regimen is of greater benefit to the women than a single-dose regimen.

There will be continued debate both in the literature and in clinical practice regarding the optimal time for administration of prophylactic antibiotics. There is currently insufficient evidence upon which to base a recommendation regarding the optimal timing of antibiotic administration. This question will not be resolved until a randomised trial of sufficient size is completed comparing pre-operative administration versus administration immediately after the cord is clamped.

Prophylactic antibiotics will reduce the incidence of endometritis following both elective and non-elective caesarean section by two-thirds to three-quarters and the incidence of wound infection by up to three-quarters. Postpartum febrile morbidity and the incidence of UTIs are also decreased. Fewer serious complications will occur. All units should have a policy that recommends the administration of prophylactic antibiotics for women undergoing caesarean section. Obstetrical units should collect information on infection rates following caesarean section as an important quality indicator.

Further placebo-controlled trials of the effectiveness of antibiotics with caesarean section are not ethically justified.[45]

### *Antibiotic Prophylaxis for Fourth-Degree Perineal Tear During Vaginal Birth*

One per cent to eight per cent of women suffer severe perineal tears after vaginal birth. These tears are more common after operative vaginal birth, especially when forceps are used. The incidence of severe perineal lacerations after the use of forceps has been reported as 21 per cent for third-degree and seven per cent for fourth-degree tears . Other risk factors include race, midline episiotomy, nulliparity, and high birth weight baby.

When a woman has a severe perineal tear (ruptured anal sphincter with or without ruptured rectal mucosa) during vaginal birth, there is thought to be an increased risk of infection. Laceration of the vagina and perineum after vaginal birth are classified as first, second, third and fourth degree. First-degree tears involve the vaginal mucosa and connective tissue. Second-degree tears involve the vaginal mucosa, connective tissue and underlying muscles. Third-degree tears involve a complete transection of anal sphincter and fourth-degree tears involve the rectal mucosa. When the rectal mucosa is ruptured, the wound is classified as contaminated or clean-contaminated. Antibiotic prophylaxis is generally used where wounds have become, or are likely to become, contaminated, such as in colorectal surgery.

A woman contracting an infection after a severe perineal tear may also be dealing with other morbidities as a result of the tear, such as haematoma, dyspareunia, incontinence and rectovaginal fistula.

### *Message*

While some authorities recommend that prophylactic antibiotics should be used for severe perineal tears, others have recommended against this course of action. As widespread use of antibiotics may contribute to antibiotic-resistant bacteria, the overuse of antibiotics is being discouraged by many groups. However, antibiotic prophylaxis is a low-cost, accessible intervention which may prevent considerable maternal morbidity. It is, therefore, important to establish the benefits of prophylactic antibiotics for preventing infection after severe perineal tears, and also to assess if there are any adverse effects on mother or child, by systematically reviewing the evidence.[46]

### *Antibiotic Prophylaxis for Operative Vaginal Delivery*

There are still some doubts about the benefit of prophylactic antibiotics in reducing postpartum infection after operative vaginal delivery. Aseptic precautions during operative vaginal delivery are thought to be enough to prevent postpartum infection.

The data are too few and of insufficient quality to make any recommendations for practice.

### *Message*

There is not enough evidence to support the use of antibiotic prophylaxis for operative vaginal delivery.

*Future research* on antibiotic prophylaxis for operative vaginal delivery is needed to clarify whether this intervention is effective in reducing postpartum morbidity. Biases should be reduced by proper methods of allocation, concealment, blinded interventions, clearly defined outcomes and consistent outcome measures. The drug regimens for future trials should be based on the principle of antibiotic prophylaxis for caesarean section with a single dose of intravenous ampicillin or first generation cephalosporins after cord clamping.[47]

## Uses in Gynaecology

### *Antibiotic Prophylaxis for Elective Hysterectomy*

Hysterectomy is one of the most commonly performed operations. Most hysterectomies are elective (non-urgent) procedures for benign gynaecological conditions, the commonest being leiomyoma (fibroids). Other common indications are endometriosis, heavy menstrual bleeding, uterovaginal prolapse and PID. The surgery can be performed abdominally, laparo-scopically or vaginally, with or without laparoscopic assistance. Even with the best surgical and postoperative care, hysterectomy is unavoidably associated with a high infection risk because the surgery breaches the genital tract, an area commonly colonised by a wide variety and large numbers of microorganisms. In addition, most women undergoing hysterectomy require an indwelling urinary catheter for the first 24 hours, which increases the risk of UTI. Common sites of infection after hysterectomy are the bladder, the pelvic floor, the cuff of tissue at the top of the vagina (vaginal vault) and the abdominal wound, while related complications include pelvic abscess, infected haematoma (accumulation of blood from the wound), septicaemia (infection of the blood) and pneumonia. Such infections are usually caused by a mixture of bacteria from the woman's own vaginal or urethral tissues, both gram-positive and gram-negative and both aerobic and anaerobic (these terms refer to the staining techniques used in identification and whether the bacteria are oxygen-dependent). The susceptibility to infection of the individual woman depends upon the effectiveness of her immune system, the virulence of the bacteria present, and the degree of tissue trauma and fluid collection resulting from surgery.

### *Message*

Antibiotic prophylaxis is now recommended in national guidelines for all types of hysterectomy, although in practice, the application of such guidelines is variable.

Although various antibiotic regimens and routes of delivery have been used, currently the most frequent practice is for a single dose of antibiotic to be given intravenously within two hours of the surgical incision, in order to facilitate optimum serum antibiotic levels during the operation. A single dose has been reported to be as effective as multiple doses, though some authors have suggested repeating the dose if the surgery is long or blood loss is high. If prophylaxis is continued postoperatively, it is recommended that the duration of therapy does not exceed 24 hours.

The type of antibiotic most commonly used is one that is active against a wide range of bacteria (broad-spectrum), such as amoxycillin/clavulanic acid (augmentin) or a cephalosporin. Cephalosporins are grouped into generations according to their antimicrobial properties, with the oldest type being termed *first generation.* Subsequent generations of these drugs have progressively widened their antibacterial coverage against gram-negative organisms, but there has been a concurrent reduction in their effectiveness against gram-positive organisms. The wide use of very BSAs greatly increases the risk of drug-resistant bacteria emerging. It is generally recommended that first or second generation cephalosporins should be used for prophylaxis, as they appear to be equally effective for this purpose, less expensive and less likely to favour drug resistance.[48]

### *Antibiotic Prophylaxis for Intrauterine Contraceptive Device Insertion*

Concern about the risk of upper genital tract infection (PID) often limits use of the intrauterine device (IUD), a highly effective contraceptive. Prophylactic antibiotic administration around the time of induced abortion significantly reduces the risk of postoperative endometritis. Since the risk of IUD-related infection is largely limited to the first few weeks to months after insertion, contamination of the endometrial cavity at the time of insertion appears to be the mechanism, rather than the IUD or string itself. Thus, antibiotic administration before IUD insertion might reduce the risk of upper genital tract infection from passive introduction of bacteria at insertion.

#### *Results*

Only four randomised controlled trials have been found; two had pilot study data available. The primary outcomes studied were PID (four reports), unscheduled visits back to the clinic (four reports), or early removals of the device (two reports). Women enrolling in the four different trials met local criteria for IUD insertion. In the African trials, IUD was less restrictive than in the other trials. The prevalence of cervical infections with *Neisseria gonorrhoeae* among participants in the Kenya trial was 3 percent, while that in the Nigerian trial was 1 percent. The prevalence of *Chlamydia trachomatis* in the cervix was higher (11% and 7%, respectively).

The Kenyan trial found a significant reduction in unscheduled visits, and the meta-analysis had an odds ratio of 0.82 (95% CI 0.70 –0.98). No other significant benefit emerged when the trials were combined.

The Kenyan trial found that doxycycline reduced the risk of PID by about one-third, which was not statistically significant (RR 0.69; 95% CI 0.32–1.5). A similar reduction in unscheduled return visits because of an IUD-related problem was statistically significant (RR 0.69; 95% CI 0.52–0.91). The Nigerian trial, which attempted to replicate the Kenyan trial, found no benefit of prophylaxis in reducing either salpingitis or unscheduled visits.

The Los Angeles trial, which focused on premature IUD discontinuation, found no overall benefit of prophylactic azithromycin (RR 1.1; 95% CI 0.7–1.8). Only one case of PID occurred in each treatment group. Similarly, the rate of unscheduled visits to the provider did not differ significantly.

The Turkish trial found no significant difference in rates of PID.

Use of prophylactic antibiotics before IUD insertion reduced the likelihood of an unscheduled visit to the provider by 18 percent, which was marginally statistically significant. No other important benefits were observed, specifically reduction in upper genital tract infection or improvement in IUD continuation rates.

The over-riding message from these four trials is that contemporary IUD use is safe, with or without use of prophylactic antibiotics. This holds true for populations with a high prevalence of sexually transmitted diseases (STDs), as is the case in much of Africa. The concern about high rates of upper genital tract infection, even in the critical early months of use, appears unwarranted. As noted by the World Health Organization, contemporary copper IUDs are among the safest and most effective reversible methods of contraception available today.

### Message

Use of prophylactic antibiotics may reduce the likelihood of an unscheduled visit back to the clinic. Authors have suggested that complaints of pain and bleeding associated with IUD use may represent subclinical endometritis. Antibiotic administration may reduce this risk and thus lead to fewer problem visits. While fewer problem-related visits will save money and reduce inconvenience, prophylaxis would probably only be cost-effective where STDs are common, as observed in the study from Kenya.

The low rate of infection or premature removals of IUDs is an important clinical news. On the other hand, the low incidence of IUD-related problems poses difficult challenges for researchers. The Kenyan trial, which enrolled over 1,800 women, had insufficient power to identify the anticipated treatment effect. In the Los Angeles trial, the investigators anticipated the low incidence of PID and focused instead on premature IUD discontuation as the primary outcome measure. In the main trial with over 1,800 participants, only two cases of salpingitis occurred.

Additional studies of prophylactic antibiotics in low-risk populations appear unjustified. In women at higher risk, further research may be considered. However, because of the low incidence of PID even in these settings, the number of women needed to treat to avert a single case of infection will be large.[49]

### *Antibiotic Prophylaxis for Medical and Surgical First Trimester-Induced Abortion*

Each year, 210 million pregnancies occur worldwide; of which, an estimated 46 million end in an induced abortion. Abortion causes 65,958 deaths and 4,652,171, the vast majority due to unsafe illegal abortions in developing countries. Infection introduced through cervical instrumentation is probably responsible for a substantial amount of this morbidity and mortality. Thirteen per cent of maternal deaths worldwide are due to unsafe abortion. A recognised iatrogenic complication of the procedure is postabortal pelvic infection, which is presumed to be due to the introduction of bacteria into the upper genital tract by surgical instruments. Infectious agents causing postabortal pelvic infection include exogenous bacteria, endogenous vaginal anaerobes or sexually transmitted cervical pathogens (*Neisseria gonorrhoeae* and *Chlamydia trachomatis*).

### *Message*

Antibiotics given prior to abortion should reduce the risk of post-abortal infective morbidity. There is, however, ongoing debate about the most effective and cost-effective method for achieving this. The possible approaches are described below.

### *Universal Antibiotic Prophylaxis*

Universal antibiotic prophylaxis means that all women undergoing termination of pregnancy (TOP) are given antibiotics around the time of surgery without carrying out tests for infection. A meta-analysis combining the results of twelve randomised controlled trials of universal antibiotic prophylaxis at the time of abortion found a reduction in the risk of subsequent pelvic infections of up to 50 per cent. This meta-analysis was based on a literature search for studies published between 1966 and 1994 using only the Medline database, which might not identify all trials and lead to bias. Furthermore, there was substantial heterogeneity between the studies, but results were combined using a fixed effect rather than the more conservative random effect model. The meta-analysis did not determine the optimal antibiotic or dosing regimen, and adverse effects were not reported.

### *Screen-and-Treat*

Combining the screen-and-treat strategy and universal antibiotic prophylaxis should prevent both short- and long-term morbidity but may increase costs to the health service. Screen-and-treat means that all women presenting for a TOP are screened for genital infections. Those with positive results are treated, preferably before the procedure. The major advantage of the screen-and-treat strategy over universal antibiotic prophylaxis is the possibility of contact tracing and treatment of sexual partners, hence reducing the risk of re-infection and reducing the reservoir of infection within the community. In addition, the screen-and-treat policy avoids the unnecessary administration of antibiotics to non-infected women, and provides an opportunity to screen for other STDs and offer counselling. However, this strategy is costly, and requires more organisation than does universal prophylaxis. Furthermore, postabortal pelvic infection can still occur due to false-negative screening tests or infections not screened for.[50]

Conclusion of Cochrane Data Base Review is summarised in Table 16.3.

**Table 16.3:** Infecting microorganisms usually associated with certain operative procedures and the prophylactic antibiotic recommendation grade A

| *Surgical procedure* | *Predominant infecting microorganism(s)* | *Recommended agent* | *Dose* | *Route* |
|---|---|---|---|---|
| Vaginal or abdominal hysterectomy | Coliforms, enterococci group B streptococci | Cefazolin | 2 g | IV |
| Caesarean section with high risk, e.g. premature rupture of membranes | As for hysterectomy | Cefazolin or<br>Cefoxitin | 1 g<br>2 g | IV<br>IV |
| Low risk-elective | | No prophylaxis | | |
| Abortion | As for hysterectomy | Cefazolin | 1 g | IV |

Some Indian studies and guidelines are also given below which match more with Indian set ups. Besides this, most of the hospitals should formulate these guidelines to avoid misuse of antibiotics. In the studies conducted at Lok Nayak Hospital, New Delhi in 1993 and 1997, single dose verses multiple dose of prophylactic antibiotics in gynae major surgery and Sulbacin (Ampicillin 1 gm with Sulbactum 0.5 gm) half an hour before caesarean section was compared with conventional ampicillin and gentamicin for 7 days. The conclusion of these studies was (1) there is no benefit of extended regimens of antibiotics for prophylactic use in gynae major surgeries (2) single injection of sulbacin was quite effective for prophylaxis.[51,52]

Another prospective randomised comparative study was conducted in the patients undergoing abdominal hysterectomy to compare postoperative morbidity with prophylactic ampicillin and a combination of ciprofloxacin and metronidazole. Ampicillin was given in 3 doses, 2 gm intramuscular (IM) along with premedication followed by 2 more doses of 1 gram each 6 hours apart (Group I). Group II received single dose of ciprofloxacin 200 mg intravenous (IV) + 500 mg metronidazole (IV) at the time of induction of anaesthesia. Postoperative morbidity in terms of febrile morbidity, UTI, vaginal cuff infection, abdominal wound infection, pelvic cellulitis, additional antibiotics and hospital stay was compared in the two groups. Overall postoperative morbidity was 65 per cent in patients receiving 3 doses of ampicillin as compared to 35 per cent in those receiving a combination of ciprofloxacin and metronidazole ($p<0.001$). Similarly, febrile morbidity of UTI was significantly reduced in group II. However, the difference in vaginal cuff infection, abdominal wound infection, hospital stay and additional antibiotics was not significant statistically.[53]

Comparison of multiple doses of ciprofloxacin with single parenteral dose was done in patients having laparoscopic sterilisation at tertiary level hospital. Single dose was effective for prophylactic purposes.[54]

A recent study from Jamnagar on use of antimicrobial in obstetrics and gynaecology with emphasis on its timing, frequency, dosage, route, duration, cost and rationality showed antimicrobials were used in 431 cases out of 453 giving an overall incidence of 95.14 per cent. Conclusion of this study was that, antimicrobial use was very high and in many cases irrational. Apart from unnecessary cost, this can increase chances of antimicrobial resistance.[55]

**Table 16.4:** Guidelines regarding antibiotic prophylaxis in obstetrics and gynaecology from King Edward Memorial Hospital and Seth Gordhandes Sunderdes Medical College[56]

| *Operation* | *Antibiotic regime* |
|---|---|
| First trimester medical termination of pregnancy (MTP) | Doxycycline ?200 mg PO the evening before operation,<br>or<br>Amoxycillin ** 500 mg IM on induction of anaesthesia |
| Dilatation and curettage (D&C) | Doxycycline ?200 mg PO the evening before operation,<br>or<br>Amoxycillin ** 500 mg IM on induction of anaesthesia |

*Contd...*

*Contd...*

| *Operation* | *Antibiotic regime* |
|---|---|
| First trimester medical termination of pregnancy (MTP) + laparoscopic sterilisation | Doxycycline ?200 mg PO the evening before operation,<br>or<br>Amoxycillin ** 500 mg IM on induction of anaesthesia |
| Laparoscopy with/without D&C | Doxycycline ? 200 mg PO the evening before operation,<br>or<br>Amoxycillin ** 500 mg IM on induction of anaesthesia |
| Hysteroscopy | Doxycycline ? 200 mg PO the evening before operation,<br>or<br>Amoxycillin ** 500 mg IM on induction of anaesthesia |
| Polypectomy with/without D&C | Doxycycline ? 200 mg PO the evening before operation,<br>or<br>Amoxycillin ** 500 mg IM on induction of anaesthesia |
| Puerperal sterilisation | Amoxycillin 500 mg IM on induction of anaesthesia |
| Cervical cerclage | Amoxycillin 500 mg IM on induction of anaesthesia |
| Obstetric forceps | Amoxycillin 500 mg IM prior to application |
| Vacuum extraction | Amoxycillin 500 mg IM prior to application |
| Episiotomy | Amoxycillin 500 mg IM prior to incision |
| Perineal tear | Amoxycillin 500 mg IM prior to suturing |
| Caesarean section | Cefazolin 2 gm IV after umbilical cord is clamped.<br>Repeat after 4 hours if the operation lasts for > 2 hours |
| Vaginal hysterectomy | Cefazolin 2 gm IV 30 min before the operation.<br>Repeat after 4 hours if the operation lasts for > 2 hours |
| Abdominal hysterectomy | Cefazolin 2 gm IV 30 min before the operation.<br>Repeat after 4 hours if the operation lasts for > 2 hours |
| Exploratory laparotomy | Cefazolin 2 gm IV 30 min before the operation.<br>Repeat after 4 hours if the operation lasts for > 2 hours |

? Not to be given to lactating women
** To be given to lactating women
Inform if * - All instructions for normal labour also to be followed.
Inform the neonatologist during 1st stage all HRP pts and on delivery.[56]

## Key Points

- Use antibiotics when the risk of infection is high or squelae is significant.
- Do not start too early or too late.
- Tissue levels should peak when incision is given. Administration must occur 30 to 45 minutes prior to incision or with the induction of anaesthesia.
- Give right antibiotic. Agents like cefazolin/cefuroxime/augmentin are quite effective.
- Give intravenous antibiotic as oral antibiotic may be unreliable.
- Effective doses should be governed by the patient's own weight, e.g cefazolin 1 gm up to weight 70 kg and 2 gm if weight is more than 70 kg.
- Use additional intraoperative dose only when necessary like procedure lasts for more than 2 to 3 hours or blood loss is high.
- Keep postoperative doses to minimum.
- Do not use the same antibiotic for therapeutic purposes, as has been used for prophylaxis.
- For therapeutic purposes, appropriate antibiotic should be used after culture report.
- Patients allergic to penicillins/cephalosporins should receive clindamycin IV.

- As far as grades of recommendations are considered, A grade recommendation for use of prophylactic antibiotic is given only for use in caesarean section, hysterectomy and induced abortion.
- Recommendations mentioned above can be considered depending on risk factors and the local policies.
- Surgical technique remains the paramount factor in preventing infection, but antibiotic prophylaxis assists the patient's host response when some bacterial contamination is inevitable.

## REFERENCES

1. Allen JL, Rampone JF, Wheeless CR. Use of prophylactic antibiotic in elective major gynecologic operations. Obstet Gynecol 1972;39:218.
2. Berger SA, Nagar H, Gordon M. Antimicrobial prophylaxis in obstetric-gynecologic surgery: a critical review. J Reprod Med 1980; 24:185.
3. Hemsell DL, Cunningham FG, Kappas S, et al. Cefoxitin for prophylaxis in premenopausal women undergoing vaginal hysterectomy. Obstet Gynecol 1980; 56:629.
4. Mickal A, Curole D, Lewis C. Cefoxitin sodium: double-blind vaginal hysterectomy prophylaxis in premenopausal patients. Obstet Gynecol 1980; 56:222.
5. Cresman WT, Hill GA, Weed JC Jr, et al. A trial of prophylactic cefamandole in extended gynecologic surgery. Obstet Gynaecol 1982;59:303.
6. Hunt TK. Surgical wound infections: an overview. Am J Med 1981;70:712-18.
7. Moss F, McNicol MW, McSwiggan DA, Miller DL. Survey of antibiotic prescribing in a district general hospital: pattern of use. Lancet 1981;2:349-52.
8. Jobe BA, Grasley A, Deveney KE, Deveney CW, Sheppard BC. *Clostridium difficile* colitis: an increasing hospital acquired illness. Am J Surg 1995; 169:480-3.
9. Hospital antibiotic control measures in the UK. Working Party of the British Society for Antimicrobial Chemotherapy. J Antimicrob Chemother 1994; 34:21-42.
10. Culver DH, Horan TC, Gaynes RP, Eykyn SJ, Littler WA, McGowan DA et al. Surgical wound infection rates by wound class, operative procedures and patient risk index. National Nosocomial Infections Surveillance System. Am J Med 1991; 91:152-7.
11. Baum ML, Anish DS, Chalmers TC, Sacks HS, Smith H, Fagerstrom RM. A survey of clinical trials of antibiotic prophylaxis in colon surgery: evidence against further use of no-treatment controls. NEJM 1981; 306;795-9.
12. Mc Gowan JE. Cost and benefit in control of nosocomial infection: methods for analysis. Rev Infect Dis 1981;3:790-7.
13. Coelle R, Glenister H, Fereres J, Bartlett C, Leigh D, Sedgwick J, et al. The cost of infection in surgical patients: a case-control study. J Hosp Infect 1993;25:239-50.
14. Lynch W, Malek M, Davey PG, Byme DJ, Napier A. Costing wound infection in a Scottish hospital. Pharmacoeconomics 1992;2:163-70.
15. Davey PG, Duncan ID, Edward D, Scott AC. Cost-benefit analysis of cephradine and mezlocillin prophylaxis for abdominal and vaginal hysterectomy. Br J Obstet Gynaecol 1988;95:1170-7.
16. Austin DJ, Kakehashi M, Anderson RM. The transmission dynamics of antibiotic-resistant bacteria: the relationship between resistance in commensal organism and antibiotic consumption. Proc R Soc Lond B Biol Sci 1997;264:1629-38.
17. Wilcox MH, Smyth ET. Incidence and impact of *Clostridium difficile* infection in the UK, 1993-1996. J Hosp Infect 1998;39:181-7.
18. Zadik PM, Moore AP. Antimicrobial associations of an outbreak of diarrhoea due to *Clostridium difficile*. J Hosp Infect 1998;39:189-93.
19. Wilcox MH, Cunniffe JG, Trundle C, Redpath C. Financial burden of hospital-acquired *Clostridium difficile* infection. J Hosp Infect 1996;34:23-30.
20. Privitera G, Scarpellini P, Ortisi G, Nicastro G, Nicolin R, de Lalla F. Prospective study of *Clostridium difficile* intestinal colonisation and disease following single dose antibiotic prophylaxis in surgery. Antimicrob Agents Chemother 1991;35:208-10.

21. Namias N, Harvill S, Ball S, McKenney MG, Salomone JP, Civetta JM. Cost and morbidity associated with antibiotic prophylaxis in the ICU. J Am Coll Surg 1999;188:225-30.
22. Martin C. Antimicrobial prophylaxis in surgery: general concepts and clinical guidelines. French Study Group on Antimicrobial Prophylaxis in Surgery, French Society of Anesthesia and Intensive Care. Infect Control Hosp Epidemiol 1994;15:463-71.
23. Classen DC, Evans RS, Pestonik SL, Horn SD, Menlove RL, Burke JP. The timing of prophylactic administration of antibiotics and the risk of surgical-wound infection. NEJM 1992;326:281-6.
24. Draft guidelines for the prevention of surgical site infection, 1998-CDC. Notice. Fed Regist1998; 63: 33167-92.
25. Ballow CH, Schentag JJ. Trends in antibiotic utilization and bacterial resistance. Report of the National Nosocomial Resistance Suveillance Group. Diagn Microbiol Infect Dis 1993;15:37S-42S.
26. McGowan JE. Cost and benefit of perioperative antimicrobial prophylaxis: methods for economic analysis. Rev Infect Dis 1991;13: 879-89.
27. Adkinson NF Jr. Risk factors for drug allergy. J Allergy Clin Immuno 1984;74: 567-72.
28. Penicillin allergy in childhood. Lancet 1989; 25: 420.
29. Idsoe O, Guthe T, Willcox RR, Weck AL de. Nature and extent of penicillin side-reactions, with particular reference to fatalities from anaphylactic shock. Bull World Health Organ 1968; 38: 159-88.
30. Sogan DD. Penicillin allergy. J Allegy Clin Immunol 1984; 74: 589-93.
31. Saxon A, Adelman DC, Patel A, Hajdu R, Calandra GB. Imipenem cross-reactivity with penicillin in humans. J Allergy Clin Immunol 1988; 82: 213-7.
32. Antimicrobial therapy for obstetric patients. Am Coll Obstet Gynecol Edu Bull 1998; 245.
33. Scher KS. Studies on the duration of antibiotic administration for surgical prophylaxis. Am Surg 1997; 63: 59-62.
34. van Dijk-van Darn MS, Moll FL, de Letter JA, Langmeijer JJ, Kuks PF. The myth of the second prophylactic antibiotic dose in aortoiliac reconstructions. Eur J Vasc Endovasc Surg 1996; 12: 428-30.
35. Vuorisalo S, Pokela R, Syrjala H. Is single-dose antibiotic prophylaxis sufficient for coronary artery bypass surgery? An analysis of peri- and postoperative serum cefuroxime and vancomycin levels. J Hosp Infect 1997; 37: 237-47.
36. Cuthbertson AM, McLeish AR, Penfold JC, Ross H. A comparison between single and double dose intravenous Timentin for the prophylaxis of wound infection in colorectal surgery. Dis Colon Rectum 1991; 63: 59-62.
37. Culver DH, Horan TC, Gaynes RP, Martone WJ, Jarvis WR, Emori TG, et al. Surgical wound infection rates by wound class, operative procedure, and patient risk index. National Nosocomial Infections Surveillance System. Am J Med 1991; 91: 152-7.
38. McDonald M, Grabsch E, Marshall C, Forbes A. Single-versus multiple-dose antimicrobial prophylaxis for major surgery: a systematic review. Aust NZ J Surg 1998; 68: 388-96.
39. Wymenga A, van Horn J, Theeuwes A, Muytjens H, Slooff T. Cefuroxime for prevention of postoperative sepsis. One versus three doses tested in a randomized multicenter study of 2651 arthroplasties. Acta Orthop Scand 1992; 63: 19-24.
40. Hall JC, Christiansen KJ, Goodman M, Lawrence-Brown M, Prendergast FJ, Rosenberg P, et al. Duration of antimicrobial prophylaxis in vascular surgery. M J Surg 1998; 175: 87-90.
41. Levy M, Egersegi P, Strong A, Tessoro A, Spino M, Bannatyne R, et al. Pharmacokinetic analysis of cloxacillin loss in children undergoing major surgery with massive bleeding. Antimicrob Agents Chemother 1990; 34: 1150-3.
42. Wollinsky KH, Buchele M, Oethinger M, Kluger P, Mehrkens HH, Marre R, et al. Influence of hemodilution on cefuroxime levels and bacterial contamination of intra- and postoperative processed wound blood during hip replacement. Beitr Infusions Transfusions Med 1996;33:191-5.
43. van Lindert AC, Giltaij AR, Derksen MD, Alsbach GP, Rozenberg-Arska M, Verhoef J. Single-dose prophylaxis with broad-spectrum penicillins (piperacillin and mezlocillin) in gynecologic oncologic surgery, with observation on serum and tissue concentrations. Eur H Obstet Gynecol Reprod Biol 1990; 36: 137-45.

44. Sue D, Salazar TA, Turley K, Guglielmo BJ. Effect of surgical blood loss and volume replacement on antibiotic pharmacokinetics. Ann Thorac Siur 1989; 47: 857-9.
45. Smaill and GJ Hofmeyr The Cochrane Database of Systematic Reviews 2005 Issue 2.
46. Buppasiri P, Lumbiganon P, Thinkhamrop J, Thinkhamrop B. Antibiotic prophylaxis for fourth-degree perineal tear during vaginal birth. (Protocol) The Cochrane Database of Systematic Reviews 2005, Issue 1. Art. No : CD005125. DOI: 10.1002/14651858.CD005125.
47. Liabsuetrakul T, Choobun T, Peeyananjarassri K, Islam M. Antibiotic prophylaxis for operative vaginal delivery. The Cochrane Database of Systematic Reviews 2004, Issue 2. Art. No.: CD004455. DOI: 10.1002/14651858. CD004455.
48. Marjoribanks J, Jordan V, Calis K. Antibiotic prophylaxis for elective hysterectomy (Protocol) The Cochrane Database of Systematic Reviews 2004, Issue 1. Art. No.: CD004637. DOI: 10.1002/14651858.CD004637.
49. Grimes DA, Schulz FK. Antibiotic prophylaxis for intrauterine contraceptive device insertion. The Cochrane Database of Systematic Reviews 2001, Issue 2. Art. No.: CD001327. DOI: 10.1002/14651858.CD001327.
50. Snieders MNE, Van Vliet HAAM, Helmerhorst FM, Low N. Antibiotic prophylaxis for medical and surgical first-trimester induced abortion. (Protocol) The Cochrane Data Systematic Reviews 2004, Issue 3. Art. No : CD005217. DOI: 10.1002/14651858.CD005217.
51. Gandhi G, Batra S. Antibiotic Prophylaxis. Paper Presented at the Xvth FIGO Congress of Gynecology and Obstetrics, Copenhagen, 1997; 3-8.
52. Batra S, Tempe A, Sachdeva P. Prophylactic antibiotics in gynae major surgery. J OBS Gynae of India, 1994; 44(3):445.
53. Arora R, Begum S, Habebeebullah S, Shashendran CH, Ravindran, Oumachigui A. Evaluation of antibiotic prophylaxis in abdominal hysterectomy. J Obstet Gynecol Ind 2001; 51(3):121-23.
54. Khera N, Sachdeva J, Batra S. Antibiotic Prophylaxis in Laparoscopic Ligation (Single Dose Parenteral Versus Multi Dose Oral Ciprofloxacin) Poster presented at the VIth World Conference of Narchi, Taj Hotel, Delhi, 20-22 September, 2002.
55. Shah BK, Shah VN, Antimicrobial use by the department of obstetrics and gynecology of a tertiary care hospital: analysis for rationality and other aspects. J Obstet Gynecol Ind 2004; 54(4):387-92.
56. www.kem.edu/dept/obstetric management-guidelines4.htm.

# Index